DRUGS, LIPID METABOLISM, AND ATHEROSCLEROSIS

ADVANCES IN EXPERIMENTAL MEDICINE AND BIOLOGY

Recent Volumes in this Series

Volume 101
ENZYMES OF LIPID METABOLISM
Edited by Shimon Gatt, Louis Freysz, and Paul Mandel

Volume 102
THROMBOSIS: Animal and Clinical Models
Edited by H. James Day, Basil A. Molony, Edward E. Nishizawa, and Ronald H. Rynbrandt

Volume 103
HOMEOSTASIS OF PHOSPHATE AND OTHER MINERALS
Edited by Shaul G. Massry, Eberhard Ritz, and Aurelio Rapado

Volume 104
THE THROMBOTIC PROCESS IN ATHEROGENESIS
Edited by A. Bleakley Chandler, Karl Eurenius, Gardner C. McMillan, Curtis B. Nelson, Colin J. Schwartz, and Stanford Wessler

Volume 105
NUTRITIONAL IMPROVEMENT OF FOOD AND FEED PROTEINS
Edited by Mendel Friedman

Volume 106
GASTROINTESTINAL HORMONES AND PATHOLOGY OF THE DIGESTIVE SYSTEM
Edited by Morton Grossman, V. Speranza, N. Basso, and E. Lezoche

Volume 107
SECRETORY IMMUNITY AND INFECTION
Edited by Jerry R. McGhee, Jiri Mestecky, and James L. Babb

Volume 108
AGING AND BIOLOGICAL RHYTHMS
Edited by Harvey V. Samis, Jr. and Salvatore Capobianco

Volume 109
DRUGS, LIPID METABOLISM, AND ATHEROSCLEROSIS
Edited by David Kritchevsky, Rodolfo Paoletti, and William L. Holmes

Volume 110
HUMAN INTERFERON: Production and Clinical Use
Edited by Warren R. Stinebring and Paul J. Chapple

DRUGS, LIPID METABOLISM, AND ATHEROSCLEROSIS

Edited by

David Kritchevsky
The Wistar Institute
Philadelphia, Pennsylvania

Rodolfo Paoletti
Institute of Pharmacology and Pharmacognosy
University of Milan
Milan, Italy

and

William L. Holmes
Division of Research
The Lankenau Hospital
Philadelphia, Pennsylvania

PLENUM PRESS • NEW YORK AND LONDON

Library of Congress Cataloging in Publication Data

International Symposium on Drugs Affecting Lipid Metabolism, 6th, Philadelphia, 1977.
Drugs, lipid metabolism, and atherosclerosis.
(Advances in experimental medicine and biology; 109)

Symposium held Aug. 29–Sept. 1, 1977; sponsored by the Council on Arteriosclerosis of the American Heart Association, etc.
Includes indexes.

1. Arteriosclerosis–Chemotherapy–Congresses. 2. Lipid metabolism–Congresses. 3. Antilipemic agents–Congresses. I. Kritchevsky, David, 1920- II. Paoletti, Rodolfo. III. Holmes, William L., 1918- IV. American Heart Association. Council on Arteriosclerosis. V. Series. VI. Title. [DNLM: 1. Lipoproteins–Metabolism. 2. Metabolism–Drug effects. 3. Lipids–Metabolism. 4. Arteriosclerosis–Drug therapy. 5. Arteriosclerosis–Metabolism. W1 AD559 v. 109/WG550 I622 1977]
RC692.I54 1977 616.1'36'061 78-14222
ISBN 0-306-40052-9

Proceedings of the Sixth International Symposium on Drugs Affecting Lipid Metabolism held in Philadelphia, Pennsylvania, August 29–September 1, 1977

Symposium sponsored by

AMERICAN HEART ASSOCIATION Council on Arteriosclerosis
INTERNATIONAL SOCIETY FOR BIOCHEMICAL PHARMACOLOGY
THE HEART ASSOCIATION OF SOUTHEASTERN PENNSYLVANIA
THE LORENZINI FOUNDATION, MILAN, ITALY

A Division of Plenum Publishing Corporation
227 West 17th Street, New York, N.Y. 10011

Printed in the United States of America

INTERNATIONAL ORGANIZING COMMITTEE

S. Bergström
L. A. Carlson
G. Fassina
W. L. Holmes
D. Kritchevsky
M. F. Oliver
R. Paoletti
G. Schettler
D. Steinberg

LOCAL ORGANIZING COMMITTEE

N. Di Tullio
W. L. Holmes
D. Kritchevsky
J. Plostnieks
G. Reichard
J. A. Story

SCIENTIFIC SECRETARIES

W. L. Holmes
R. Paoletti

PROGRAM CHAIRMAN

D. Kritchevsky

SECRETARY TO ORGANIZING COMMITTEE

Mrs. C. Hyatt

The Organizing Committee gratefully acknowledges the contributions of the following organizations:

ABBOTT LABORATORIES, North Chicago, Illinois
AMERICAN CYANAMID COMPANY – LEDERLE LABORATORIES DIVISION, Pearl River, New York
AYERST LABORATORIES, New York, New York
BRISTOL LABORATORIES, Syracuse, New York
CIBA-GEIGY CORPORATION, Ardsley, New York
CUTTER LABORATORIES, INC., Berkeley, California
THE DOW CHEMICAL COMPANY, Indianapolis, Indiana
ELI LILLY AND COMPANY, Indianapolis, Indiana
G. D. SEARLE AND COMPANY – SEARLE LABORATORIES DIVISION, Chicago, Illinois
ICI UNITED STATES INCORPORATED, Wilmington, Delaware
THE KROC FOUNDATION, Santa Ynez, California
MC NEIL LABORATORIES, INC., Fort Washington, Pennsylvania
MERCK AND COMPANY, Rahway, New Jersey
NATIONAL DAIRY COUNCIL, Rosemont, Illinois
ORTHO PHARMACEUTICAL CORPORATION, Raritan, New Jersey
PARKE, DAVIS AND COMPANY, Detroit, Michigan
THE PROCTER AND GAMBLE COMPANY, Cincinnati, Ohio
SANDOZ, INC., East Hanover, New Jersey
SCHERING CORPORATION, Bloomfield, New Jersey
SMITH, KLINE AND FRENCH LABORATORIES, Philadelphia, Pennsylvania
SUMITOMO CHEMICAL COMPANY, Osaka, Japan
TRAVENOL LABORATORIES – FLINT DIVISION, Deerfield, Illinois
THE UPJOHN COMPANY, Kalamazoo, Michigan
WARNER-LAMBERT COMPANY, Morris Plains, New Jersey
WYETH LABORATORIES, Philadelphia, Pennsylvania

Preface

This volume comprises the proceedings of the Sixth International Symposium on Drugs Affecting Lipid Metabolism. Since the first of these symposia in 1960 these triennial meetings have been devoted to the exploration of new ideas, new data and new concepts related to lipid metabolism and atherosclerosis. The Sixth Meeting was particularly stimulating in this regard. The concept of the "protective" action of HDL was thoroughly explored within the framework of its molecular biology with data on its epidemiological as well as its in vitro mechanism(s) of action being discussed. The action of drugs on arterial and HDL metabolism was also discussed as were newer aspects of platelet aggregation, especially as related to prostaglandins. New ground was also broken in discussions of lipid mobilization and mechanisms of hypocholesteremia.

We are indebted to the many organizations who contributed generously to the support of this meeting. Among the sponsors, the assistance of the Lorenzini Foundation was especially helpful. As in all meetings of this type, the hard work of the local organizing committee was instrumental in its success. We are grateful to Mrs. Caroline Hyatt and Mr. Ralph Hollerorth for their invaluable help in the secretariat. We are also deeply indebted to Miss Jane T. Kolimaga for her expert assistance in the preparation of this volume.

David Kritchevsky
Rodolfo Paoletti
William L. Holmes

Contents

DRUGS, LIPID MOBILIZATION AND PLATELETS

CHOLESTEROL METABOLISM IN MAN

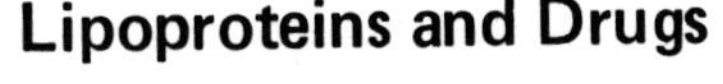

Lipoproteins and Drugs

LIPOPROTEIN METABOLISM - NEW INSIGHTS FROM CELL BIOLOGY

Daniel Steinberg, M.D., Ph.D.

Division of Metabolic Disease, University of California San Diego, La Jolla, California, U.S.A.

The primary purpose of this paper is to review some of the recent developments in our understanding of how lipoproteins are metabolized by peripheral cells. Studies utilizing cultured mammalian cells promise to enhance considerably our insights into factors regulating steady-state levels of lipoproteins in the plasma compartment and, at least potentially, our insights into the cellular basis for atherogenesis. Quite possibly we may see the development of new modalities of pharmacologic intervention based on a better understanding of how lipoproteins are degraded by or modified by interactions with peripheral cells. Research in this area is still at an early stage of development but progress is being made rapidly. Those of us interested in the role of lipids in atherogenesis and in the possibilities for preventive intervention should be aware of the opportunities to capitalize on the new findings as they come along. Before turning to the cellular level, however, we should establish the context by briefly reviewing current concepts of lipoprotein metabolism *in vivo*.

LIPOPROTEIN METABOLISM *IN VIVO*

The liver is generally accepted to be the major source of the plasma lipoproteins. Undoubtedly the intestine makes some contribution as well but in man that contribution is probably quantitatively minor. The fate of chylomicrons, well studied in the rat, has not been fully established in man. To what extent do they contribute to the very low density, low density and high density lipoprotein fractions (VLDL, LDL and HDL)? Does chylomicron and/or VLDL clearance play a role in atherogenesis as proposed by Zilversmit (1)? To what extent is the intestine an important source of lipoprotein apoproteins? None of these questions has been satisfactorily answered in man. Clearly it would be premature to set aside the intestine as a source of materials of importance in overall lipoprotein metabolism and atherogenesis. The information available does not permit any firm conclusions and we shall not attempt to deal with this question further today.

The primary lipoproteins secreted by the liver are VLDL and HDL. In normal human subjects most or all of the circulating LDL can be accounted for as a product of VLDL metabolism i.e. relatively rapid degradation of VLDL by lipoprotein lipase giving rise to an intermediate density lipoprotein (IDL) and then LDL as a more slowly metabolized "end product" (2-6). In the rat, IDL (or VLDL "remnant") is rapidly removed by the liver (7) but its fate in man is uncertain. There is now direct and indirect evidence that the liver can under some circumstances secrete LDL directly into the plasma compartment. In patients with familial hypercholesterolemia the daily transport of apoprotein B in the LDL fraction (d 1.019 - 1.063) has been found to exceed the transport of apoprotein B in the VLDL fraction ($d<1.006$) (8,9). As much as 50% of the LDL apo B may have an origin other than VLDL. Recently it has been reported that the isolated perfused liver of the pig may directly secrete LDL (10,11). It now appears that not all of the apo B in VLDL must obligatorily be converted to LDL prior to its disappearance from the plasma compartment i.e. the net daily transport of apo B in VLDL can exceed that in LDL (9). Another recent finding worth noting is that changes in transport of triglycerides in VLDL need not parallel changes in apo B transport in VLDL (12). During carbohydrate-induction the transport of triglycerides can increase (along with an increase in steady-state plasma levels of VLDL triglycerides) with either no increase or a much smaller increase in apo B transport. Evidently on a high carbohydrate diet the triglyceride:apo B ratio in the secreted VLDL is increased i.e. larger, triglyceride-rich particles are secreted (13).

These findings should help to rationalize some seeming paradoxes in the hyperlipoproteinemias. As long as we assumed that all VLDL must be converted to LDL and that all LDL had its origin in VLDL, it was difficult to explain hyperlipoproteinemic patterns with widely different ratios of VLDL to LDL and to explain some of the complex responses to dietary and drug interventions. If LDL can be directly secreted we can see how LDL levels can be increased without changes in VLDL levels or rates of VLDL secretion. If not all VLDL apo B must be converted to LDL we can see how VLDL levels can be increased as a result of overproduction (including overproduction of VLDL apo B) without necessarily affecting LDL levels or LDL transport. Finally, if VLDL triglyceride transport can be increased without concomitant increase in VLDL apo B transport, we can see how VLDL (triglyceride) levels can be increased as a result of overproduction without affecting LDL levels or LDL transport.

Interest in HDL metabolism and its regulation has increased considerably with the accumulation of epidemiologic evidence that the risk of coronary heart disease varies inversely with HDL cholesterol levels (14-17). As shown by Hamilton and coworkers (18), HDL is secreted from perfused rat livers in the form of a disc-shaped particle with a high ratio of free cholesterol to ester cholesterol and a high content of arginine-rich protein (apo E). It is presumably converted to the form found at steady-state through the action of plasma lecithin-cholesterol acyltransferase (19) and shifts in apoprotein composition effected by interchanges with other lipoprotein fractions. It should be stressed that the designation "HDL" can be ambiguous. The fraction isolated in the density range 1.063-1.21 is not homogeneous. Subfractions can be recognized by analytic ultracentrifugation (20). More importantly, the fraction includes subpopulations of molecules with different apoprotein patterns. Mahley and coworkers have shown that the heterogeneity is further increased in cholesterol-fed animals (21), a population of molecules rich in cholesterol and in apo E increasing. This is especially relevant, as discussed below, to the interactions between LDL and HDL metabolism and possibly to the "antiatherogenic" role of HDL.

The major apoproteins in the HDL fraction in man are apo A-I and apo A-II and the occurrence of apo E has just been discussed. In addition HDL binds the several classes of C apoproteins, serving as a reservoir from which these can be readily exchanged into VLDL or chylomicrons (22,23). Since apo A-I and C-I are activators for lecithin-cholesterol acyltransferase (24) and apo C-II an activator for lipoprotein lipase (25), HDL-associated apoproteins could play a regulatory role in overall lipoprotein metabolism. The precise role of this "apoprotein reservoir" function in normal subjects and in hyperlipoproteinemic subjects remains to be established.

EXTRAHEPATIC DEGRADATION OF LIPOPROTEINS

It has been the general view that LDL must be degraded in the liver. At first glance this seems an unavoidable conclusion because extrahepatic tissues (with the quantitatively minor exceptions of the adrenal cortex and the gonads) do not have any significant capacity to degrade or eliminate cholesterol. All that is absolutely required, however, is that the _cholesterol moiety_ of the LDL ultimately make its way back to the liver for excretion. The _apoprotein moiety_ of the LDL (and probably the other lipid components) could in principle be degraded outside the liver. In fact there is now evidence from several directions that, at least in some species, most of the degradation of LDL apoprotein takes place extrahepatically.

The first evidence for this was provided by the work of Sniderman _et al._(26), who showed that the rate of the degradation of intravenously injected ^{125}I-LDL in swine was not reduced by total hepatectomy. In intact swine the injected LDL showed a biphasic disappearance, the initial more rapid phase being attributable to equilibration with an extravascular pool of LDL. Postmortem tissue distribution studies indicated that much of this extravascular pool resided in the liver. If the liver were the exclusive or predominant site of degradation, there should be little or no disappearance of labeled LDL after hepatectomy. Instead the disappearance rate was as great as or greater than the rate in the same animal studied prior to hepatectomy. Similar results were obtained in hepatectomized dogs. Furthermore, in swine the net plasma level of LDL protein fell progressively after hepatectomy and at the same rate as ^{125}I-LDL, eliminating the possibility that the labeled LDL might not be a valid tracer and, additionally, indicating that under the conditions of the experiment there was little or no extrahepatic contribution to the plasma LDL fraction. These results do not rule out some hepatic contributions to LDL apoprotein degradation but strongly suggest that, in the species studied, it is small.

Table 1

COMPARISON OF LDL DEGRADATION RATES IN CELL CULTURE AND *IN VIVO*

	µg/mg/h	mg/kg/24h
Swine: Plasma LDL protein about 30 mg/dl; estimated lymph LDL protein about 3 mg/dl (30 µg/ml)		
Aortic smooth muscle cells	0.4	60
Whole swine *in vivo*	-	8-21
Man: Plasma LDL protein about 80 mg/dl; estimated lymph LDL protein about 8 mg/dl (80 µg/ml)		
Skin fibroblasts	0.5-0.6	75-90
Arterial smooth muscle cells	0.5	75
Umbilical vein endothelium*	0.4	60
Whole man *in vivo*	-	10-20

*Data of Stein and Stein (62).

If the proposal that LDL apo B is degraded peripherally is correct, it must follow that some or many peripheral cell types have a relatively high capacity for degrading LDL. A weighted average would have to be comparable to the rates of LDL degradation observed *in vivo*. Our first cell culture studies to test this corollary hypothesis were done with smooth muscle cells derived from swine aorta (27). The degradation of ^{125}I-LDL was followed by determining the rate of appearance of labeled TCA-soluble products in the medium. The results indicated that with LDL presented at a concentration 10% of that of plasma LDL - a concentration approximately that in lymph (28) - the degradation rate per milligram of cell proteins was actually in excess of the degradation rate *in vivo* expressed the same way. As shown in Table 1, the rate of LDL degradation in several human cell lines is similarly high enough to be compatible with the hypothesis that all or most of LDL degradation *in vivo* occurs extrahepatically.

HDL degradation is still assumed to be primarily hepatic. Studies of the fate of ^{125}I-HDL in the rat show that at least some degradation occurs in the liver (29) but the data available do not justify conclusions about the quantitative importance of the liver. In

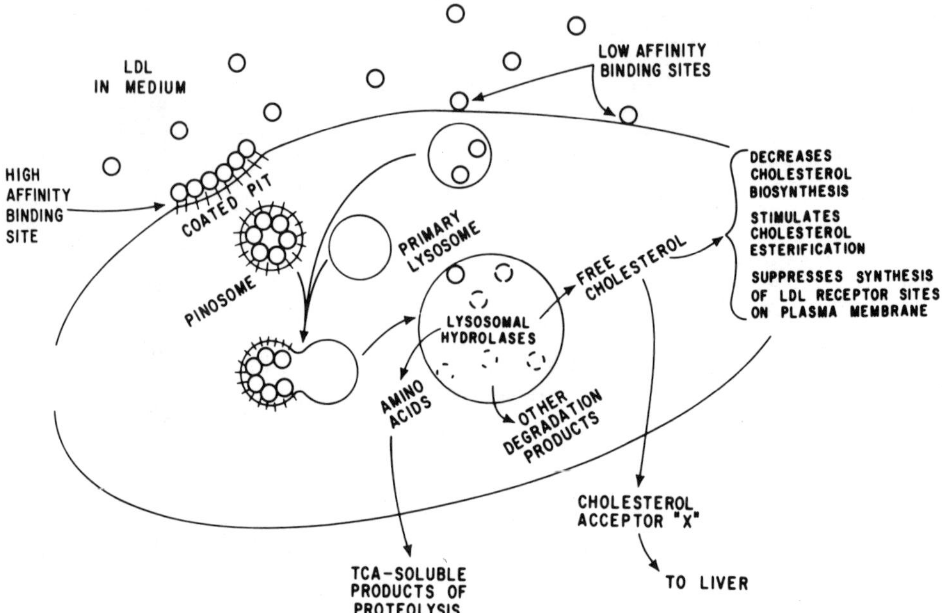

Figure 1: Schematic diagram summarizing current concepts of binding, internalization and degradation of LDL by peripheral cells.

culture, cells of extrahepatic origin (fibroblasts, smooth muscle cells, endothelial cells) do degrade HDL (30-32). The rates of degradation of human HDL by human fibroblasts are actually high enough to suggest that much or all of HDL turnover could be accounted for by peripheral degradation if all the peripheral tissue shared the capacity of fibroblasts to degrade HDL (30). Conversely the rate of HDL degradation by perfused rat liver (presented at concentrations equal to those in rat plasma) is reported to be less than 10% the rate of HDL degradation in the intact rat (33).

MECHANISMS OF LDL DEGRADATION BY ISOLATED CELLS IN CULTURE

A scheme summarizing current concepts of uptake and degradation of LDL by peripheral cells is presented in Figure 1. The initial binding of LDL to the cell surface is of two types. The central importance of the high affinity binding at specialized receptor areas of the plasma membrane has been clearly documented by the seminal studies of Brown, Goldstein and coworkers at Dallas (34-36). Their demonstration that high affinity binding sites are deleted or nonfunctional in cells cultured from patients with homozygous familial hypercholesterolemia (HFH) (34) and that the number of high affinity sites is reduced by approximately 50% in cells from heterozygotes (35) has opened new vistas in research on LDL metabolism. Using LDL coupled covalently to ferritin as an electron opaque marker, Anderson, Goldstein and Brown showed that LDL-ferritin complexes (at low concentrations) bind predominantly, although not exclusively to specialized areas of the membrane designated "coated pits" (36). Dr. Cheng-Ming Chang in our laboratory has confirmed this finding using the double antibody ("sandwich") method in which the ferritin marker is coupled not directly to the LDL but to the second antibody (first antibody, rabbit anti-LDL; second antibody, goat anti-rabbit gamma globulin) (37). This avoids the possible objection that the large ferritin molecule (MW about 5×10^5) might alter LDL binding. Most of the bound LDL was localized at "coated pits" but a significant amount was distributed on the membrane at nonspecialized sites as in the studies of Anderson *et al* (36). The possible importance of this low affinity binding in LDL catabolism is discussed below.

LDL bound to the cell membrane is thus internalized as the membrane invaginates to form endocytotic vesicles (Fig. 1). These vesicles fuse with primary lysosomes and there the rich collection of lysosomal acid hydrolases go to work to degrade the several components of the LDL. The protein moiety is degraded to free amino acids or very small peptides which leave the cell and enter the medium as trichloroacetic acid-soluble end products. The cholesterol esters are hydrolyzed by lysosomal acid lipase and the free cholesterol released then influences several key processes. Endogenous cholesterol synthesis is suppressed (38,39). This is a relatively slow response and is mediated primarily by suppression of *de novo* synthesis of the enzyme 3-hydroxy-3-methylglutaryl CoA (HMG CoA) reductase (39). The possibility that the effect is mediated by a more polar metabolite of cholesterol rather than cholesterol itself has been suggested (40). At the same time there is a striking increase in the rate of esterification of free cholesterol by acyl CoA cholesterol transferase (ACAT) (41) and a decrease in the number of high affinity binding sites for LDL on the cell surface (42). The latter effect has obvious importance as a means by which the cell can potentially regulate the uptake of LDL according to its requirement for cholesterol (43). Whether such regulation of receptor number actually plays an important role in regulation of LDL uptake in normal individuals is not established. The fact that HFH patients, who lack the high affinity receptor, have strikingly elevated LDL levels certainly speaks for such a role. However, these patients also overproduce LDL (44). Studies of human lymph show that the levels of LDL to which peripheral cells are exposed in normal individuals actually exceed the levels needed to saturate the high affinity receptors (28). This would be expected to keep the number of receptors suppressed to a very low value and yet these are normal individuals with normal circulating LDL levels. Further studies are needed before the cell culture data can be put into context in the *in vivo* system.

The evidence supporting the schema shown in Figure 1 is extensive. Degradation of LDL is blocked by chloroquin, a known inhibitor of lysosomal enzyme activity (45). The possibility that some LDL degradation may occur at the surface of the cell has been examined in our laboratory by covalently linking ^{125}I-LDL to large Sepharose beads (40-190 μ diameter) to prevent internalization (46). Even though cell-bead contact was maximized, no TCA-soluble degradation products could be detected. Moreover there was no suppression of endogenous cholesterol synthesis, ruling out the possibility that LDL-receptor interaction might trigger a "second messenger" type of system.

Goldstein *et al.* showed that fibroblasts from patients with cholesterol ester storage disease or Wolman's disease (lysosomal acid lipase deficiency) internalize and degrade LDL normally but fail to suppress HMG CoA reductase (47). Williams *et al.* in our laboratory studied fibroblasts from patients with I-cell disease, an inherited disorder in which there are multiple lysosomal hydrolase deficiencies (48). Studies of homogenates showed that acid cholesterol ester hydrolase activity was markedly reduced (49). As shown in Figs. 2 and 3 degradation of LDL protein was defective and there was a concomitant deficiency in LDL regulation of sterol synthesis. However, free cholesterol added to the medium suppressed sterol synthesis as effectively as it did in normal cells, showing that the mechanism for suppression was functional if enough free sterol could be provided.

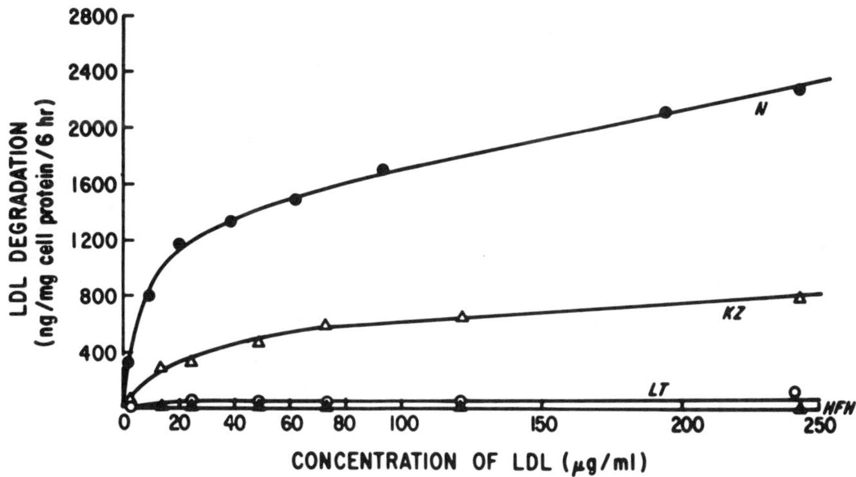

Figure 2: Degradation of ^{125}I-LDL by normal human skin fibroblasts (N), by fibroblasts from a patient with homozygous familial hypercholesterolemia (HFH) and by cell lines from patients with I-cell disease (LT, KZ). Preconfluent monolayers were incubated for 18 hours in a medium containing lipoprotein-deficient serum, washed and then incubated with lableled LDL at the indicated concentrations for 6 hours. Degradation was determined from measurements of the non-iodide, trichloroacetic acid-soluble ^{125}I in the medium (48, 58).

After a 6-hour incubation of I-cell fibroblasts with ^{125}I-LDL one finds that the washed cells contain a large amount of TCA-precipitable ^{125}I, presumably internalized but as yet undegraded ^{125}I-LDL. Whether or not patients with I-cell disease have a deficiency in LDL degradation *in vivo* is not known. They may progressively build up intracellular concentrations of LDL until the absolute degradation rate equals that of normal individuals. However, it is of interest that the plasma cholesterol levels of some children with I-cell disease is elevated (Williams, Miller, Weinstein and Steinberg, unpublished data). The elevation is modest (200-300 mg/dl) compared to the levels in HFH patients. It is possible that the hypercholesterolemia is in fact due to a partial defect in peripheral LDL degradation and that the elevation is

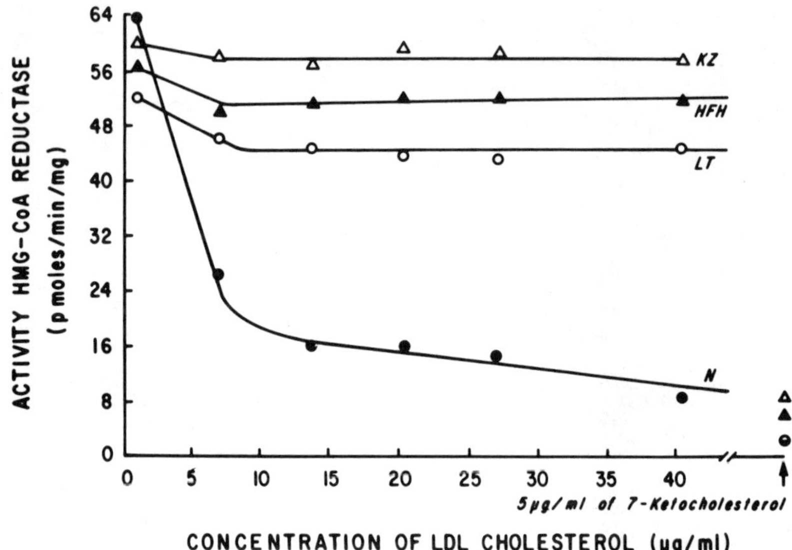

Figure 3: Suppression of the activity of 3-hydroxy-3-methylglutaryl coenzyme A reductase after 6-hour incubation in the presence of LDL at the concentrations indicated. Normal fibroblasts (N) showed the expected suppression of activity but there was little or no suppression in either cells from homozygous familial hypercholesterolemic subjects (HFH) or cells from patients with I-cell disease (KZ, LT).

not more marked than it is because hepatic lipoprotein production in these patients can be suppressed; in HFH patients lipoprotein production not only shows no suppression but, as mentioned above, is even greater than it is in normal subjects.

SPECIFICITY OF THE HIGH AFFINITY RECEPTOR

Because VLDL shared with LDL the ability to suppress HMG CoA reductase, whereas HDL had little or no effect, it was at first assumed that apoprotein B was the key element in recognition. However, Assman, Brown and Mahley found that an HDL subfraction accumulating in cholesterol-fed animals, a fraction they designated HDL_C, was fully as effective as LDL in suppressing

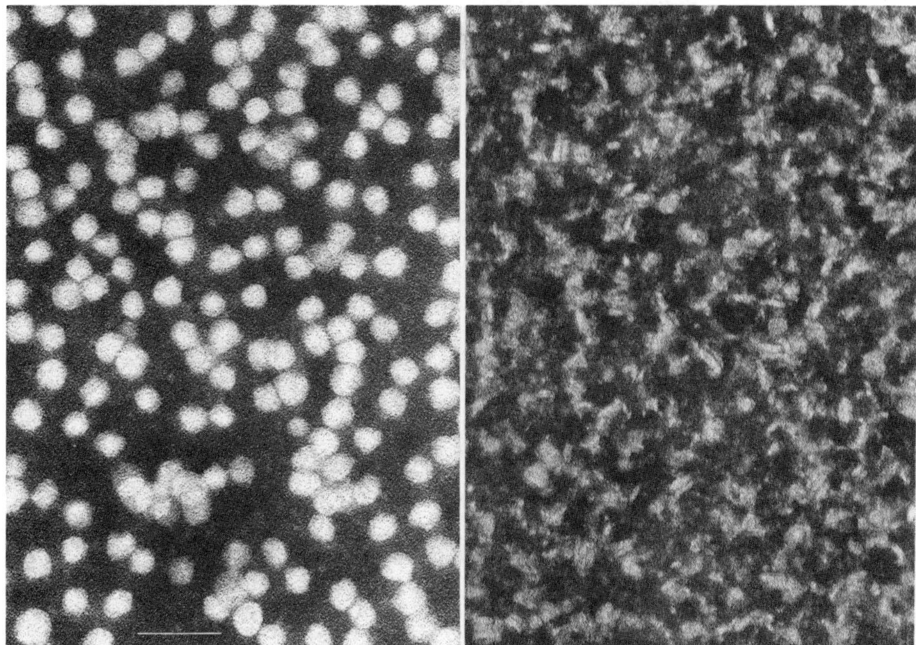

Figure 4: Electron microscopic appearance of native LDL (left) and of LDL from which non-polar lipids had been extracted by the method of Gustafson (52) (right). Bar represents 500 Å.

reductase activity in cultured aortic smooth muscle cells (50). Further studies in collaboration with Brown and Goldstein showed that HDL_C competed very effectively with LDL for binding and degradation by normal human fibroblasts and failed to effect fibroblasts from HFH patients (51). Since HDL_C contains no apoprotein B, this raised the question of what properties it had in common with LDL that led to the observed results.

The diameter of HDL_C is significantly greater than that of normal HDL and it was suggested that this might be a significant variable in lipoprotein-receptor interaction. That possibility now seems unlikely in view of some studies in our laboratory on the ability of a radically modified LDL to interact with the receptor (46). Native human LDL was treated by a modification of the heptane extraction procedure described by

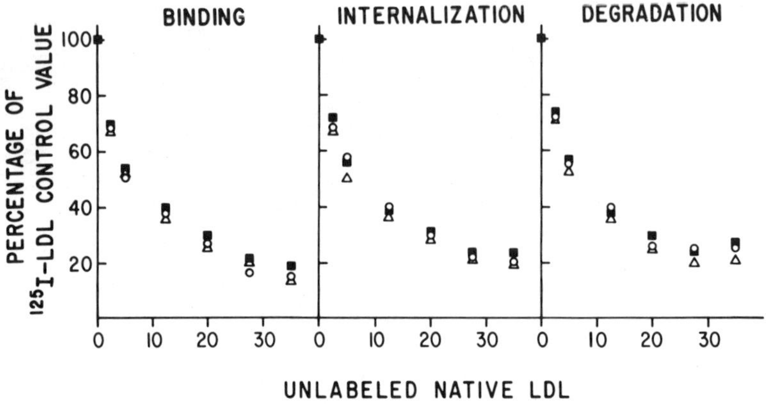

Figure 5: Comparison of the ability of native LDL and of "cholesterol-free" LDL [extracted by the method of Gustafson (52)] to compete with native ^{125}I-LDL for binding, internalization and degradation by normal human skin fibroblasts. Values for binding, internalization and degradation of native ^{125}I-LDL in the absence of added competing lipoproteins is arbitrarily assigned a value of 100. Competition by unlabeled native LDL is indicated by the solid squares; competition by two preparations of "cholesterol-free" LDL are shown by the open circles and open triangles.

Gustafson (52). This procedure leads to the removal of 99% of the cholesterol and cholesterol ester (and also the triglyceride) without significant loss of phospholipid or apoprotein. The appearance of the LDL before and after the lipid extraction is shown in Fig. 4. There has been an obvious and dramatic change in the size and shape of the LDL molecule. Nevertheless, this radically modified LDL competes with native LDL on an equal basis for binding to fibroblasts as shown in Fig. 5. The binding, internalization and degradation of native ^{125}I-LDL was determined when it was added alone or in the presence of increasing concentrations either of unlabeled native LDL or our extracted, cholesterol-free LDL. There clearly was no discrimination between the native and the modified LDL despite the radical change in molecular size and lipid content. The protein moiety of the cholesterol-free LDL was labeled with ^{125}I and its binding compared directly with that of ^{125}I-labeled native LDL. The binding curves were virtually superimposable. Furthermore, the binding of both forms of LDL was markedly reduced - to about the same extent - in fibroblasts from a patient with HFH (46). These results show that the recognition of LDL by the receptor is relatively unaffected by even such a radical alteration in molecular size, shape and chemical composition and that the apoprotein is in some way presumably the key to cell recognition.

LOW AFFINITY BINDING OF HDL AND LDL AND ITS SIGNIFICANCE

Over the past few years our laboratory has examined the uptake and degradation of HDL by several cell types - pig smooth muscle cells (27,30), human skin fibroblasts (31) and rabbit aortic endothelium (32) - and compared its handling with that of LDL. Such a comparison is shown for human fibroblasts in Fig. 6. The binding of HDL was only slightly less than that of LDL but HDL was much more slowly internalized and degraded. Replotting the data as in Fig. 7 brings out an important qualitative difference in the way the cell handles these two lipoproteins. In Fig. 7 internalization and degradation are plotted not against concentrations in the medium but against the amount of HDL or LDL bound to the cell surface. (In 37° incubations, binding of both HDL and LDL occurs fairly rapidly and then plateaus.) In the case of LDL the internalization and degradation both show sharp inflection points when plotted this way. This implies that the probability of a molecule of LDL being internalized (and then degraded) is considerably greater for those molecules bound at low medium concentrations, presumably bound to high affinity binding sites. In contrast, the relationship is essentially linear for HDL i.e. there is no such inflection. The implication is that the probability of internalization is no greater for those molecules bound at low concentration than for those molecules bound at high concentration i.e. that there are few if any high affinity sites and/or that internalization from all sites occurs at the same rate.

During the past year we have also examined other aspects of cellular HDL metabolism and compared them to LDL metabolism (53). Brown and Goldstein had previously shown that treatment of fibroblasts with pronase destroyed the high affinity sites for binding of LDL (54). We confirmed that finding for LDL binding to normal cells. Binding of HDL, however, was not affected by pronase

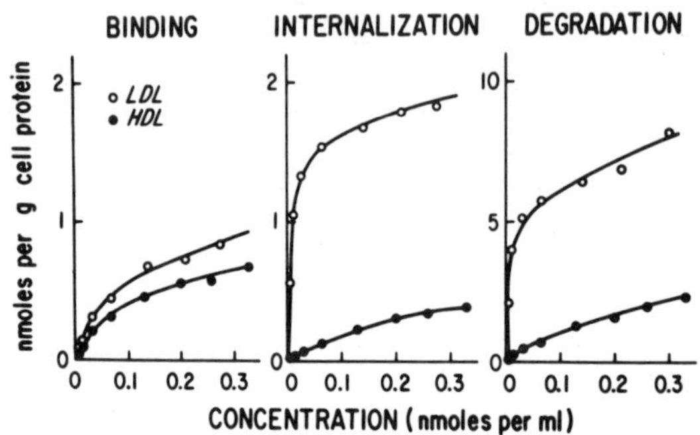

Figure 6: A comparison of the binding, internalization and degradation of ^{125}I-LDL (O) and ^{125}I-HDL (●) by normal human fibroblasts at 37°. After an 18 hour incubation in medium containing 5% lipoprotein-deficient serum, fresh medium was added containing 5% lipoprotein-deficient serum and the indicated concentrations of ^{125}I-LDL (355 cpm/ng) or ^{125}I-HDL (specific activity, 561 cpm/ng). After a further 18 hour incubation at 37° the cells were harvested and the extent of binding, internalization and degradation determined as previously described (53).

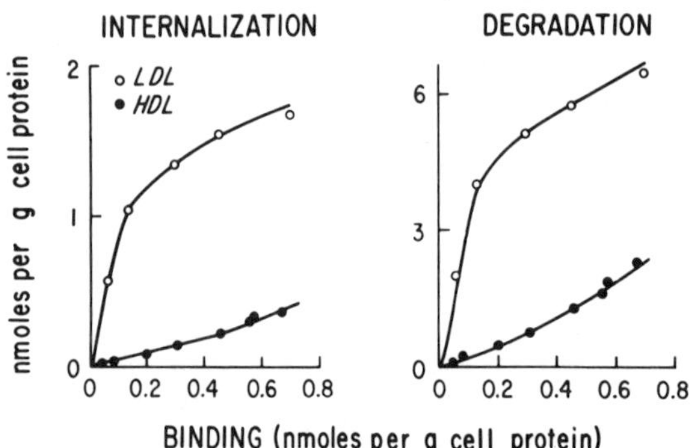

Figure 7: Relationship of internalization (left) and degradation (right) to surface binding for ^{125}I-LDL (O) and ^{125}I-HDL (●) after incubation at different concentrations (LDL from 3.5 to 69 μg/ml; HDL from 0.7 to 33 μg/ml) with normal fibroblast monolayers for 18 hours at 37°.

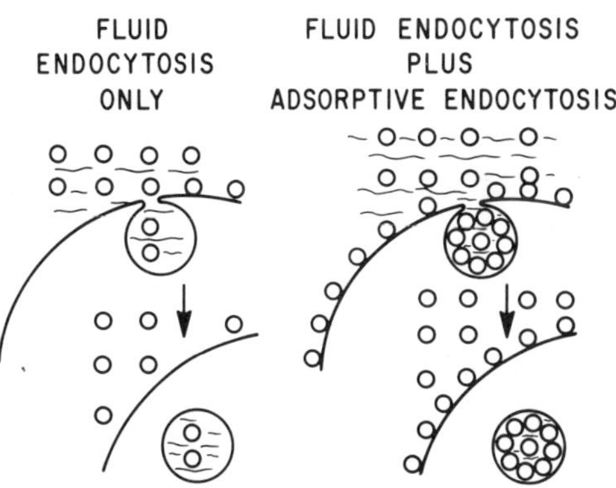

Figure 8: Diagramatic representation of the mechanisms involved in fluid or bulk endocytosis (left) and adsorptive endocytosis (right). In the former, only the number of molecules in free solution are internalized with the droplet of medium contained in the endocytotic vacuole. In the latter, there is in addition the internalization of molecules adsorbed on to the cell membrane invaginating to form the endocytotic vacuole.

treatment; in cells from HFH patients the binding of LDL was well below that seen with normal cells and pronase treatment had no effect on binding of either LDL or HDL.

Another property of the LDL receptor demonstrated by the Dallas group is that incubation of normal cells in the absence of LDL leads to an increase in the density of LDL receptor sites and, conversely, incubation in the presence of high concentrations of LDL leads to a decrease in the number of binding sites (42). We confirmed this finding (53) but found no analogous regulation of HDL binding. After a 24-hour incubation of normal cells in the absence of lipoprotein there was a 2- to 3-fold increase in LDL binding sites and this was prevented by incubating in the presence of cyclohexamide or cholesterol. In HFH fibroblasts there was no induction of LDL binding on incubation in the absence of lipoprotein. In the case of HDL there was no induction of binding sites and no effect of cholesterol and this was true both for normal fibroblasts and HFH fibroblasts.

Finally, we have compared HDL metabolism in normal

fibroblasts and HFH fibroblasts (55). Degradation of HDL was slightly decreased in the HFH fibroblasts (about 20%) whereas degradation of LDL in HFH fibroblasts was decreased by 90-95%.

We have tried to gain further insight into the nature of the difference between the cell's handling of LDL and HDL by considering the mechanisms available for endocytotic uptake. All cells are constantly taking up surrounding medium and its solutes at some rate by the process of fluid endocytosis. As shown in Fig. 8 (left) each endocytotic vacuole pinches off a tiny droplet of medium and with it the solutes contained therein at the same concentration as that present in the surrounding medium. If any of the solute of interest is adsorbed onto the cell surface then each endocytotic vacuole will contain, in addition to the solute taken up by fluid endocytosis, an additional number of molecules due to their binding to the cell surface that invaginates (Fig. 8, right). Thus the sum of fluid endocytosis and adsorptive endocytosis will exceed that attributable to fluid endocytosis alone. Fluid endocytosis can be measured in terms of the uptake of labeled sucrose from the medium because sucrose does not bind to the cell surface. Once inside the lysosome sucrose cannot be degraded and leaks out very slowly (56,57). Our approach to calculating fluid and adsorptive endocytosis is described in detail elsewhere (31). What we have done is first to calculate the total uptake of labeled lipoprotein by adding together that found in the cell at the end of the incubation (internalized) and that which has undergone degradation during the course of the incubation, making the assumption that all that has been degraded had to first enter the cell, as discussed above. Fluid endocytosis was measured from measurements of sucrose clearance. Finally, we measured the binding of the labeled lipoprotein to the cell surface and used stereologic parameters published by Steinman, Brodie and Cohn (57) to calculate adsorptive endocytosis. Results of one such calculation for HDL and for LDL are shown in Table II. For an incubation with HDL at 1 μg of HDL protein/ml (first line) the calculated uptake by fluid endocytosis was 3.4 ng/mg cell protein over the 18-hour incubation i.e. the sucrose clearance was about 3.4 μl/mg cell protein in the 18 hours. The calculated uptake by adsorptive endocytosis was 26 ng and the sum of the two, 29 ng. The observed total uptake was 24 ng. For LDL incubated at the same molar concentration (and using the same stereologic parameters) the value for uptake by fluid endocytosis was

Table II

COMPARISON OF OBSERVED LIPOPROTEIN UPTAKE WITH THE CALCULATED SUM OF UPTAKE BY FLUID ENDOCYTOSIS AND ADSORPTIVE ENDOCYTOSIS

Labeled Lipoprotein in Medium	Observed Surface Binding[a] (ng/mg)	Calculated Uptake (ng/mg)			Observed Lipoprotein Uptake (ng/mg)
		By Fluid Endocytosis[b]	By Adsorptive Endocytosis[c]	Sum[d]	
HDL, 1 μg/ml	6	3.4	26	29	24
HDL, 50 μg/ml	120	170	530	700	530
HDL, 250 μg/ml	325	850	1,436	2,286	1,475
LDL, 5 μg/ml	48	17	212	2,975	2,975
LDL, 250 μg/ml	505	850	2,236	3,086	6,400

[a] Mean value for binding at 37°.

[b] Mean value for sucrose clearance (3.4 μl/mg cell protein per 18 hr) x concentration of lipoprotein in medium (ng/μl).

[c] Density of lipoproteins binding to cell surface (ng/μm^2) x total area of cell surface internalized in 18 hr due to pinocytosis (μm^2/mg cell protein per 18 hr). Cell surface area was calculated assuming a mean cell diameter of 25 μm and using the formula proposed by Steinman, Brodie and Cohn (57) to estimate true surface area ($3\pi D^2$). From cell counts and cell protein measurements, 1 mg cell protein represents about 2.5×10^6 cells. Mean surface area and volume of pinocytotic vessels were assumed to be 0.162 μm^2 and 0.00847 μm^3, respectively, as reported by Steinman, Brodie, and Cohn (57) for the mouse fibroblast L cell line.

[d] Sum of observed internalization and degradation over 18 hr.

Table III

OBSERVED LDL UPTAKE VERSUS CALCULATED UPTAKE BY FLUID AND ADSORPTIVE ENDOCYTOSIS: COMPARISON OF NORMAL CELLS AND HFH CELLS[a]

Medium LDL Conc. (μg/ml)	Observed LDL-bound (ng/mg)	CALCULATED UPTAKE By fluid endocytosis[b] (ng/mg cell protein/18 h)	CALCULATED UPTAKE By adsorptive endocytosis[c] (ng/mg cell protein/18 h)	Sum	OBSERVED UPTAKE (internalized and degraded) (ng/mg/18 h)
Normal Cells					
0.5	14.9±1.2	1.8	70	72	308±37
2.5	61.4±5.1	9	287	296	1349±114
12.5	218 ±20.8	45	1019	1064	3125±301
HFH Cells					
0.5	7.9±0.40	1.8	24	26	16.8±1.0
2.5	36 ±3.7	9	110	119	106±6.1
12.5	193 ±8.7	45	593	638	530±25

[a] Cells were incubated 18 h at 37°, quadruplicate dishes at each concentration of ^{125}I-LDL. Average protein content per dish: normal cells, 443 μg; HFH cells, 304 μg.

[b] A value of 3.6 μl/mg cell protein/18 h was used for these calculations. Observed values were: normal cells, 3.40±0.30 (S.D.; n=14); HFH cells, 3.53±0.48 (S.D.; n=8).

[c] Calculations as described in legend to Table II. Mean cell diameter of 25 μm was assumed for normal cells but 31 μm for HFH cells. The larger value for HFH cells is based on the observed lesser number of cells per dish at confluency (58).

17 ng, the value for adsorptive endocytosis was 212 ng and the sum was 229 ng. This contrasts with the observed total uptake which was some 10 times greater. In other words, one can adequately account for HDL uptake on the basis of fluid and adsorptive endocytosis making the assumption that the HDL is bound randomly over the surface and that there is no specialized mechanism for its rapid uptake. In contrast, the uptake of LDL is far in excess of that expected unless there were some focal binding and some specialized process for more rapid internalization from such specialized binding sites. We showed that the greater uptake of LDL is not due to stimulation of generalized endocytosis since the rate of clearance of sucrose (fluid endocytosis) was not affected by high concentrations either of LDL or HDL. One has to conclude that LDL must be bound to some localized sites and that endocytosis must occur more rapidly from those sites. The results are consonant with the electron microscopic findings of Anderson, Brown and Goldstein that LDL is selectively and specifically bound to specialized areas of the cell surface (36) and lead to the further conclusion that endocytosis at these sites must be more rapid than endocytosis at other sites on the cell membrane.

In an earlier paper from this laboratory we reported studies on an HFH line with a gross defect in internalization and degradation of LDL (58), in agreement with the findings of Goldstein and Brown (54). However, the difference in surface binding, determined by trypsin treatment of the monolayer, was less striking than the difference in degradation. Subsequent studies in this laboratory (53) and in Dallas (59) show that this cell line is in fact "receptor negative" i.e. lacks high affinity receptors. We now believe the binding to these HFH cells does in fact represent binding to low affinity sites as shown by our more recent studies on the nature of the binding sites summarized above (53) and as shown by data on fluid and adsorptive endocytosis shown in Table III (55). The results, using the same assumptions applied in studies of normal cells, show that total uptake is in good agreement with that calculated for fluid endocytosis and random (nonfocal) adsorptive endocytosis. As in the case of HDL uptake by normal cells, it is not necessary to postulate selective, more rapid uptake of LDL bound to HFH cells i.e. there need not be any specialized process involved. However, -- and this is the key point -- the measured uptake is well in excess of the uptake that can be attributed to fluid endocytosis alone (column 6 versus column 3). We conclude that a significant element in the uptake of LDL by HFH cells is uptake from low affinity binding sites. Furthermore, both in normal fibroblasts and in HFH fibroblasts the overall rate of LDL degradation increases with the concentrations of LDL in the medium even to the highest levels studied - far above the LDL level needed to saturate the high affinity receptors on the normal cells. We conclude that both in normal cells and in HFH cells uptake from low affinity sites contributes to LDL degradation. In HFH cells, of course, all the observed degradation is attributable to low affinity uptake. In normal cells exposed to low LDL levels (below 50μg/ml) low affinity degradation will be a small component but at levels above 100 μg/ml it may become the dominant mode. Thus when endothelial integrity is breached and plasma enters the artery wall, low affinity uptake may become a critical element in atherogenesis.

HDL-LDL INTERACTIONS

In closing, let me briefly review some recent findings with regard to the interactions between HDL and LDL. These findings are perhaps of special interest because of emerging data establishing HDL as a negative risk factor in atherosclerosis (14-17). Carew, Weinstein, Hayes and Steinberg (30) showed that the binding, uptake and degradation of LDL by pig smooth muscle cells was inhibited by the presence of high concentrations of HDL in the medium. With Dr. Norman E. Miller we have since made similar observations in human fibroblasts (53). In both cell lines we showed that HDL could prevent LDL-induced increases in net cell cholesterol content. Incubation with high concentration of HDL alone had no significant effect on cell cholesterol content. Incubation with high concentrations of LDL alone caused a statistically significant increase in cell cholesterol content. When the incubation medium included both LDL and HDL at these same concentrations the increment in cell cholesterol content was much less. This past year Dr. John P.D. Reckless working with us in La Jolla studied the metabolism of lipoproteins by cultured rabbit endothelial cells, an established cell line from rabbit aortic endothelium generously given to us by Dr. Vincenzo Buonassisi of our Department of Biology (60). The same general phenomenon of HDL inhibition of LDL metabolism was shown with this cell line and again it was possible to show that HDL could prevent LDL induced increases in net cell cholesterol content (32).

What is the nature of this HDL-LDL interaction? Above we have reviewed our data indicating that the binding sites for HDL are qualitatively quite distinct from at least the high affinity binding sites for LDL. If the binding sites are distinct, the interaction would seem to be paradoxical. We have pointed out, however, that the number of LDL molecules displaced is small relative to the total number of HDL molecules bound to the cell at the high medium concentrations of HDL used to demonstrate the competition. Recent studies by Mahley and Innerarity (61) suggest that the interaction can in fact be attributed to a minor subfraction of HDL, the fraction containing arginine-rich protein (apoprotein E). Using canine HDL, they confirm that HDL does interfere with LDL binding and degradation. However, by precipitating with heparin-manganese they could resolve the HDL into a fraction containing no detectable apo E and a fraction rich in apo E. The former did not compete with LDL while the latter was many times more effective than the original, unfractionated HDL. Thus, it appears very likely that it is a subfraction of HDL molecules - those containing apo E - that is responsible for the HDL-LDL interaction. The "protective" effect of a high HDL level in man could thus be due to either the action of HDL inhibiting uptake of LDL, and thus reducing the rate of delivery of cholesterol to the cells in the artery wall, or the action of HDL functioning as an acceptor of cholesterol, and thus facilitating "reverse cholesterol transport" (19,27), or both. However, other mechanisms or additional mechanisms may be operative _in vivo_.

ACKNOWLEDGEMENTS

The original studies from the author's laboratory were supported by NIH Research Grants: HL-14197 awarded by the National Heart, Lung, and Blood Institute; GM-17702 awarded by the National Institute of General Medical Sciences; NS-08246 awarded by the National Institute of Neurological and Communicative Disorders and Stroke, PHS/DHEW.

REFERENCES

1. Zilversmit, D.B.
Circ. Res. 33: 633 (1973)
2. Havel, R.J., Felts, J.M. and Van Duyne, C.M.
J. Lipid Res. 3: 297 (1962)
3. Havel, R.J.
Metabolism 10: 1031 (1961)
4. Quarfordt, S.H., Frank, A., Shames, D.M., Berman, M. and Steinberg, D.
J. Clin. Invest. 49: 2281 (1970)
5. Bilheimer, D.W., Eisenberg, S. and Levy, R.I.
Biochim. Biophys. Acta 260: 212 (1972)
6. Sigurdsson, G., Nicoll, A. and Lewis, B.
J. Clin. Invest. 56: 1481 (1975)
7. Faergeman, D. and Havel, R.J.
J. Clin. Invest. 55: 1210 (1975)
8. Soutar, A.K., Myant, N.B. and Thompson, G.R.
Atherosclerosis 28: 247 (1977)
9. Janus, E., Wooten, R., Nicoll, A., Turner, P. and Lewis, B.
Circulation 56 (Part II): III-21 (1977)
10. Nakaya, N., Chung, B.H. and Taunton, O.D.
J. Biol. Chem. 252: 5258 (1977)
11. Nakaya, N., Chung, B.H., Patsch, J.R. and Taunton, O.D.
J. Biol. Chem. 252: 7530 (1977)
12. Melish, J., Le, N.A., Ginsberg, H., Brown, W.V. and Steinberg, D.
Circulation 56 (Part II): III-5 (1977)
13. Ruderman, N.B., Richards, K.C., Valles, V. and Jones, A.I.
J. Lipid Res. 9: 613 (1968)
14. Miller, G.J. and Miller, N.E.
Lancet I: 16 (1975)
15. Castelli, W.P., Doyle, J.T., Gordon, T., Hames, C., Hulley, S.B., Kagan, A., McGee, D., Vicic, W. and Zukel, W.J.
Circulation 52: 11 (1975)
16. Rhoads, G.G., Gulbrandsen, C.L. and Kagan, A.
New England J. Med. 294: 293 (1976)
17. Miller, N.E., Førde, O.H., Thelle, D.S. and Mjøs, O.D.
Lancet I: 965 (1977)
18. Hamilton, R.L., Williams, M.C., Fielding, C.J. and Havel, R.J.
J. Clin. Invest. 58: 667 (1976)
19. Glomset, J.A.
Am. J. Clin. Nutr. 23: 1129 (1970)

20. Anderson, D.W., Nichols, A.V., Pan, S.S. and Lindgren, F.T.
Circulation 56 (Part II): III-57 (1977)
21. Mahley, R.W., Weisgraber, K.H., Innerarity, T., Brewer, H.B., Jr., and Assman, G.
Biochemistry 14: 2817 (1975)
22. Eisenberg, S., Bilheimer, D.W. and Levy, R.I.
Biochim. Biophys. Acta 280: 94 (1972)
23. Havel, R.J., Kane, J.P. and Kashyap, M.L.
J. Clin. Invest. 52: 32 (1973)
24. Fielding, C.J., Shore, R.G. and Fielding, P.E.
Biochem. Biophys. Res. Commun. 46: 1493; (1972); Soutar, A.K., Garner, C.W., Barker, H.N., Sparrow, J.T., Jackson, R.L., Gotto, A.M. and Smith, L.C.
Biochemistry 14: 3057 (1975)
25. LaRosa, J.C., Levy, R.I., Herbert, P., Lux, J.E. and Fredrickson, D.S.
Biochem. Biophys. Res. Commun. 41: 59 (1970)
26. Sniderman, A.D., Carew, T.E., Chandler, J.G. and Steinberg, D.
Science 183: 526 (1974)
27. Weinstein, D.B., Carew, T.E. and Steinberg, D.
Biochim. Biophys. Acta 424: 404 (1976)
28. Reichl, D., Simons, L.A., Myant, N.B. Pflug, J.J. and Mills, G.L.
Clin. Sci. Mol. Med. 45: 313 (1973)
29. Rachmilewitz, D., Stein, O., Roheim, P.S. and Stein, Y.
Biochim. Biophys. Acta 270: 414 (1972)
30. Carew, T.E., Koschinsky, T., Hayes, S.B. and Steinberg, D.
Lancet I: 1315 (1976)
31. Miller, N.E., Weinstein, D.B. and Steinberg, D.
J. Lipid Res. 18: 438 (1977)
32. Reckless, J.P.D., Weinstein, D.B. and Steinberg, D.
Circulation (Suppl. II) 54: 56 (1976);
Reckless, J.P.D., Weinstein, D.B. and Steinberg,D.
J. Lipid Res., in press
33. Sigurdsson, G., Simon-Pierre, N. and Havel, R.J.
Circulation 56 (Part II): III-4 (1977)
34. Brown, M.S. and Goldstein, J.L.
Proc. Natl. Acad. Sci. USA 71: 788 (1974)
35. Brown, M.S. and Goldstein, J.L.
Science 185: 61 (1974)
36. Anderson, R.G.W., Goldstein, J.L. and Brown, M.S.
Proc. Natl. Acad. Sci. USA 73: 2434 (1976)
37. Chang, C.M. and Steinberg, D., unpublished observations

38. Williams, C.D. and Avigan, J.
Biochim. Biophys. Acta 260: 413 (1972)
39. Brown, M.S., Dana, S.E. and Goldstein, J.L.
J. Biol. Chem. 249: 789 (1974)
40. Kandutsch, A.A. and Chen, H.W.
J. Biol. Chem. 248: 8408 (1973)
41. Goldstein, J.L., Dana, S.E. and Brown, M.S.
Proc. Natl. Acad. Sci. USA 71: 4288 (1974)
42. Brown, M.S. and Goldstein, J.L.
Cell 6: 307 (1975)
43. Brown, M.S. and Goldstein, J.L.
Science 191: 150 (1976)
44. Simons, L.A., Reichl, D., Myant, N.B. and Mancini, M.
Atherosclerosis 21: 283 (1975)
45. Goldstein, J.L., Brunschede, G.Y. and Brown, M.S.
J. Biol. Chem. 250: 7854 (1975)
46. Steinberg, D., Nestel, P.J., Weinstein, D.B., Remaut-Desmeth, M. and Chang, C.M.
Biochim. Biophys. Acta, in press
47. Goldstein, J.L., Dana, S.E., Faust, J.R., Beaudet, A.L. and Brown, M.S.
J. Biol. Chem. 250: 8487 (1975)
48. Williams, J.C., Weinstein, D.B. and Steinberg, D.
Circulation 56: **III-99 (1977)**
49. Pittman, R.C., Williams, J.C., Miller, A.L. and Steinberg, D.
Clin. Res., in press
50. Assman, G., Brown, B.G., and Mahley, R.W.
Biochemistry 14: 3996 (1975)
51. Bersot, T.P., Mahley, R.W., Brown, M.S. and Goldstein, J.L.
J. Biol. Chem. 251: 2395 (1976)
52. Gustafson, A.
J. Lipid Res. 6: 512 (1965)
53. Miller, N.E., Weinstein, D.B., Carew, T.E., Koschinsky, T. and Steinberg, D.
J. Clin. Invest. 60: 78 (1977)
54. Goldstein, J.L. and Brown, M.S.
J. Biol. Chem. 249: 5153 (1974)
55. Miller, N.E., Weinstein, D.B. and Steinberg, D.
J. Lipid Res., in press
56. Becker, G. and Ashwood-Smith, M.J.
Exp. Cell Res. 82: 310 (1973)
57. Steinman, R.M., Brodie, S.E. and Cohn, Z.A.
J. Cell Biol. 68: 665 (1976)
58. Stein, O., Weinstein, D.B., Stein, Y. and Steinberg, D.
Proc. Natl. Acad. Sci. USA 73: 14 (1976)
59. Brown, M.S. and Goldstein, J.L.
Cell 9: 663 (1976)

60. Buonassisi, V. and Root, M.
Biochim. Biophys. Acta 385: 1 (1975)
61. Mahley, R.W. and Innerarity, T.L.
J. Biol. Chem. 252: 3980 (1977)
62. Stein, O. and Stein, Y.
Biochim. Biophys. Acta 431: 363 (1976)

LIPOPROTEIN METABOLISM IN MAN

G. Schlierf, P. Oster, D. Lang, H. Raetzer,
B. Schellenberg and C.C. Heuck

Klinisches Institut für Herzinfarktforschung,
Medizinischen Universitätsklinik Heidelberg,
Heidelberg, Germany

In the majority of us middle-aged males in the post-prandial state, right now pancreatic and plasma lipases are working to dispose of the fatty parts of our breakfast aided by carbohydrate stimulated insulin incretion. At the vascular endothelium the rising VLDL and IDL compete for binding sites with LDL and the HDL as "guards" may be fighting adverse effects of tobacco smoke, hopefully assisted by yesterday evening's glass of beer. This would, in shorthand, describe "human lipoprotein metabolism, 1977."

In trying to present more material on the vast topic I am honored and embarrassed at the same time since there are, in the audience, many colleagues who by their amount of work and experience in the field could do a better job for this expert group. In attempting to review briefly areas of acute interest:

1. a dynamic view of human lipoprotein metabolism is presented which is sketchy in many areas and which contains a considerable amount of speculation in others. In this metabolic scheme the vulnerable intersections are pointed out, where disturbances are known to occur and where therapeutics may be acting.

2. factors will be summarized known to affect plasma lipoprotein concentrations with particular emphasis on diet and HDL since such factors must be considered before effects of drugs can be evaluated.

HUMAN LIPOPROTEIN METABOLISM

Lipid transport, in man, serves to move food energy from stomach to storage and from the adipose bank to tissues such as muscle. In addition, "used" lipid components of body cells, in particular cholesterol which cannot be broken down in the periphery, are carried to the liver for breakdown and excretion. Specific proteins help to solubilize the lipids for transport and to regulate catabolic processes by activating or inhibiting lipolytic enzymes.

Approximately 140 g fat as triglycerides enter the body each day (1), are digested and packed into chylomicrons. Assuming a mean content of 3% cholesterol in these particles, almost 5 g of cholesterol are used for this purpose only 300 mg of which are from dietary cholesterol. The remainder comes from enterohepatic circulation of biliary cholesterol (1-1.5 g) (2) and from local sources. Bile also contributes phospholipids for the chylomicron coat.

Entrance of chylomicrons into the blood stream is followed by uptake of apolipoprotein C from the HDL fraction. It results in alimentary lipemia the magnitude and duration of which is affected, among other factors, by the amount and kind of fat, the amount and kind of carbohydrate in the food and the physical activity of the individual. About 18 of each 24 hour period is occupied by food-related fluctuations in plasma triglycerides or triglyceride-rich lipoproteins, respectively (3).

Immediately upon entry of chylomicrons into the circulation their catabolism is initiated (Fig. 1) by attack of "lipoprotein lipases" which appear to be located at the capillary endothelium; of these "adipose tissue lipoprotein lipase" is activated by apolipoprotein C II and inhibited by C III (4). Thus, the chylomicrons carry with them material which regulates their catabolism. At the same time, phospholipase A activity breaks down coat lecithin. Free cholesterol exchanges with HDL and is esterified by LCAT. HDL also accepts apolipoprotein C. When chylomicrons become depleted of triglycerides, lecithin, free cholesterol and apolipoprotein, they become smaller and relatively enriched with cholesterol ester and apolipoprotein B (5).

Chylomicron triglycerides are predominantly hydrolyzed. Part of their triglyceride fatty acids enter the

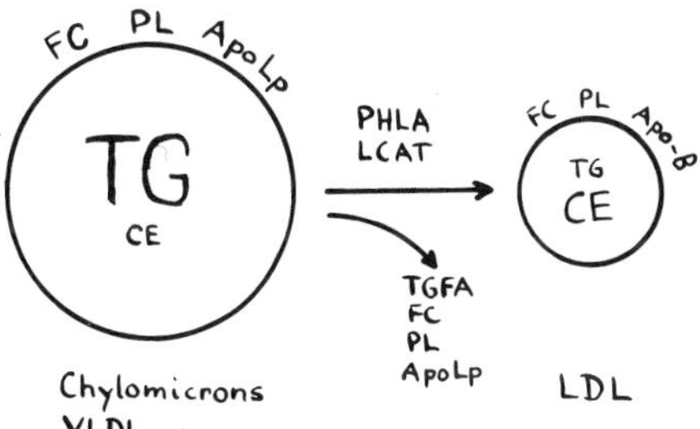

Figure 1: Metabolism of triglyceride-rich lipoproteins. Chylomicrons and VLDL are broken down by "postheparin lipolytic activity" (lipoprotein lipases). LCAT is also involved. The final product is LDL.

Abbreviations: FC=free cholesterol, PL=phospholipids, ApoLP=Apolipoproteins, TG=triglycerides, CE=cholesterol ester, PHLA=postheparin lipolytic activity, LCAT=lecithin cholesterol acyl transferase, TGFA=triglyceride fatty acids.

FFA pool; a great part is incorporated into adipose tissue triglycerides for temporary or even more or less permanent storage (fig. 2). The proportion of FFA used for storage and oxidation, respectively, is dependent on the metabolic state of the individual, high glucose and insulin levels favoring deposition of triglycerides in adipose tissue. The enzymatic breakdown of chylomicrons is disturbed in familial hyperchylomicronemia (type I-HLP) (6) and in some patients with type V hyperlipoproteinemia.

In a matter of minutes (t/2 of chylomicrons is around 10') chylomicrons have, by depletion of triglycerides, phospholipids, free cholesterol and apolipoproteins, become "remnants" which may be taken up by the liver or catabolized further in the bloodstream. Here hepatic lipoprotein lipase is postulated to be effective. There may also be interaction of remnants with vascular endothelium as Dr. Zilversmit may tell this audience in more detail. The half-life of "remnants" is very short. In normal subjects, they cannot be found in more than trace amounts in the fasting state. A disturbed catabolism of such remnants appears to underlie Type III hyperlipoproteinemia (7).

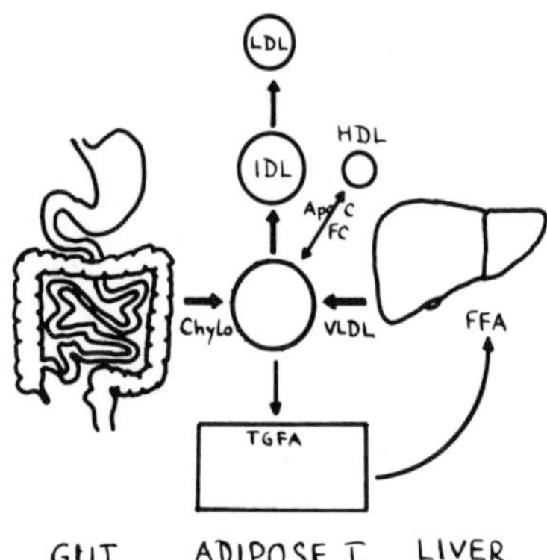

Figure 2: Metabolism of lipoproteins in man. Chylomicrons and VLDL are broken down to IDL and LDL. HDL donates and accepts from chylomicrons and VLDL apolipoproteins and lipids. Triglyceride fatty acids enter adipose tissue for storage, free fatty acids are liberated from adipose tissue and are oxidized or enter the liver to be repacked into VLDL.

Abbreviations: LDL=low density lipoproteins, IDL=intermediate density lipoproteins, TGFA=triglyceride fatty acids, HDL=high density lipoproteins, ApoC=apolipoprotein C, FC=free cholesterol, VLDL=very low density lipoproteins, FFA=free fatty acids.

Endogenous triglyceride transport is directed from the liver to the periphery and occurs via VLDL (figure 2) Increased VLDL secretion and/or impaired catabolism are characteristic of the state of positive energy balance and, at least for a limited period of time, for high carbohydrate feeding. Alochol also appears to increase VLDL synthesis. In obesity, increased VLDL transport and elevated FFA levels are signs of a "futile cycle" of energy liberation, repacking and storage. The half life of VLDL is 2-4 hr, the turnover has been estimated to be in the area of 48 g/day. The mechanisms for the breakdown of VLDL may be similar to those operating with chylomicrons (5) and there may be competition for catabolizing enzymes (8). The metabolic disturbances of endogenous hyperlipemia (Type II-b and IV-HLP) are considered to reside in the above areas.

The preliminary "end-product" of intravascular lipoprotein catabolism is LDL containing still most of the chylomicron and VLDL cholesterol (fig. 1). It has been estimated that the catabolism of chylomicrons could account for 10-50% of the circulating LDL, the remainder may come from VLDL. Direct (hepatic) synthesis of LDL has also not been excluded. LDL carry approximately 80% of the total plasma cholesterol in normal adults. Their half-life has been calculated at 2.5 days. There is no noticeable diurnal fluctuation of this fraction which the human metabolic machinery has problems to catabolize. LDL breakdown, according to present knowledge, can occur in the liver and in other body tissues among which fibroblasts have been studied extensively (9). By way of extracellular binding and intracellular uptake of LDL-cholesterol these cells regulate their own cholesterol synthesis and deliver LDL cholesterol for "out of town" shipment by HDL. LDL-binding and catabolism is defective in familial hypercholesterolemia (type II-HLP).

The triad comprising HDL, cell membranes and LCAT appears to function as a scavenger system by which membrane cholesterol becomes HDL free cholesterol which in turn is esterified by LCAT and thus as a completely apolar lipid can become a core component of lipoproteins. It has already been mentioned that the LCAT system hereby participates in the breakdown of chylomicrons and VLDL in accordance with the rise of LCAT activity during alimentary lipemia (10).

HDL, in addition, carry surplus apolipoproteins for chylomicron and VLDL formation. They also inhibit entry of LDL (and perhaps VLDL) into endothelial cells, an aspect which has attained significant popularity in recent months. The half-life of HDL has been estimated at approximately 5 days; the catabolism occurs in the liver.

A significant but often neglected lipid fraction is plasma FFA, which exhibit the greatest turnover of the plasma lipids amounting to approximately 160 g/day. FFA-levels, under a variety of circumstances determine hepatic FFA uptake and VLDL synthesis and thus are important determinants of plasma triglyceride and lipoprotein levels. The elusive role of "stress" on plasma lipid levels should be mediated by excessive FFA liberation and several lipid lowering drugs are thought to operate by inhibition of lipolysis. On the other hand, the FFA-VLDL cycle may be interrupted at the level of adipose tissue and form the pathogenetic basis of some hypertriglyceridemias (type IV HLP) (11).

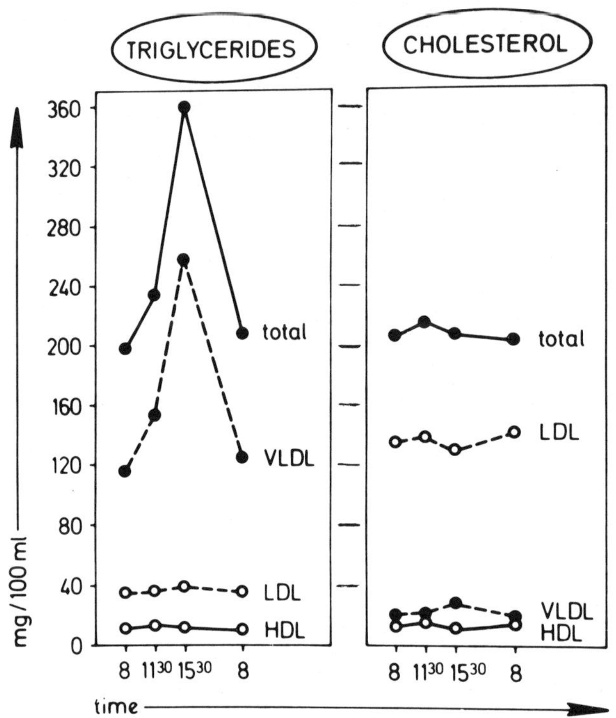

Figure 3: Diurnal plasma lipoproteins in patients with endogenous hypertriglyceridemia (n=10) on prudent diet.

Plasma concentrations of the three main lipoprotein classes during a 24-hour period with controlled food intake are shown in figure 3 for patients with endogenous hypertriglyceridemia. VLDL fluctuate with incoming dietary fat while LDL and HDL remain unchanged. A qualitatively similar pattern is seen in normal subjects.

Most studies of plasma lipids and lipoproteins in man have been performed in the "fasting state" 12 to 14 hours after the last meal. Compared to postprandial metabolic activities, this "fasting state" is considered to be relatively stable. However, in "normal" as well as in hyperlipemic subjects, plasma lipids will show marked changes upon prolonged fasting. VLDL fall within a few days to very low levels. LDL rise significantly (fig. 4) with maximal values after 1 week and then return to low levels. HDL (fig. 5) in this group of

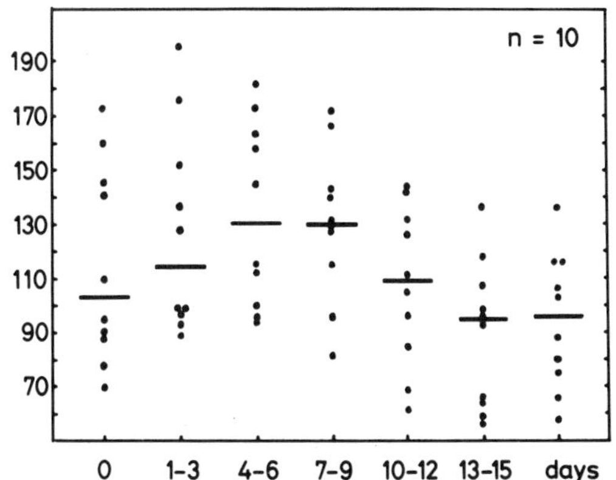

Figure 4: LDL cholesterol with prolonged fasting (16-18 days) in 10 obese subjects. Individual values and medians are given.

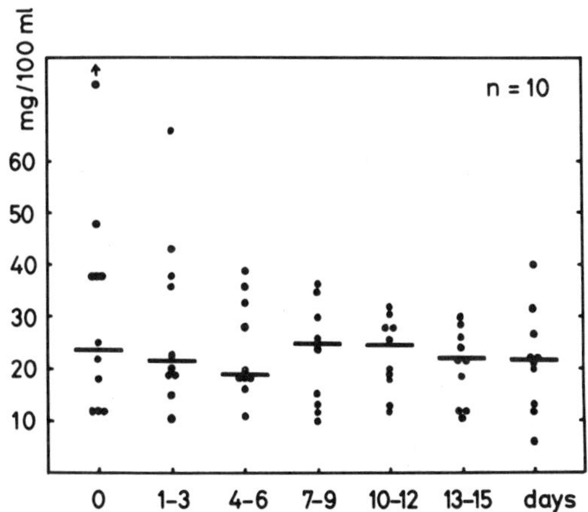

Figure 5: HDL cholesterol with prolonged fasting (16-18 days) in 10 obese subjects. Individual values and medians are given.

sex	female	>	male
age	old	>	young (♂)
race	Negro	>	White
	Eskimo		
weight	lean	>	obese

Figure 6

Hyperlipidemia	↓
Diabetes	(↓)
Hemodialysis	↓
CHD	↓
Porphyria	↑
Pesticides	↑
Smoking	(↓)
Exercise	↑

Figures 6 and 7: Factors affecting HDL-cholesterol, condensed from references 12-19.

markedly obese, are quite low and remain so for the period of observation (16-18 days).

FACTORS AFFECTING LIPOPROTEIN AND IN PARTICULAR HDL CONCENTRATION

Let us now return to normal fasting conditions, 12-14 hours after the last meal and consider some factors which affect lipoprotein concentrations. Figures 6 and 7 review "endogenous" factors affecting plasma lipoproteins. The opinions summarized in the figures are not uniform and reflect those of the references given (see legends).

The effect of exercise on HDL concentration is, in addition, exemplified by figure 8 from Dr. Wood's

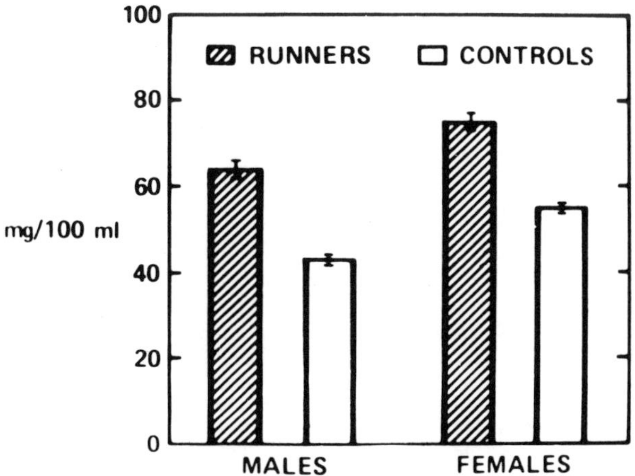

Figure 8: Plasma HDL cholesterol (mean ± SE) in male and female long distance runners (20).

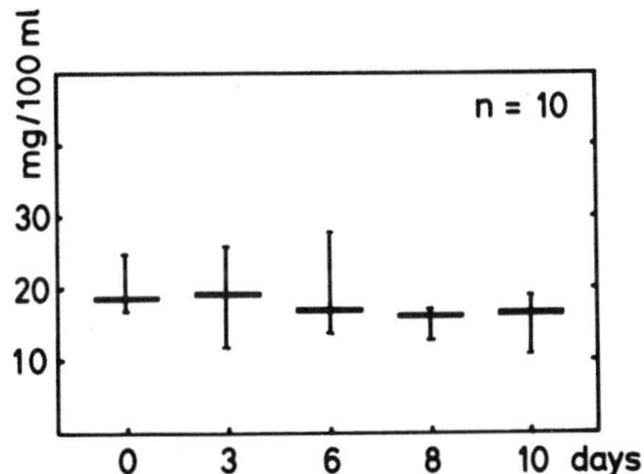

Figure 9: HDL cholesterol with prudent diet in 10 patients with endogenous hypertriglyceridemia (type IV hyperlipoproteinemia). Medians and 75 percentiles are given.

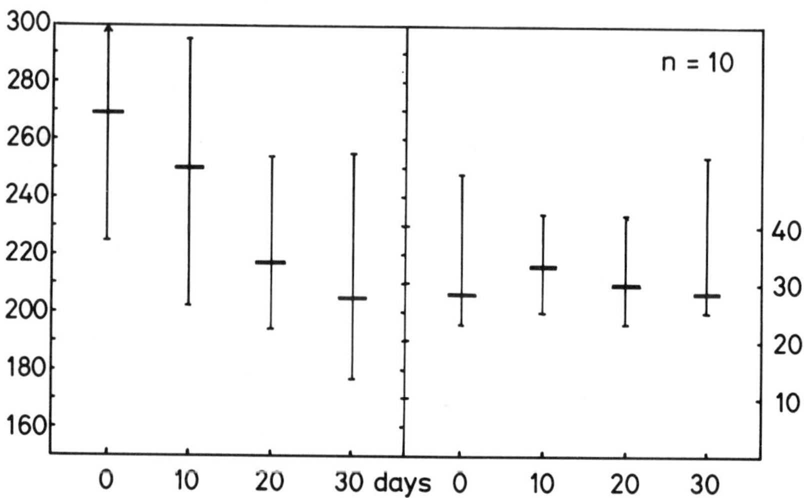

Figure 10: LDL and HDL cholesterol with prudent diet in 10 patients with familial hypercholesterolemia (type II hyperlipoproteinemia) (mg/100 ml). Medians and 75 percentiles are given.

experience with long-distance runners. Other authors have shown that different HDL concentrations between the physically active and inactive are not inherent characteristics but can be modified by the introduction or omission of exercise (21-22).

What does therapy, in particular diet, do to low HDL levels? Figure 9 shows our experience with prudent diet in type IV hyperlipoproteinemia. While, in this admittedly brief period, triglycerides were returned close to normal, there was no change in HDL concentrations.

Figure 10 shows corresponding data in familial type II hyperlipoproteinemia. While LDL fell markedly during the 30 days of therapy, there was likewise no change of the (low) HDL levels. Long-term experience (3) with dietary management of children and adolescents with familial type II-hyperlipoproteinemia have yielded similar results. In accordance are observations of Vessby et al (23) on the failure of (low) HDL levels in hyperlipoproteinemias to respond to diet therapy.

	VLDL	LDL	HDL
Calories	↑	(↑)	(↓)
Protein	?	↓ veget. ↑ animal	↑ low prot. fish?
Fat, satur.	↓	↑	(↓)
unsat.	↓↓	↓	(↑)
Cholesterol	–	↑	(↑)
Carbohydrate	↑ tempor.	↓	↓
Alcohol	↑	↓	↑

Data condensed from references 24 and 26-33. Arrows in parentheses indicate that some contradictory evidence is available.

	VLDL	LDL	HDL
Clofibrate	↓	↑ or ↓	(↑)
Nicotinic acid	↓	↓	↑
D-Thyroxin	(↓)	↓	–
Colestyramin	(↑)	↓	–
Contraceptives	↑	(↑)	(↓)

References pertinent to data in Table 2: General review (34), Clofibrate (35), Nicotinic acid (36,37), D-thyroxine (38), Cholestyramine (39), contraceptives (40), fiber (pectin) (41).

There is one dietary modification which markedly affects HDL cholesterol levels, namely, high carbohydrate, low fat feeding. This is associated with marked changes in HDL composition: ApoA decreases and HDL triglycerides increase as published by Schonfeld et al (24) and by Levy et al (25) who also found an increased HDL turnover with high carbohydrate diet. It is not known whether or not these effects on HDL are persistent or reversible such as carbohydrate induction of hypertriglyceridemia. Likewise it is not known whether such altered HDL behave like normal HDL with regard to receptor binding as a substrate for LCAT etc.

Table 1 summarizes dietary effects on plasma lipoprotein concentrations in the human from a number of studies which are referenced in the legend. There are a significant number of unexplored or controversial areas in this field. Thus information on the effects of dietary protein is scanty. The HDL raising effect of a low protein diet has been taken from an experiment in monkeys and the effects of fish consumption on HDL have only been surmised from a study in vegetarians. Likewise, the effects of carbohydrates, amount and kind, are still far from clarified and so is the matter of alcohol and blood lipoproteins.

In summary, a multitude of internal and external factors and of the latter prominently diet and exercise determine the "individual" lipoprotein pattern. These factors must be carefully controlled before drugs affecting lipoproteins (table 2) can be evaluated.

ACKNOWLEDGEMENT

This study was supported by Deutsche Forschungsgemeinschaft, SFB 90-K4.

REFERENCES

1. Ernährungsbericht 1976. Ed. Deutsche Gesselschaft für Ernährung, Frankfurt am Main, 1976.
2. Grundy, S.M.
J. Clin. Invest. 55: 269 (1975)
3. Schlierf, G., G. Vogel, C.C. Heuck, P. Oster, H. Raetzer, B. Schellenberg
MSchr. Kinderheilk. 125: 770 (1977)

4. Augustin, J., G. Middelhoff and W.V. Brown
In: Fettstoffwechsel. G. Schettler, H. Greten, G. Schlierf and D. Seidel, editors, Springer Verlag, 1976, p. 219
5. Eisenberg, S. and R.I. Levy.
In: Advances in Lipid Research, Volume 13, R. Paoletti and D. Kritchevsky, editors, Academic Press, New York, 1975, pp. 2-80
6. Greten, H. and W.V. Brown
In: Fettstoffwechsel. G. Schettler, H. Greten, G. Schlierf and D. Seidel, editors, Springer Verlag, 1976, p. 267
7. Chait, A., J.D. Brunzell, J.J. Albers and W.R. Hazzard.
Lancet I: 1176 (1977)
8. Brunzell, J.D. W.R. Hazzard, D. Porte, Jr., and E.L. Bierman
J. Clin. Invest. 52: 1578 (1973)
9. Goldstein, J.L.,M.J.E. Harrod and M.S. Brown
Amer. J. Hum. Genet. 26: 199 (1974)
10. Rose, H.G. and J. Juliano
J. Lab. Clin. Med. 89: 524 (1977)
11. Carlson, L.A. and G. Walldius
Europ. J. Clin. Invest. 6: 195 (1976)
12. Bagdade, J.D. and J.J. Albers
New Engl. J. Med. 296: 1436 (1977)
13. Bang, H.O., J. Dyerberg and A.B. Nielson
Lancet I: 1143 (1971)
14. Castelli, W.P., J.T. Doyle, T. Gordon, C.G. Hames, M. Hjortland, S.B. Hulley, A. Kagan, and W.J. Zukel
Lancet II: 153 (1977)
15. Castelli, W.P., J.T. Doyle, T. Gordon, C.G. Hames, M.C. Hjortland, S.B. Hulley, A. Kagan and W.J. Zukel
Circulation 55: 767 (1977)
16. Gordon, T., W.P. Castelli, M.C. Hjortland, W.B. Kannel and T.R. Dawber
Am. J. Med. 62: 707 (1977)
17. Miller, G.J. and N.E. Miller
Lancet I: 16 (1975)
18. Mjos, O.D., D.S. Thelle, O.H. Forde and H. Vik-Mo
Acta Med. Scand. 201: 323 (1977)
19. Rhoads, G.G., C.L. Gulbrandsen and A. Kagan
New Engl. J. Med. 294: 293 (1976)
20. Wood, P.D.S.
Kronberg Conference, May, 1977
21. Lopez, S.A., R. Vial, L. Balart, and G. Arroyave
Atherosclerosis 20: 1 (1974)
22. Hoffman, A.A., W.R. Nelson and F.A. Goss
Am. J. Cardiol. 20: 516 (1967)

23. Vessby, B., H. Lithell and I.-B. Gustafsson
Postgrad. Med. J. 51: 52 (1975)
24. Schonfeld, G., S.W. Weidman, J.L. Witztum, and R.M. Bowen
Metabolism 25: 261 (1976)
25. Levy, R.I., C.B. Blum and E.J. Schaefer
In: Lipoprotein Metabolism, H. Greten, editor, Springer-Verlag, Berlin, 1976, p. 56
26. Bagdade, J.D., W.R. Hazzard, and J. Carlin
Metabolism 19: 1020 (1970)
27. Connor, W.E.
In: Cerebrovascular Diseases, P. Scheinberg, editor, Raven Press, New York, 1976, p. 121
28. Hulley, S.B., W.S. Wilson, M.I. Burrows, and M.Z. Nichaman
Lancet II: 551 (1972)
29. Sacks, F.M., W.P. Castelli, A. Donner and E.H. Kass
New Engl. J. Med. 292: 1148 (1975)
30. Spritz, N. and M.A. Mishkel
J. Clin. Invest. 48: 78 (1969)
31. Srinivasan, S.R., B. Radhakrishnamurthy, E.R. Dalferes, L.S. Webber and G.S. Berenson
Proc. Soc. Exper. Biol. Med. 154: 102 (1977)
32. Vessby, B., H. Hedstrand and U. Olsson
Uppsala J. Med. Sci. 81: 71 (1976)
33. Vessby, B. and H. Lithell
Artery 1: 63 (1974)
34. Levy, R.I.
Ann. Rev. Pharmacol. Toxicol. 17: 499 (1977)
35. Carlson, L.A., A.G. Olsson, L. Orö, S. Rössner, and G. Walldius
In: Atherosclerosis III, G. Schettler and A. Weizel, editors, Springer-Verlag, Berlin, 1974, p. 768
36. Olsson, A.G., L. Orö, and S. Rössner
Atherosclerosis 19: 61 (1974)
37. Carlson, L.A., A.G. Olsson and D. Ballantyne
Atherosclerosis 26: 603 (1977)
38. Rakow, A.D., H.U. Klör, E. Küter, H.H. Ditschuneit, and H. Ditschuneit
Atherosclerosis 24: 369 (1976)
39. Levy, R.I., D.S. Fredrickson, N.J. Stone, D.W. Bilheimer, W.V. Brown, C.J. Glueck, A.M. Gotto, P.N. Herbert, P.O. Kwiterovich, T. Langer, J. LaRosa, S.E. Lux, A.K. Rider, R.S. Shulman, and H.R. Sloan
Ann. Int. Med. 79: 51 (1973)
40. Rössner, S., U. Larsson-Cohn, L.A. Carlson and J. Boberg
Acta Med. Scand. 190: 301 (1971)

41. Durrington, P.N., C.H. Bolton, A.P. Manning, and M. Hartog
Lancet _II_: 394 (1976)

RELATIVE ATHEROGENICITY OF DIFFERENT PLASMA LIPOPROTEINS

Donald B. Zilversmit*

Division of Nutritional Sciences and Section of Biochemistry, Molecular and Cell Biology, Division of Biological Sciences, Cornell University, Ithaca, New York, U.S.A.

Atherosclerosis has been described by many as a multifactorial disease. This description had left me with the uneasy feeling that it says very little. Although it is true that a multitude of risk factors has been established (1,2) it is equally true that most diseases are not the result of a single cause, but are instead a combination of necessary and permissive conditions that disturb the homeostasis of a living organism.

Among the factors that are prominent in the etiology of atherosclerosis are the serum lipids or serum lipoproteins. From the standpoint of predicting the number of coronary events in a given population, it appears that the quantity of one or more serum lipoproteins is no better than the total serum cholesterol (3). Yet to investigators of this disease it seems unlikely that the cholesterol of every lipoprotein is equally involved in the production of raised lesions in the large arteries. It is the purpose of this presentation to summarize our knowledge about the involvement of individual lipoprotein fractions in the atherogenic process. In addition, I wish to present some of our recent studies on the possible involvement of chylomicrons and chylomicron remnants in atherogenesis.

---

* Career Investigator of the American Heart Association

LOW- AND VERY LOW- DENSITY LIPOPROTEINS

In 1966 Gofman *et al* (4) reviewed the evidence for the proposal that the prevalence of coronary heart disease is more closely related to the concentration of serum low- and very low-density lipoproteins (Sf 0-12 and Sf 12-400) than to total serum cholesterol. This issue was hotly debated in the ten preceding years after a cooperative study came to the conclusion that, for the purpose of prediction, differences between the two measures were inconsequential, and did not warrant the use of the much more elaborate and expensive ultracentrifugal techniques (5). Moreover, one should consider that people, living in areas in which coronary heart disease is common, carry most of their serum cholesterol in the low density ($1.019<d<1.063$) or beta lipoprotein fraction. Thus, in these populations the amount of total serum cholesterol primarily reflects the cholesterol in this low density fraction. The belief continues, however, that the low density lipoprotein fraction is the principal atherogenic factor in serum. This belief is strengthened by studies on individuals with inherited hyperlipidemias and premature coronary heart disease in many of whom the low density lipoprotein fraction is elevated (6). However, a systematic study of hyperlipidemic patients with premature atherosclerotic disease (6,7,8,9, 10) established categories of hyperlipidemia that were not simply a manifestation of elevated low density lipoprotein levels. Premature coronary heart disease is common in people with combined hyperlipidemia in which both low and very low density lipoproteins are increased (7). According to some investigators an increase in serum triglycerides or very low density lipoproteins alone is associated with coronary heart disease, although others have minimized this relationship. In addition, the relatively rare condition of dysbetalipoproteinemia, in which very low density lipoproteins enriched in cholesteryl ester are elevated, a predisposition to arteriosclerosis and peripheral vascular disease is well established (6). It seems likely, by the way, that a large portion of the very low density lipoproteins in this condition stem from partially degraded chylomicrons, which appear to accumulate as chylomicron remnants (11).

The interpretation of these findings is to some extent simplified by the knowledge that the structure, transport, and metabolism of the various lipoproteins are interrelated. In addition to the sharing of apolipoproteins, it seems now likely that the low density lipoproteins are derived from very low density lipoproteins

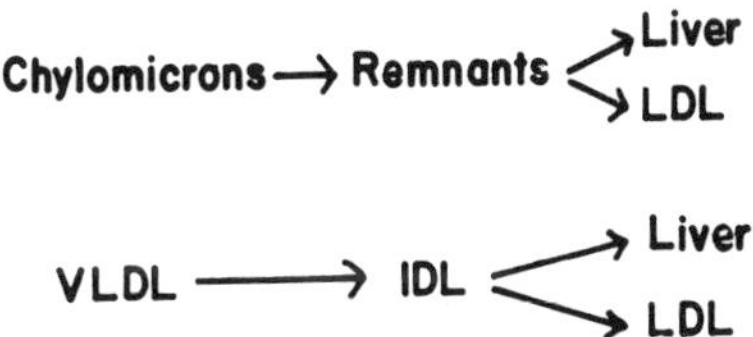

Figure 1: Stepwise degradation of chylomicrons and very low density lipoproteins. VLDL: d<1.006, IDL: 1.006<d<1.019, LDL: 1.019<d<1.063.

(Figure 1) and possibly chylomicrons (12,13). The observations that more apolipoprotein B is found in atheromatous lesions than in normal aortas (14,15) and that large amounts are present in areas of diffuse intimal thickening (16,17) probably means that low density lipoproteins are taken up by the arterial wall. These findings are also consistent with the uptake of very low density lipoproteins and chylomicron remnants. That such uptake probably takes place, is inferred from the presence of apolipoprotein C in arterial lesions (15). It is supported also by the uptake of these various lipoprotein fractions by arterial smooth muscle cells in culture (18,19,20,21).

HIGH DENSITY LIPOPROTEINS

Even a brief summary of epidemiological studies would be remiss in not alluding to the possible inverse relationship of high density lipoproteins and coronary heart disease. Although such an inverse relationship was described more than 25 years ago (22), and although an inverse relation between the serum concentrations of high density lipoprotein with those of low density- or very low density-lipoprotein, has been repeatedly observed, (see refs 23 and 24) it was not until fairly recently that a possible causal relationship became evident. This relationship is based on cell culture studies, showing that high density lipoprotein or apolipoprotein in the incubation medium accelerates the egress of cholesterol from the cell (19,25,26,27). *In vivo*, this mechanism could be coupled (Figure 2) to the continued depletion of high density lipoprotein cholesterol by the lecithin:cholesteryl acyl transferase as

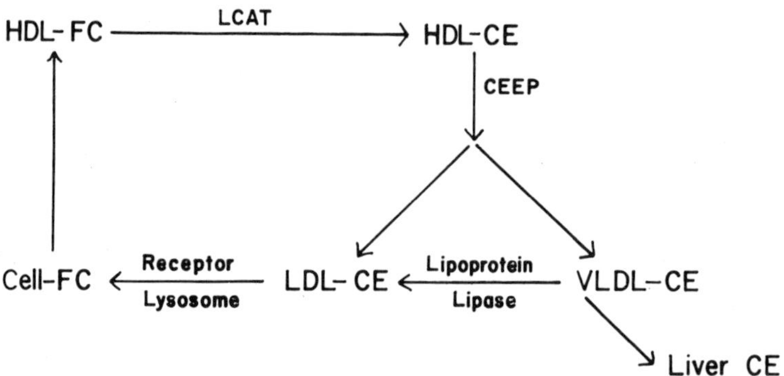

Figure 2: Possible roles of HDL, lecithin:cholesterol acyl transferase (LCAT) and cholesteryl ester exchange protein (CEEP) in cholesterol removal from cells.

proposed by Glomset (28), and possibly by the transfer of cholesteryl esters from high density lipoproteins to other serum lipoprotein fractions by means of a cholesteryl ester exchange protein which is present in human serum (unpublished observations) as well as in serum of normal and of hypercholesterolemic rabbits (29).

In this connection, it is interesting that most mammals that do not show tendencies to develop atherosclerosis, have relatively low serum cholesterol concentrations and relatively high proportions of high density lipoproteins. In a recent study we showed that even in mink, in which the total serum cholesterol averaged 200-500 mg/dl over a period up to 8 years, 80% of which was in the high density lipoprotein fraction, no intimal thickening or microscopic lipid accumulation was discovered (30). It is possible, of course, that arteries of mink are highly resistant to cholesterol infiltration, but it seems more likely that a high serum cholesterol concentration *per se* is not harmful to the arterial system when that cholesterol is mostly present in the high density lipoprotein fraction. It is also of interest that premenopausal women, who show markedly lower rates of coronary heart disease than do men in the same age group, also have somewhat higher serum high density lipoprotein concentrations (23).

Table 1

LOCALIZATION OF LIPOPROTEIN LIPASE ACTIVITY IN THE BOVINE AORTA

Sections I, II and III are parallel to the intimal surface: I representing mostly intimal cells, II and III media.

	Experiment I		Experiment II	
	LPL spec. act. (units[a]/mg)	Total act. (units)	LPL spec.act. (units/mg)	Total act. (units)
Section I	20	190	20	190
Section II	11	630	7	270
Section III	5	504	3	216

[a] One unit equals one nmole FA released/hr. The activity values represent triolein hydrolysis that was inhibitable by protamine sulfate (1 mg/ml). (From ref. 31)

CHYLOMICRON REMNANTS

It is usually assumed that chylomicrons are not athergenic because persons with chylomicronemia are not in the postabsorptive condition do not appear to suffer from premature atherosclerosis. However, this reasoning cannot be applied to the chylomicron remnants, since these patients appear to have a deficiency of lipoprotein lipases (6) and presumably an impaired mechanism for remnant formation. The remnants are much smaller than the original chylomicrons. They have lost most of their triglyceride and a large portion of the C apolipoproteins. Compared to the chylomicron, they are enriched in cholesteryl ester. As was mentioned before, the cholesteryl ester of the chylomicron remnant is readily taken up by isolated smooth muscle cells. It is not known whether or not chylomicron remnants can be produced at the endothelial surface of a large artery, in an analogous manner to which they are produced in contact with the endothelium of capillaries. We have shown (Table 1),

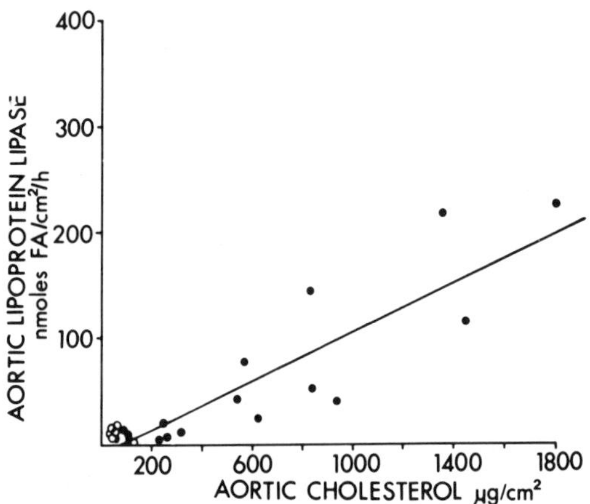

Figure 3: Aortic lipoprotein lipase vs aortic cholesterol in cholesterol-fed rabbits (from ref. 33).

however, that bovine aorta contains lipoprotein lipase (31,32) not only at or near the endothelial surface, but also deeper in the media (31). We have also demonstrated (Figure 3) that in the cholesterol-fed rabbit, aorta lipoprotein lipase increases linearly with the amount of aortic cholesterol (33). In these aortas the lipoprotein lipase appears to be closely associated with the intimal lesion, because the media localized below the lesion is not particularly enriched with lipoprotein lipase (Table 2). One may speculate that the increased amount of lipoprotein lipase in the atheromatous aorta is related to the uptake of chylomicron cholesterol by this organ. This hypothesis is supported by the finding that lipoprotein lipase in mammary gland (34) is involved, not only in the uptake of triglyceride FA but also in the uptake of chylomicron cholesterol. These observations, coupled to the previously reported (Figure 4) high influx of plasma esterified cholesterol into more extensively involved atheromatous aortas of cholesterol-fed rabbits (35-37), strengthens the concept that the chylomicron cholesterol and cholesteryl ester can be incorporated directly into the arterial lesion with the aid of the local lipoprotein lipase.

It is not clear at the moment whether the degradation of chylomicron triglyceride takes place at the arterial endothelium or whether the lipase contained in the subendothelial region (4) may be more effective. If the latter, the current concept that endothelial

Table 2

LIPOPROTEIN LIPASE IN LESIONS OF RABBIT AORTAS AND IN SUBINTIMA

Aorta	Cholesterol $\mu g/cm^2$	Lipoprotein Lipase*
1. Lesion	1889	332
1. Subintima	363	10
2. Lesion	1036	58
2. Subintima	121	0

* nmoles FA released cm^2/h
Subintima is from the same area as the lesion (from ref. 33).

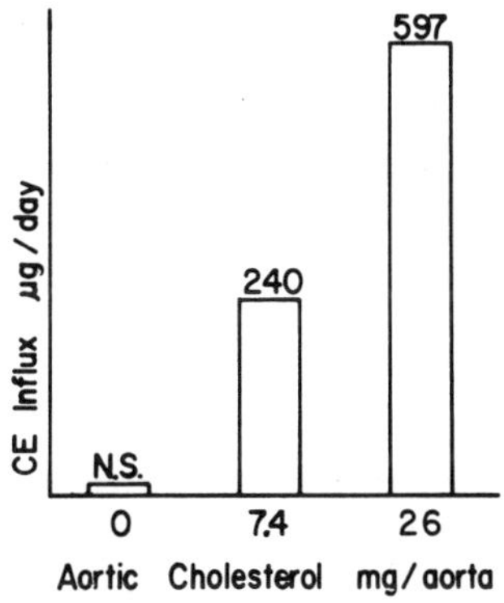

Figure 4: Cholesteryl ester influx in normal and atheromatous aortas (from refs. 36 and 37).

injury precedes the formation of arterial lesions (38) may act by making the subendothelial lipoprotein lipase accessible to the chylomicrons.

There are other reasons why chylomicron cholesterol could be a direct precursor of the arterial cholesterol. Even if the degradation of chylomicrons to chylomicron remnants on the arterial surface does not directly contribute to the cholesterol in the lesions, it seems likely that chylomicron remnants produced elsewhere could attach to the arterial lining and be ingested by pinocytosis. This type of mechanism has been proposed by Hülsmann and Jansen (39), and would be compatible with the observation of Hazzard *et al* that in broad beta disease (phenotype III) the very low density lipoprotein fraction is composed in part of chylomicron remnants (11).

ORIGIN OF VERY LOW DENSITY LIPOPROTEIN IN CHOLESTEROL-FED RABBITS

I do not need to emphasize that the rabbit responds to a cholesterol-rich diet with hypercholesterolemia and a rapid development of atheromatous lesions. It seemed, therefore, that this animal might be particularly suitable for answering questions about the origin of the hyperlipidemia induced by dietary cholesterol and fat.

In our experiments (40) we used New Zealand white rabbits that were fed for 2-4 days 100 g of Purina Laboratory Rabbit Chow, supplemented with 500 mg of cholesterol and 2.7 g of vegetable oil per day. Figure 5 shows a lipoprotein cholesterol profile for the first 48 h period. The increase in the $d>1.006$ fraction, which consists primarily of low and intermediate density lipoproteins, appears to be delayed by approximately 9 h after the first cholesterol-containing meal. The $d<1.006$, very low density lipoprotein fraction, on the other hand, increases promptly. The increase halts about 12 h after feeding and then continues in response to the second cholesterol-containing meal. These events are compatible with a mechanism that involves an influx of cholesterol-containing chylomicrons or chylomicron remnants and a somewhat delayed conversion of these lipoproteins to the low density fraction.

In order to clarify this interpretation we have used radiolabeled retinol to label chylomicrons and their remnants. The virtue of retinol is that, upon absorption,

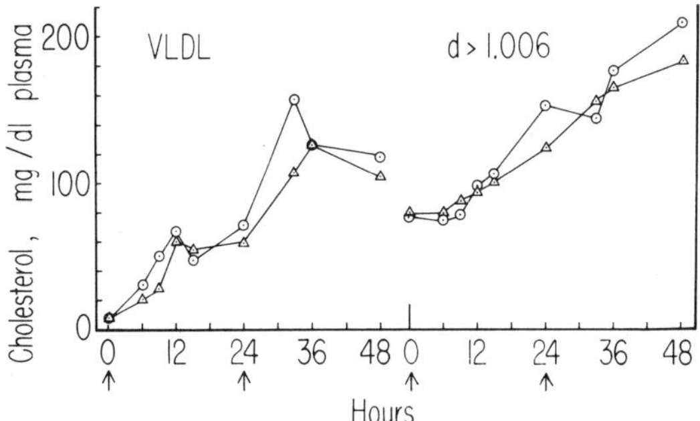

Figure 5: Lipoprotein profiles in two rabbits fed 500 mg cholesterol at 0 and 24 hours. (From ref. 40) 0)

it is carried in the esterified form, largely by chylomicrons and remains part of the chylomicron remnant, until the latter is taken up by the liver. At that point, the retinol ester is hydrolyzed and, at least in part, resecreted in combination with retinol binding protein (41). By the use of this label it is possible, therefore, to differentiate between chylomicron remnants, which contain the labeled retinol, and very low density lipoproteins secreted by liver, which are free of labeled retinol.

Thoracic duct lymph chylomicrons, labeled with [^{3}H]retinyl esters, were obtained from donor rabbits fed the ^{3}H-labeled dose in a cholesterol-containing meal (40). After injection of labeled chylomicrons into rabbits fed the control diet, or a diet containing 500 mg of cholesterol per day for 4 days, the disappearance curves were seen to differ markedly (Figure 6). In the control rabbits, the injected dose and subfractions of very low density lipoproteins were cleared rapidly, whereas in the cholesterol-fed recipient, clearance of all retinol-labeled fractions was slow. Similar studies with chylomicrons labeled with [^{3}H]cholesterol ester showed the same characteristics. Calculations based on the specific activities of the cholesterol ester in the very low density lipoprotein subfractions revealed that at least two-thirds of the very low density cholesterol ester is derived from chylomicrons and probably represents chylomicron remnants. For the purpose of this discussion it is not important why the cholesterol-rich chylomicron remnants are not readily cleared. Ross and Zilversmit (40) assumed that the delay in clearance was

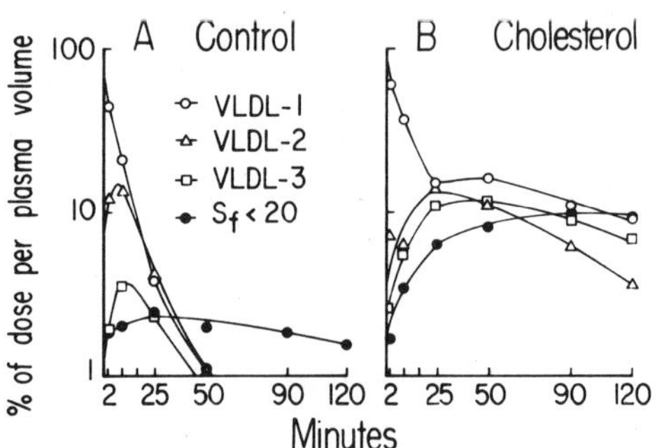

Figure 6: Disappearance of intravenously injected [^{3}H] retinyl ester labeled chylomicrons. One rabbit was fed stock diet (A) and one was fed 500 mg of cholesterol per day for 4 days. VLDL 1,2 and 3 are fractions with particle diameters 75 nm, 49-75 and 23-49 nm respectively (From ref. 40).

associated with an impairment of liver function in the recipient animal or with a saturable removal mechanism. Rodriquez et al (42,43,44) on the other hand appear to favor a difference in lipoprotein composition as the principal factor. From the point of view of the atherogenic potential of chylomicrons it is of interest, however, that in an animal that is very sensitive to the development of experimental arterial lesions, the principal lipoprotein fraction that accumulates in the bloodstream represents partially degraded chylomicrons.

Although similar data obtained in other animal species are not available, one might consider the possibility that in other species as well an accumulation of chylomicron remnants could account for an appreciable fraction of the atherogenic effect of certain diets. Both in humans (11) and in the cholesterol-fed rabbit (40,45) it appears that chylomicron remnants are very low density particles, rich in cholesteryl ester and arginine-rich apolipoprotein or apo E lipoprotein) and exhibiting beta electrophoretic mobility. A similar type of particle has also been observed in the serum of swine (46), dogs (47), rats (48) and monkeys (49) subjected to atherogenic regimens. Even if in humans that eat a moderately high cholesterol diet, remnants do not ordinarily appear in postabsorptive blood samples, one wonders what impact the nascent chylomicron remnants, either circulating in the blood stream or formed on the arterial surface, might have on the development of arterial lesions.

It is unfortunate that most of the available serum lipid determinations in humans are limited to the post-absorptive condition. Although it is probably true that serum cholesterol concentrations are affected little by the postprandial influx of chylomicrons, the serum triglyceride concentrations are greatly affected by the absorptive state. The statement that "the vast majority of hypertriglyceridemias encountered are endogenous and carried in the Sf_{20-400} pre-beta lipoprotein (3) ignores the persistence of postprandial hypertriglyceridemia throughout most of the day, at least in North Americans. Apparently, the prolonged exposure of arteries to chylomicrons and their remnants is not thought to be of any consequence for atherosclerosis. Yet it would appear from the animal studies cited here and elsewhere (50-52), that cholesterol-rich chylomicron remnants should not be ignored as an atherogenic factor.

There is one additional study in rabbits (53) that may bear on the question of relative atherogenicity of chylomicron remnants versus endogenously synthesized very low density and low density lipoproteins. In this study we pair-fed two groups of rabbits: group one on a semipurified diet of casein and sucrose with a minimal but sufficient amount of polyunsaturated fatty acid, and group two on a cholesterol-containing commercial diet. The second group of animals received equal calories and variable amounts of dietary cholesterol so as to maintain the total serum cholesterol in the two groups at equal levels, varying between 250 and 650 mg/dl. Rabbits on the semisynthetic diet transported relatively more cholesterol in the form of low density lipoproteins, whereas rabbits on the cholesterol-containing diet showed more beta-migrating, very low density lipoproteins, which most likely are chylomicron remnants (40), in their blood serum. Assessment of aortic atherosclerosis by scoring the extent of lesions, measuring aortic cholesterol or by microscopic evaluation, failed to show significant differences. Apparently, arteries exposed largely to cholesterol in the form of chylomicron remnants and those exposed to lipoproteins synthesized by the liver, show equal rates of atherogenesis.

SUMMARY

Originally, data from the Framingham study appeared to show that serum lipoprotein fractions were no better in predicting coronary heart disease than the total serum cholesterol. More recently, the concentration of high density lipoprotein has been shown to exhibit a strong negative correlation with coronary heart disease, especially in the older age groups in which total serum cholesterol shows little or no correlation with clinical events. Biochemical mechanisms that might clarify the role of high density lipoprotein in atherogenesis are forthcoming. Another aspect of the lipoprotein-atherogenesis question pertains to the possible role of chylomicrons. Animal experiments show that cholesterol feeding is frequently accompanied by an increase in beta-migrating, very low density lipoproteins which appear to be chylomicron remnants. The atherogenic effect of serum low- and very low-density lipoproteins, including chylomicron remnants, appears to depend more on their contribution to the total cholesterol concentration than to their origin in liver versus intestines.

ACKNOWLEDGEMENT

This investigation was supported by National Institutes of Health research grant HL 10933 from the National Heart, Lung and Blood Institute, United States Public Health Service.

REFERENCES

1. Report of the Inter-Society Commission for Heart Disease Resources.
   Circulation 42: A-55 (1970)
2. Stamler, J., Berkson, D.M. and Lindberg, H.A.
   In: The Pathogenesis of Atherosclerosis, R.W. Wissler, J.C. Geer and N. Kaufman, editors.
   Williams and Wilkins, Baltimore, 1972, pp. 41-119.
3. Kannel, W.B.
   Amer. J. Clin. Nutr. 24: 1074 (1971)
4. Gofman, J.W., Young, W. and Tandy, R.
   Circulation 34: 679 (1966)
5. Technical group of the Committee on Lipoproteins and Atherosclerosis and the Committee on Lipoproteins and Atherosclerosis of the National Advisory Heart Council. Circulation 14: 691 (1956)

6. Fredrickson, D.S. and Levy, R.I.
In: The Metabolic Basis of Inherited Disease, J.B. Stanbury, J.B. Wyngaarden and D.S.Fredrickson, editors, McGraw-Hill, New York, 1972, pp. 545-614
7. Goldstein, J.L., Hazzard, W.R., Schrott, H.G., Bierman, E.L. and Motulsky, A.G.
J. Clin. Invest. 52: 1533 (1973)
8. Carlson, L.A., Ekelund, L.G. and Olsson, A.G.
Lancet II: 1 (1975)
9. Bloch, A., Dinsmore, R.E. and Lees, R.S.
Lancet I: 928 (1976)
10. Crepaldi, G., Fellin, R., Briani, G., Baggio, G., Manzato, E. and Veronese, R.
Atherosclerosis 26: 593 (1977)
11. Hazzard, W.R. and Bierman, E.L.
Metabolism 25: 777 (1976)
12. Sigurdsson, G., Nicoll, A. and Lewis, B.
J. Clin. Invest. 56: 1481 (1975)
13. Eisenberg, S. and Levy, R.I.
In Advances in Lipid Research, Volume 13, R. Paoletti and D. Kritchevsky, editors, Academic, New York, 1975, p. 1-89
14. Hoff, H.F., Heideman, C.L., Gaubatz, J.W., Gotto, A.M., Erickson, E.E. and Jackson, R.L.
Circ. Res. 40: 56 (1977)
15. Hoff, H.F., Jackson, R.L. and Gotto, A.M.
In Atherosclerosis Drug Discovery. Advances in Experimental Medicine and Biology, Volume 67, C.E. Day, editor, Plenum, New York, 1976, pp.109-120
16. Smith, E.B. and Smith, R.H.
In Atherosclerosis Reviews, Volume I, Raven, New York, 1976, pp. 119-136
17. Smith, E.B.
In Advances in Lipid Research, Volume 12, R. Paoletti and D. Kritchevsky, editors, Academic, New York, 1974, pp. 1-49
18. Bierman, E.L. and Albers, J.J.
Ann. N.Y. Acad. Sci. 275: 199 (1976)
19. Stein, O., Vanderhoek, J. and Stein, Y.
Atherosclerosis 26: 465 (1977)
20. Bierman, E.L. and Albers, J.J.
Biochim. Biophys. Acta 388: 198 (1975)
21. Albers, J.J. and Bierman, E.L.
Artery 2: 337 (1976)
22. Barr, D.P., Russ, E.M. and Eder, H.A.
Am.J. Med. 11: 480 (1951)
23. Gordon, T., Castelli, W., Hjortland, M.C., Kannel, W.B. and Dawber, T.R.
Am. J. Med. 62: 707 (1977)

24. Miller, G.J. and Miller, N.E.
Lancet I: 16 (1975)
25. Bailey, J.M.
Exp. Cell Res. 37: 175 (1965)
26. Burns, C.H. and Rothblat, G.H.
Biochim. Biophys. Acta 176: 616 (1969)
27. Stein, O., Vanderhoek, J., Friedman, G. and Stein, Y.
Biochim. Biophys. Acta 450: 367 (1976)
28. Glomset, J.A.
Am. J. Clin. Nutr. 23: 1129 (1970)
29. Zilversmit, D.B., Hughes, L.B. and Balmer, J.
Biochim. Biophys. Acta 409: 393 (1975)
30. Zilversmit, D.B., Clarkson, T.B. and Hughes, L.B.
Atherosclerosis 26: 97 (1977)
31. DiCorleto, P.E. and Zilversmit, D.B.
Proc. Soc. Exp. Biol. Med. 148: 1101 (1975)
32. Henson, L.C. and Schotz, M.C.
Biochim. Biophys. Acta 409: 360 (1975)
33. Corey, J.E. and Zilversmit, D.B.
Atherosclerosis 27: 201 (1977)
34. Zinder, O., Mendelson, C.R., Blanchette-Mackie, E.J. and Scow, R.O.
Biochim. Biophys. Acta 431: 526 (1976)
35. Newman, H.A.I. and Zilversmit, D.B.
J. Biol. Chem. 237: 2078 (1962)
36. Zilversmit, D.B.
Ann. N.Y. Acad. Sci. 149: 710 (1968)
37. Zilversmit, D.B. and Hughes, L.B.
Atherosclerosis 18: 141 (1973)
38. Ross, R. and Glomset, J.A.
New Engl. J. Med. 295: 369-377, 420-425 (1976)
39. Hülsmann, W.C. and Jansen, H.
In Energy, Regulation and Biosynthesis in Molecular Biology, Walter de Gruyter, Berlin, 1974, pp. 322-335
40. Ross, A.C. and Zilversmit, D.B.
J. Lipid Res. 18: 169 (1977)
41. Smith, J.E., Muto, Y., Milch, P.O. and Goodman, D.S.
J. Biol. Chem. 248: 1544 (1973)
42. Rodriguez, J.L., Ghiselli, G.C., Torreggiani, D. and Sirtori, C.R.
Atherosclerosis 23: 73 (1976)
43. Rodriguez, J.L., Catapano, A., Ghiselli, G.C. and Sirtori, C.R.
Atherosclerosis 23: 85 (1976)

44. Rodriguez, J., Catapano, A., Ghiselli, G.C. and Sirtori, C.R.
In Atherosclerosis Drug Discovery. Advances in Experimental Biology and Medicine, Volume 67, C.E. Day, editor, Plenum, New York, 1976, pp. 169-189
45. Shore, V.G., Shore, B. and Hart, R.G.
Biochemistry 13: 1579 (1974)
46. Mahley, R.W., Weisgraber, K.H., Innerarity, T., Brewer, H.B. and Assman, G.
Biochemistry 14: 2817 (1975)
47. Mahley, R.W., Weisgraber, K.H. and Innerarity, T.
Circ. Res. 35: 722 (1974)
48. Mahley, R.W. and Holcombe, K.S.
J. Lipid Res. 18: 314 (1977)
49. Mahley, R.W., Weisgraber, K.H. and Innerarity, T.
Biochemistry 15: 2979 (1976)
50. Zilversmit, D.B.
Circ. Res. 33: 633 (1973)
51. Zilversmit, D.B.
Am. J. Card. 35: 559 (1975)
52. Zilversmit, D.B.
Ann. N.Y. Acad. Sci. 275: 138 (1976)
53. Ross, A.C., Minick, C.R. and Zilversmit, D.B.
Circulation, in press

A NEW APPROACH TO THE INVESTIGATION OF DRUGS AFFECTING LIPOPROTEINS

R. Paoletti, C.R. Sirtori, G.C. Ghiselli and R. Fumagalli

Institute of Pharmacology and Pharmacognosy and Center E. Grossi Paoletti for Atherosclerosis Research, University of Milan, Milan, Italy

The results of some recent epidemiological studies, notably the Coronary Drug Project (CDP), on the preventive effect of drugs affecting lipid metabolism against atherosclerosis and some of its complications such as myocardial infarction, have prompted, during the last few years, a careful reassessment of the goals and end-points in investigating drugs interfering with tissue and plasma lipids and lipoproteins. The Coronary Drug Project (1,2,3), involving over 5,000 patients, gave on the whole negative results.

Clofibrate and nicotinic acid were tested against a placebo in a double-blind protocol. The findings are summarized in Tables 1 and 2. The effects of the two drugs on cardiovascular morbidity and mortality were negligible; there was also a significant incidence of side effects, particularly with clofibrate, some of which may be explained on the basis of the drug's mechanisms of action, some others are of less clear origin, and possibly of doubtful clinical significance (4).

The results of the CDP should probably not be wholly ascribed to a therapeutic inefficacy of the two hypolipidemic agents tested. The modest reduction of plasma lipid levels in the treated groups may suggest an insufficient adherence to drug treatment. It should be noted that no plasma drug levels were measured in the CDP. In addition to this, hyperlipidemia may not be the most significant risk factor in the secondary prevention of

Table 1

CLOFIBRATE (CPIB), NICOTINIC ACID (NA) AND PREVENTION OF CORONARY HEART DISEASE (data from the Coronary Drug Project, 1975)

	Placebo	CPIB (1.8 g/day)	NA (3.0g)
Total patients	2,789	1,103	1,110
% Mortality:			
Total	20.9	20.0	21.2
Cardiovascular	18.9	17.3	18.8
Lipid changes (% of pretreatment levels)			
Cholesterol	+0.3	-6.2	-9.6
Triglycerides	+6.7	-15.6	-19.4

Table 2

CLOFIBRATE (CPIB), NICOTINIC ACID (NA) AND PREVENTION OF CORONARY HEART DISEASE (data from the Coronary Drug Project, 1975)

% Mortality	Placebo	CPIB	NA
Pretreatment cholesterol (mg/dl)			
< 250	19.7	20.4	21.5
> 250	22.3	19.6	20.8
Pretreatment triglycerides (mEq/L)[a]			
< 5	20.9	18.5	21.7
> 5	20.9	21.4	20.7

[a] 5 mEq/L = 147.4 mg/dl.

coronary heart disease. Analysis of the placebo group in the CDP indicated that the first six risk factors in secondary cardiovascular mortality cannot be corrected by drugs of this type (5). Among these risk factors are in fact: ST segment depression, cardiomegaly on x-ray, and presence of Q waves on EKG. Plasma cholesterol is only the seventh risk factor, lack of exercise the tenth, cigarette smoke the 13th; hypertriglyceridemia was not classified among the first 20 risk factors.

In spite of these considerations, and in spite of the positive results of a similar study with the anion exchange resin colestipol (6), the CDP was a strong incentive to revise the current beliefs in the pathogenesis of atherosclerosis and in the role of plasma lipids in the development and reversal of the atherosclerotic lesions and the onset of complications. It stimulated, in fact, further research on the specific roles for some lipoprotein classes in the process of lipoprotein deposition and removal from the arterial walls (7).

NEW APPROACHES IN DRUG INVESTIGATION

The attempts to control the formation of atherosclerotic lesions and to facilitate their regression are clearly the main scope of the present pharmacological investigations through a better use of the already known drugs or the design and the investigation of new compounds. Carlson _et al_ (8) have recently observed in 558 survivors of myocardial infarction that a combination of 2 g of clofibrate and 3 g of nicotinic acid daily may reduce in a statistically significant way the number of non-fatal myocardial infarctions (38 in the control and 19 in the treated group) over a period of about 4 years. A fairly constant serum lipid lowering has been observed in the treated group: cholesterol drop was between 15 and 20%, and that of triglycerides around 30%. In spite of the fact that the total mortality or that related to ischemic heart disease was not modified by the treatment, the number of not fatal reinfarctions was reduced by 50%. This more recent study may encourage the use of intensive serum lipid-lowering treatment as a mean to reduce the clinical complications of atherosclerosis. However it is most important to concentrate the efforts on drugs with well-defined mode of action, with the hope to obtain a more effective and possibly sequential chemotherapy on one or more of the steps leading to the atherosclerotic lesions and their complications. Some new agents have been already found to be active on specific patterns, such as the ratio between high density lipoproteins (HDL) and low and very low density lipoproteins (LDL and VLDL) in plasma, drugs and natural compounds active on the uptake of lipoproteins by the arterial walls, and drugs able to modify the lipoprotein composition in order to obtain less atherogenic macromolecules.

Drugs Modifying Lipoprotein Distribution

The VLDL and LDL lipoproteins are considered definite risk factors. The presence in the atherosclerotic lesions of apoproteins B and C-III, major components of circulating VLDL and LDL, has been demonstrated with immunological techniques (9). Studies on the lipoprotein profile of patients with and without coronary heart disease (CHD) have reported a negative correlation between plasma levels of HDL and the incidence of CHD (10, 11). Similar findings have been reported in different populations by comparing patients with similar plasma cholesterol levels but differing in the incidence of CHD (12,13). These findings are also in agreement with the relative immunity to CHD of pre-menopausal women whose HDL concentrations are some 30-60% higher than those of male counterparts (14). The protective effect of HDL would explain the prolonged life-expectancy of persons with familial hyper-α-lipoproteinemia (15,16). It is important to note that the level of plasma HDL-cholesterol is not correlated with that of total blood cholesterol, nor with that of LDL or VLDL-cholesterol (17). In addition, when elevated total blood cholesterol is associated with α-hyperlipoproteinemia, no clinical manifestations of atherosclerosis are observed (18,19). Experimental studies have demonstrated that the mink, with a high percentage of total plasma cholesterol bound to HDL (80%), is protected against arterial lesions (20). The protective effect of HDL may be related to its interaction with lecithin-cholesterol acyl-transferase (LCAT) in plasma, providing a mechanism for the removal of free cholesterol from peripheral tissues, such as the arterial walls, and its transport as cholesteryl esters to the liver (21,22). Addition of HDL indeed facilitates removal of cholesterol from atherosclerotic tissue (23), or from cultured cells (24,25). A second mechanism for HDL activity has been identified by Carew _et al_ (26). HDL binds to the surface of porcine aortic smooth muscle cells as effectively as LDL, but is internalized and degraded much more slowly. The presence of HDL in the medium partially inhibits uptake and degradation of LDL, and also partially suppresses the net increment in cell sterol content induced by LDL. It is therefore evident the need for drugs specifically active in increasing circulating HDL or improving the ratio between HDL and VLDL + LDL. Schurr _et al_ (27) have recently demonstrated that none of the commonly used hypocholesteremic drugs, such as clofibrate, nicotinic acid, probucol, d-thyroxine, estrone and diethyl-stilbestrol, exhibit a specific hypo-β-lipoproteinemic effect. A new hypolipidemic drug, more potent than clofibrate in lowering serum and liver lipids in animal studies, has been however recently described (28). This compound, Procetofen (the isopropyl ester of p-(4'-chlorobenzoyl) phenoxy-2-methyl-2-propionic acid), increases HDL concentrations in plasma of rabbits kept on a hyperlipidemic diet and normalizes the ratio between HDL and VLDL+LDL (28). Clofibrate, under the same experimental conditions, does not modify this ratio. Procetofen also lowers serum cholesterol in type II patients by 25-30% and triglycerides by 45-50% in hypertriglyceridemic patients (29,30). Preliminary ultracentrifugation studies confirm that the drug decreases specifically VLDL and LDL cholesterol, thus favouring the HDL/VLDL+LDL ratio (28).

Drugs Affecting Lipoprotein Uptake by the Arterial Wall

"*In vitro*" investigations have shown that sulfated mucopolysaccharides (MPS) inhibit the binding of LDL to arterial tissue (31). Exogenous MPS or MPS-like compounds may provide binding sites to LDL. In this way the mucopolysaccharide-lipoprotein complex on the arterial surface (32) is avoided. Investigations carried out in our laboratory (33) using a sulfated mucopolysaccharide of duodenal origin (glucuronylglycosaminoglycansulfate, 3-GS) (34) have shown "*in vivo*" and "*in vitro*"a potent inhibitory effect on lipoprotein uptake. In "*in vivo*" experiments the uptake of ^{125}I-VLDL from hypercholesteremic rabbits (HC) has been tested at the level of the aortic walls and a significant reduction of the uptake of radioactivity has been found 1 and 2 hours after the injection of 3-GS in the hypercholesteremic rabbits. By an extraction technique (35) it was demonstrated that the radioactivity was more than 90% protein-bound.

The "*in vitro*" experiments have been carried out by using the aortic glycoprotein fraction, recently described by Camejo *et al* (36), which has been demonstrated to specifically bind cholesterol-rich lipoproteins from rabbit. This arterial-lipoprotein complexing factor (ALCF) was isolated from aortas of cholesterol-fed rabbits. The ALCF was incubated with HC-VLDL, then the complexes were separated by ultracentrifugation and the cholesterol content determined (37). 3-GS was added in increasing concentrations at the beginning of the incubation time, and a linear inhibiting effect was observed over a wide range of concentrations.

These results indicate that 3-GS, by significantly inhibiting the interaction of HC-VLDL with the arterial wall in rabbits, reduces the inherent atherogenicity of this lipoprotein fraction (38,39). 3-GS may exert a competitive effect on arterial polyanions for lipoprotein binding sites, thus making lipoproteins unavailable for arterial deposition. Recent data by Goldstein _et al_ (40) also indicate that sulfated MPS may actively release LDL bound to cell-surface receptors in cultured human fibroblasts. These data provide therefore some evidence for the antiatherosclerotic effect of sulfated MPS.

Among the agents inhibiting the formation of atherosclerotic plaques in experimental animals, only one has also shown a definite effect on regression of preestablished atherosclerosis. This compound is lecithin, when infused intravenously (41). This effect has been shown in rabbits (42,43) and in baboons (44). Stafford and Day (45) have more recently shown that in SEA quail, when grossly visible atherosclerosis was developed by using an atherogenic diet, an intravenous administration of a solution of polyunsaturated soya phosphatides continued weekly for 3 months induced a regression of preestablished plaques and of the arterial cholesterol levels, without any effect on circulating cholesterol. The prevailing hypothesis on the mode of action of phospholipids is a possible solubilization of tissue cholesterol, facilitating its transport into plasma. Lecithin in fact greatly facilitates resorbtion of cholesterol from subcutaneous implants (46). Polyunsaturated lecithin also increases aortic cholesterol-esterase activity in baboons (44). Free cholesterol can be more readily transported across cell membranes and out of the cells. These phospholipids may also prevent the deleterious effects of excess membrane cholesterol on membrane functions, which may lead to cell lysis and necrosis (47). Phospholipids might also inhibit the interaction between LDL and polyanions (48), a factor for the trapping of LDL in arteries (49).

Pharmacological Modifications of Apoprotein Composition

The treatment with biguanide (Metformin) of rabbits fed a high cholesterol diet does not modify the dietary induced hypercholesteremia, but it exerts a protective effect on the arterial wall (50). These morphological observations have prompted Sirtori _et al_ (51) to investigate the plasma lipid and lipoprotein composition in

Metformin treated hypercholesteremic rabbits. The VLDL composition of these animals shows a considerable modification of the lipid fraction (a significant increase of phosphatidyl-inositol) and of the apoprotein composition. Recent data from our laboratory (52) indicate that this atherogenic lipoprotein fraction shows a decreased content of arginine-rich apoprotein and an increase of apo AI. By using polyacrylamide sodium dodecyl sulfate fractionation, the presence of albumin has been also demonstrated. This protein represents 4.9% of apo-VLDL (d<1.006) in hypercholesteremic (HC) rabbits treated with Metformin (Met) versus 0.85% in HC animals.

The aortic uptake of VLDL, labelled with ^{125}Iodine, obtained from HC and HC + Met rabbits and reinjected into normal rabbits, has been investigated by Rodriguez _et al_ (53). The data indicate an uptake of HC + Met-VLDL which is only 0.017 against an uptake of 0.083%/g for HC-VLDL from animals not protected by Metformin, and very similar to that of labelled VLDL from normal rabbits.

In agreement with the hypothesis by Ross and Zilversmit (54) on the metabolic significance of hypercholesteremia in rabbits, these data suggest the formation of a non-atherogenic VLDL fraction. Recent studies in our laboratory evidentiate a more rapid turnover of HC + Met-VLDL when compared with HC-VLDL. After injection of labelled HC-VLDL and respectively HC + Met-VLDL into normal rabbits, the plasma radioactivity decay associated with the tetramethylurea insoluble portion of VLDL (apo B) has been followed. Our preliminary data are reported in Table 3.

Table 3

HALF LIVES (HOURS) OF VLDL-APO B AFTER INJECTION INTO CONTROL ANIMALS OF ^{125}I-LABELLED VLDL (d<1.006) OBTAINED EITHER FROM HYPERCHOLESTEREMIC (HC) OR HYPERCHOLESTEREMIC+METFORMIN (HC+MET) TREATED RABBITS

	t 1/2 α	t 1/2 β
HC	2.3	20.2
HC + Met	0.5	9.5

In every experiment the radioactivity decay shows biphasic curves, in agreement with the recent finding of Kushwaha and Hazzard (55). The observation of a lipoprotein distribution in HC+Met rabbits (Table 4a and 4b) more similar to control animals, i.e., characterized by a higher level of "terminal" lipoproteins (LDL), further supports the hypothesis of an improved VLDL clearance in Metformin treated rabbits.

Table 4a

PLASMA LIPOPROTEIN DISTRIBUTION (mg/dl) IN FASTED RABBITS FED A STANDARD CHOW (CONTROL) AND CHOLESTEROL-RICH DIET (HC) WITH OR WITHOUT 135 mg/Kg/day OF METFORMIN (HC+MET) ($\overline{x}$ ± SE from 6 animals/group)

	Control	HC	HC+Met
VLDL ($d<1.006$)	100.7±11.3	681.5±28.5	580.3±41.2
IDL ($1.006<d<1.019$)	71.6±10.5	425.6±40.7	405.4±46.7
LDL ($1.019<d<1.063$)	56.5± 8.5	246.5±32.7	325.2±34.6
HDL ($1.063<d<1.21$)	126.5±17.9	116.9±10.7	98.9±15.2

Table 4b

LIPOPROTEIN QUANTITATIVE INTERRELATIONS DETERMINED FROM THE RATIO OF THEIR PLASMA CONCENTRATIONS AS REPORTED IN TABLE 4a ($\overline{x}$ ± SE from 6 animals/group)

	Control	HC	HC+Met
$\frac{VLDL}{IDL}$	1.53±0.1	1.61±0.1	1.39±0.2
$\frac{IDL}{LDL}$	1.23±0.1	1.83±0.2*	1.37±0.2

*$p<0.05$ as compared to controls

The apo VLDL components of patients with type III hyperlipoproteinemia has been investigated in detail by Sirtori et al (56), who have shown variation of the arginine-rich and AI apoproteins induced by Metformin treatment similar to what observed in HC+Met rabbits. Also in these cases the presence of albumin in VLDL has been observed.

These experimental and clinical data might suggest why Metformin protects the rabbit arterial wall even in presence of high plasma cholesterol levels. However the molecular and cellular sites of action of the drug are not yet clarified.

Metformin acts on the lipoprotein metabolism independently of its anti-hyperglycemic effect as suggested by Sirtori et al (56), and by Stout et al (57) using Phenformin, a chemically and pharmacologically related drug. Concerning the main site of action, recent observations in our laboratory indicate that lipoproteins obtained from lymph of HC+Met rabbits show an apoprotein pattern different from that of lymph lipoproteins of HC rabbits, with a strict increase of AI, a clear indication of a direct activity on the lipoprotein assembly in the intestinal wall.

A NEW DIETARY APPROACH

Many attempts have been made during the last decades to substitute or potentiate the effects of drugs in the control of dyslipidemias in animal and man with diets low in fats or rich in polyunsaturated fatty acids (58, 59). Only recently the possible role of vegetable proteins versus animal proteins have been reinvestigated in animals and clinical studies. The treatment of human hypercholesteremia with a soybean protein diet, i.e. with total substitution of the animal proteins in the diet with a soybean textured product (60), has provided new perspectives for the clinical treatment of the most difficult forms of hyperlipidemia as well as a new tool for the study of the dietary control of the cholesterol absorption-excretion processes. The investigations carried out in our Clinical Center, and now totalling 42 in-patients, have generally indicated the efficacy of this diet (Table 5).

The most recent trials have analysed the effects of variations of the lipid content and composition of the soybean diet on the cholesterol responses and on the

Table 5 - Overall results of the 42 in-patient studies with the soybean protein diet (3 weeks of treatment following different protocols)

Patients	Total cholesterol mg/dl $\bar{x} \pm$ SEM		LDL cholesterol mg/dl $\bar{x} \pm$ SEM		Tryclycerides mg/dl $\bar{x} \pm$ SEM		VLDL cholesterol mg/dl $\bar{x} \pm$ SEM	
	Start	End	Start	End	Start	End	Start	End
Type II A	346.0 ±21.8	288.8[b] ±23.7	277.8 ±21.2	224.3[c] ±23.0	134.0 ± 7.3	118.9 ± 8.5	27.8 ±1.7	30.4 ±2.7
Type II B	325.6 ±15.4	261.9[c] ±10.2	232.6 ±13.5	181.2[c] ± 9.5	245.8 ±15.8	220.9 ±24.0	55.5 ±4.4	46.5[a] ±5.2
Type II B - III	336.7 ±20.4	247.5[d] ±19.3	190.0 ±35.3	135.2[d] ±26.3	347.5 ± 6.8	288.0[b] ±19.2	110.0 ±14.2	86.2 ±13.6
Grand Totals	337.4 ±12.9	269.9[d] ±13.4	252.1 ±13.2	199.4[d] ±13.4	196.9 ±13.2	173.9 ±13.8	46.2 ±4.4	41.9 ±3.7

a: $p < 0.05$ b: $p < 0.01$ c: $p < 0.001$ d: $p < 0.0001$ vs Start values

Type II A: 22 patients, 16 M and 6 F, age 9-67 yrs, including 2 homozigous patients

Type II B: 16 patients, 8 M and 8 F, age 39-68 yrs

Type II B-III: 4 patients, 2 M and 2 F, age 46-67 yrs

From Sirtori et al. (to be published)

Table 6 - Effect of a semisynthetic low cholesterol diet on plasma cholesterol and fecal steroids in rabbits

Type of protein in the diet	Time on diet (weeks)	Plasma cholesterol mg/dl $\bar{x} \pm$ SEM	Fecal excretion (mg/Kg/day) $\bar{x} \pm$ SEM Neutral steroids	Bile acids
Diet 1 - Casein	16	400 ± 98	3.6 ± 0.5	4.4
Diet 2 - Casein replaced by soya bean meal	16	212 ± 51	6.2 ± 0.8	5.3
		$p < 0.01$	$p < 0.01$	

- Six adult New Zealand white male rabbits followed the two diets in sequence
- Bile acids were determined in pools of feces from all animals

From Fumagalli et al. (64)

alterations of lipoprotein composition induced by the different regimens. The most interesting findings have been an increase of VLDL cholesterol levels after switching from a soybean diet of high P/S (2.7) to a similar diet with a 0.1 P/S. Present studies in our laboratory are being focussed on the mechanism of the hypocholesteremic effect of soy protein. A short study on two in-patients (two weeks of strictly soybean diet and two weeks of soybean + meat) showed a marked cholesterol decrease in the first two weeks and a return to base-line after the second two weeks, thus indicating that the protein component of the diet, as suggested by most Authors (61, 62) and denied by some (63), is probably responsible for the hypocholesteremic effect.

Animal studies have been of particular help in suggesting the mode of action of soy proteins. Fumagalli _et al_ (64) have in fact demonstrated, in a dietary experiment with rabbits fed a semi-synthetic, low cholesterol diet, that switching from a casein to a soy protein diet, causes a dramatic reduction (about 50%) of plasma cholesterol levels (Table 6). Analysis of the fecal steroid pattern shows that the change of the dietary protein does not modify the excretion of bile acids, but it almost doubles fecal neutral steroids. This effect is similar to that previously reported in man with clofibrate (65).

This short review of investigations carried out in many laboratories points to the new possibilities opened to the practical therapeutic applications of the more recent studies in the biochemical pharmacology of dyslipidemias. These results underline how the recent advances in molecular and cell biology of lipoproteins are of immediate interest for the pharmacological and possibly clinical applications.

REFERENCES

1. Coronary Drug Project, Research Group. J. Amer. Med. Assoc. 220: 996 (1972)
2. Coronary Drug Project, Research Group. J. Amer. Med. Assoc. 226: 652 (1973)
3. Coronary Drug Project, Research Group. J. Amer. Med. Assoc. 231: 360 (1975)
4. Sirtori, C.R., A. Catapano, and R. Paoletti. In: Atherosclerosis Reviews, R. Paoletti and A.M. Gotto, Jr., editors, Raven Press, New York, Volume 2, 1977, pp. 113-153.

5. Stamler, J.
In: Atherosclerosi , R. Paoletti and C.R. Sirtori, editors, Casa Editrice Ambrosiana, 1977, pp. 873-955
6. Dorr, A.E., W.B. Martin, and W.A. Freyburger.
In: Lipids, Lipoproteins, and Drugs, D. Kritchevsky, R. Paoletti and W.L. Holmes, editors, Volume 63, Advances in Experimental Biology and Medicine, Plenum, New York, 1975, p. 447.
7. Paoletti, R., A. Catapano, G.C. Ghiselli, and C.R. Sirtori.
In: Atherosclerosis IV, G. Schettler, Y. Goto Y. Hata, and G. Klose, editors, Springer-Verlag, Berlin, 1977, pp. 517-527.
8. Carlson, L.A., M. Danielson, I. Ekberg, B. Klintemar, and G. Rosenhamer.
Atherosclerosis 28: 81 (1977)
9. Hoff, H.F., R.L. Jackson, and A.M. Gotto, Jr.
In: Atherosclerosis Drug Discovery, Volume 67, Advances in Experimental Biology and Medicine, C.E. Day, editor, Plenum, New York, 1976, pp. 109-120
10. Miller, G.J. and N.E. Miller
Lancet 1: 16, (1975)
11. Miller, G.J.
CVD Epidemiology Newsletter, Am. Heart Assoc. 21: 36 (1976)
12. Wiklund, O., A. Gustafson, and L. Wilhelmsen
Artery 1: 399 (1975)
13. Oliver, M.F., I.A. Nimmo, M. Cooke, L.A. Carlson, and A.G. Olsson
Europ. J. Clin. Invest. 5: 507 (1975)
14. Levy, R.I., C.B. Blum, and E.J. Schaefer
In: Lipoprotein Metabolism, H. Greten, editor, Springer-Verlag, Berlin, 1976, pp. 56-64
15. Glueck, C.J., R.W. Fallat, F. Milett, P. Gartside, R.C. Elston, and R.C.P. Go
Metabolism 24: 1243 (1975)
16. Glueck, C.J., P. Gartside, R.W. Fallat, J. Sielski, and P.M. Steiner
J. Lab. Clin. Med. 88: 941 (1976)
17. Rhoads, G.G., C.L. Gulbrandsen and A. Kagan
New Engl. J. Med. 294: 293 (1976)
18. Avogaro, P. and G. Cazzolato
Atherosclerosis 22: 63 (1975)
19. Glueck, C.J., R.W. Fallat, F. Milett, P.M. Steiner
Arch. Intern. Med. 135: 1025 (1975)
20. Zilversmit, D.B., T.B. Clarkson and L.B. Hughes
Atherosclerosis 26: 97 (1977)

21. Hamilton, R.L.
In: Pharmacological Control of Lipid Metabolism, Volume 26, Advances in Experimental Medicine and Biology, W.L. Holmes, R. Paoletti and D. Kritchevsky, Plenum, New York, 1972, pp. 7-24
22. Glomset, J.A.
J. Lipid Res. 9: 155 (1968)
23. Bondjers, G. and S. Bjorkerud
Artery 1: 3 (1976)
24. Stein, O. and Y. Stein
Biochim. Biophys. Acta 326: 232 (1973)
25. Stein, O. and Y. Stein
Biochim. Biophys. Acta 431: 347 (1976)
26. Carew, T.E., S.B. Hayes, T. Koschinsky, and D. Steinberg
Lancet I: 1315 (1976)
27. Schurr, P.E., J.R. Schultz and C.E. Day
In: Atherosclerosis Drug Discovery, Volume 67, Advances in Experimental Medicine and Biology, C.E. Day, editor, Plenum, New York, 1976, pp. 215-229
28. Wülfert, E., personal communication
29. Rouffy, J. and B. Chanu, these proceedings (abstract)
30. Fromentin, M., D. Gautier, and R. Bon
Gaz. Med. France 83: 1459 (1976)
31. Day, C.E., J.R. Powell, and R.S. Levy
Artery 1: 126 (1975)
32. Berenson, G.S., S.R. Srinivasan, P.J. Dolan, and B. Radhakrishnamurthy
Circulation 44: II-6 (1971) (abstract)
33. Sirtori, C.R., A. Catapano, G.C. Ghiselli, and R. Malinow
Artery 2: 390 (1976)
34. Bianchini, P., B. Osima, R. Casetta, G. Bramanti, and C. Mostacci
Giorn. Arterioscl. 3: 327 (1967)
35. Klimov, A.N., A.D. Denisenko and E.Y.A. Magracheva
Atherosclerosis 19: 243 (1974)
36. Camejo, C., A. Lopez, H. Vegas, and H. Paoli
Atherosclerosis 21: 77 (1975)
37. Abell, L.L., B.B. Levy, B.B. Brodie and F.E. Kendall
J. Biol. Chem. 195: 357 (1952)
38. Rodriguez, J.L., G.C. Ghiselli, D. Torreggiani, and C.R. Sirtori
Atherosclerosis 23: 73 (1976)
39. Shore, V.G., B. Shore, and R.G. Hart
Biochemistry 13: 1579 (1974)
40. Goldstein, J.L. S.K. Basu, G.Y. Brunschede, and M.J. Brown
Cell 7: 85 (1976)

41. Friedman, M., S.D. Byers, and R.H. Rosenman
Proc. Soc. Expt. Biol. Med. 95: 586 (1957)
42. Adams, C.W.M., Y.H. Abdulla, O.B. Bayliss, and R.S. Morgan
J. Path. Bact. 94: 77 (1967)
43. Patelski, J., D.E. Bowyer, A.N. Howard, I.W. Jennings, C.J.R. Thorne, and G.A. Gresham
Atherosclerosis 12: 41 (1970)
44. Howard, A.N., J. Patelski, D.E. Bowyer, and G.A. Gresham
Atherosclerosis 14: 17 (1971)
45. Stafford, W.W. and C.E. Day
Artery 1: 106 (1975)
46. Adams, C.W.M. and R.S. Morgan
J. Path. Bact. 94: 73 (1967)
47. Papahadjopoulos, D.
J. Theoret. Biol. 43: 329 (1974)
48. Day, C.E. and R.S. Levy
Artery 1: 150 (1975)
49. Levy, R.S. and C.E. Day
In: Atherosclerosis, Proceedings of the Second International Symposium, R.J. Jones, editor, Springer-Verlag, New York, 1970, pp. 186-189
50. Agid, R., G. Marquie, and M. Lafontan
Journees de Diabetologie 259, (1975)
51. Sirtori, C.R., A. Catapano, G.C. Ghiselli, A.L. Innocenti and J. Rodriguez
Atherosclerosis 26: 79 (1977)
52. Sirtori, C.R., A. Catapano, G.C. Ghiselli, B. Shore, and V. Shore
In: Protides and Biological Fluids, Pergamon, Oxford, Vol. 25, in press, 1978
53. Rodriguez, J., A. Catapano, G.C. Ghiselli, and C.R. Sirtori
In: Atherosclerosis Drug Discovery, Volume 67, Advances in Experimental Medicine and Biology, C.E. Day, editor, Plenum, New York, 1976, pp.169-189
54. Ross, A.C. and D.B. Zilversmit
J. Lipid Res. 18: 169 (1977)
55. Kushwaha, R.S. and W.R. Hazzard
Circulation 56: II-22 (1977)
(abstract)
56. Sirtori, C.R., E. Tremoli, M. Sirtori, F. Conti, and R.Paoletti
Atherosclerosis 26: 583 (1977)
57. Stout, R.W., J.D. Brunzell, D. Porte, Jr., and E.L. Bierman
Metabolism 23: 815 (1974)

58. Keys, A., J.T. Anderson, and F. Grande
Metabolism 14: 747 (1965)
59. Keys, A., J.T. Anderson and F. Grande
Metabolism 14: 759 (1965)
60. Sirtori, C.R., E.Agradi, E. Conti, O. Mantero, and E. Gatti
Lancet I: 275 (1977)
61. Hamilton, R.M.G. and K.K. Carroll
Atherosclerosis 24: 47 (1976)
62. Kritchevsky, D., S.A. Tepper , D.E. Williams, and J.A. Story
Atherosclerosis 26: 397 (1977)
63. Helms, P.
Lancet I: 805 (1977)
64. Fumagalli, R., R. Paoletti and A.N. Howard
Life Sci., 1978, in press
65. Grundy, S.M., E.H. Ahrens, Jr., G. Salen, P.H. Schreibman, and P.J. Nestel
J. Lipid Res. 13: 531 (1972)

NEW HYPOLIPIDEMIC DRUGS

William L. Bencze

Research Department, Pharmaceuticals Division,
CIBA-GEIGY Ltd., Basel, Switzerland

The past 12 months have been an encouraging period for the development of new hypolipidemic agents. The Food and Drug Administration approved the drugs Probucol from Dow Chemical Company and Colestipol-HCl from Upjohn Company as official hypolipidemic agents.

The approval is no guarantee for the survival of the new drugs. Marion Finkel (1), an official of the FDA, outlined the requirements that must be furnished during the postmarketing period: 1) Longterm safety must be demonstrated, as well as 2) Evidence of clinical effectiveness, reduction of xanthomata, size of arterial plaques, morbidity and mortality must be established within a specified time period, e.g. 10 years.

This brief review will address itself to the survey of a few compounds which emerged during the past three years. The substances may not convey revolutionary ideas. They have, however, a great value if they, ever so slightly, modify our thinking about and our approach to atherosclerosis.

CLOFIBRATE ANALOGS

The phenoxysubstituted acids still serve as tempting templates for the synthesis of almost inexhaustible variations of clofibrate analogs.

Among 31 analogs prepared in the Laboratories Fournier-Dijon in France, compound LF-178 has been selected for further development (2). In the rat, LF-178

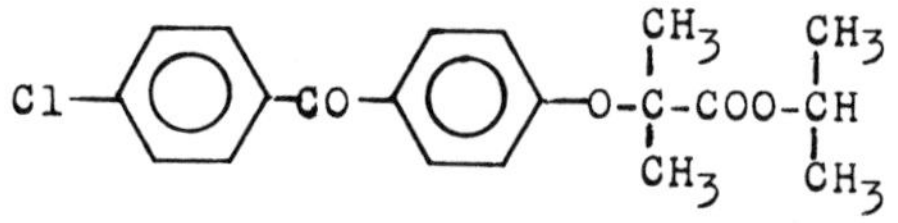

LF 178 Lipanthyl Procetofen

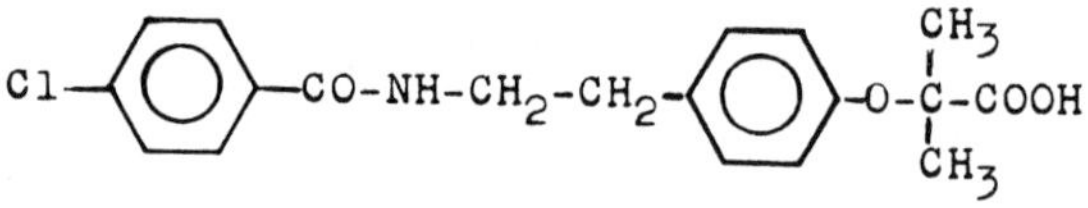

BM 15,075 Bezafibrate

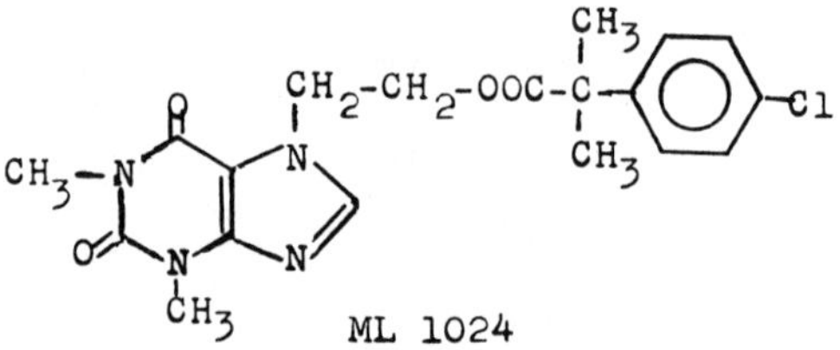

ML 1024

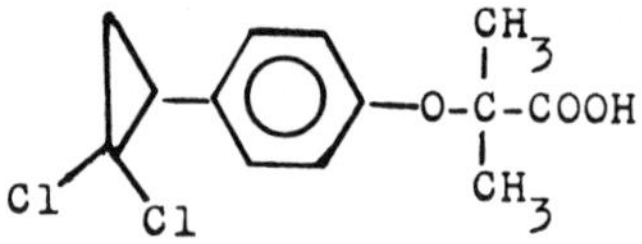

WIN 35,833 Ciprofibrate

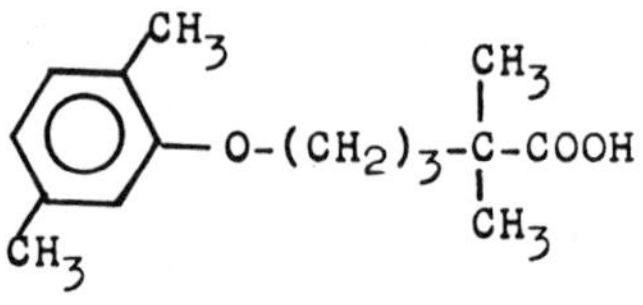

Gemfibrozil

Figure 1: Clofibrate Analogs

was about six times more active than clofibrate. The drug appeared to be highly active in a multicenter clinical trial comprising 393 patients. The mean depression of plasma cholesterol level exceeded 26% and that of the triglycerides 60% after six months of treatment (3).

Bezafibrate, BM-15,075 (Boehringer Mannheim, Germany) at a dose of 0.6 g/day lowered serum levels of very low density lipoprotein, cholesterol and triglycerides in all types of hyperlipoproteinemia in 29 patients (4).

The theophilline derivative, ML-1024 lowered plasma cholesterol concentration in a group of minipigs by 68% after six months of treatment. Triglyceride values remained within normal range in this species but were reduced in the rat (5).

Ciprofibrate, WIN-35833, is a hypolipidemic agent developed by the Winthrop Laboratories (6).

Gemfibrozil is a potent triglyceride lowering agent in monkeys, dogs and rats. A preliminary clinical trial indicated that gemfibrozil is an effective medication for the treatment of Types IIb and IV hyperlipoproteinemia. On a weight for weight basis the drug was ten times more potent than clofibrate (7).

CYCLIC CLOFIBRATE ANALOGS

Witiak and his colleagues created a set of cyclized clofibrate analogs, although not by simple ring closure (8-13).

Among the bicyclic clofibrate analogs A,F and G, the 6-chlorochromane derivative F compared most favorably with the parent compound. Substance F lowered both serum cholesterol and triglyceride levels in the Triton hyperlipemic rat (8). The benzodioxane analog G exhibits mainly hypotriglyceridemic activity, while the dihydrobenzofuran analog A diminishes the serum cholesterol concentration (8).

The tricyclic substance B containing a lactone ring, was less active than clofibrate. In contrast to clofibrate it did not cause hepatomegaly, whereas the reduced hemiacetal derivative D exhibited most of the properties of clofibrate, including the increase in liver weight (9).

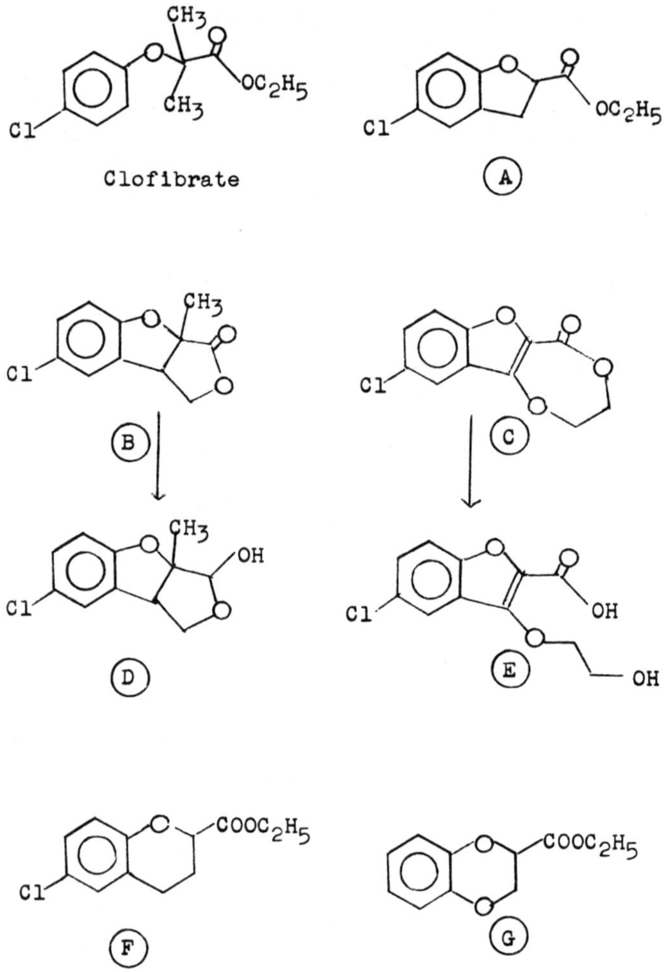

Clofibrate

A

B

C

D

E

F

G

Figure 2: Cyclized Clofibrate Analogs

The dioxepino-benzofuran analog C reduced the plasma lipid levels in the hyperlipidemic rat back to normal values. The hydrolyzed open acid form E was inactive (10). Minute chemical structural changes resulted in substantial alterations of the activity profile in this series of clofibrate analogs.

COMPOUNDS AFFECTING LIPOPROTEINS

In the Norwegian municipality Tromsoe 6595 men, aged 20-49, have been examined for a period of 2 years. This group of young men represented 83% of all such subjects living in the township of Tromsoe, which is known to have a high incidence of coronary heart disease. Of the eight variables measured, high density lipoprotein-cholesterol appeared to be the most reliable criterion for the prediction of incipient coronary heart disease. Coronary risk was increasing with decreasing HDL-cholesterol concentration (14).

The search for hypolipidemic agents that are capable of decreasing serum VLDL and LDL and increasing HDL, has been going on for a good many years. Clofibrate has been known to reduce serum VLDL in many patients and to elicit a compensatory rise in LDL. Pichardo _et al_ however, have found that clofibrate is a potent plasma cholesterol and beta-lipoprotein (LDL) lowering agent in a good portion of patients with familial Type II hyperlipoproteinemia. Only in some patients, who did not respond to clofibrate treatment was there an increase in plasma LDL concentration (15).

Oral administration of U-41792 to rats fed an atherogenic diet caused a reduction of plasma VLDL and LDL lipoprotein levels to normal values, while it raised the HDL level to above the normal values (16,17).

Sirtori _et al_ treated 30 patients with stable hypertriglyceridemia (Types IIb, III and IV) with metformin. In the 18 responding patients metformin was found to enhance VLDL metabolism without causing a compensatory rise in LDL levels (18).

Cayen et al (19) studied the hypolipidemic activity of the synthetic estrogen Dibenzylcyclooctanone (DBCO). Oral doses of 0.3-30 mg/kg/day of DBCO elicited a hypocholesterolemic response in the rat. The decrease in serum cholesterol level was due primarily to a lowering of cholesterol in the serum HDL fraction. According to the Tromsoe study, this kind of hypocholesterolemic shift is the ominous signal in man for an impending myocardial infarction. Consequently, we are faced here with a most undesirable hypocholesterolemic agent.

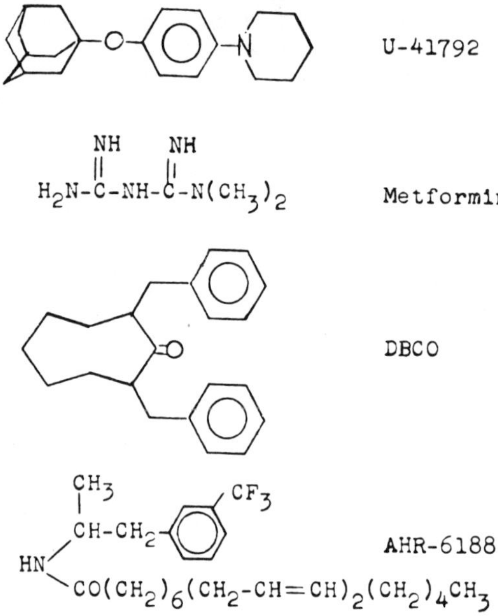

U-41792

$H_2N\text{-}C(=NH)\text{-}NH\text{-}C(=NH)\text{-}N(CH_3)_2$ Metformin

DBCO

$HN(CH(CH_3)\text{-}CH_2\text{-}C_6H_4CF_3)\text{-}CO(CH_2)_6(CH_2\text{-}CH{=}CH)_2(CH_2)_4CH_3$ AHR-6188

Figure 3: Compounds Affecting Lipoproteins

Estrogens usually elicit a hypocholesterolemic action, but do cause a rise in plasma triglyceride concentration. This was not the case in the study described by Chait *et al* (20). The authors injected labeled VLDL from a donor who was a Type IV patient into another patient having broad-beta-disease (Type III hyperlipoproteinemia). Ethinylestradiol therapy, 1μg/kg/day, resulted not only in a decrease in plasma cholesterol but also in the triglyceride levels.

The hypocholesterolemic agent AHR 6188 has been developed in the A.H. Robins Research Laboratories. The compound is the linoleic acid amide of norfenfluramine, an anorexic amphetamine derivative. AHR 6188 has been reported to decrease low density and increase high density serum lipoproteins in a dose-dependent fashion when added to an atherogenic diet of the rat (21).

INHIBITORS OF LIPID ABSORPTION

While the fenfluramine derivative AHR-6188 of Robins Laboratories did not affect serum triglycerides but reduced serum cholesterol levels in the rat, the French variation of fenfluramine, compound 780-SE, has been found to lower serum triglyceride levels and to have an erratic or no effect on serum cholesterol concentration in the rat. In man 780-SE reduced also serum cholesterol concentration. The compound has been reported to cause a reduction of liver weight and to restore insulin sensitivity to a normal value in genetically obese rats. The French workers claimed that 780-SE inhibited triglyceride absorption (22).

Among the numerous N-substituted linoleamide derivatives developed in Japan, moctamide has been reported to inhibit the rise of serum cholesterol levels in healthy male volunteers who consumed 9 egg yolks daily for 14 days in addition to their ordinary meals. The mean elevation of serum cholesterol levels due to the egg yolk was 11.4% (23). Kritchevsky et al concluded that the mechanism of the hypocholesterolemic action of moctamide appeared to involve the inhibition of cholesterol absorption (24).

Dietary-induced hypertriglyceridemia in the rat has been inhibited by Bayer's N,N'-bis-(10-undecenoyl)-propyleendiamine (25).

Tiadenol, bis-(hydroxyethylthio)1,10-decane, 2.4 g/day was administered orally to patients with Type IIa hyperlipoproteinemia for a period of 3 months. A marked hypocholesterolemic response was observed (26).

Esterification of Tiadenol with p-chlorophenoxyisobutyric acid furnished the diester Tiafibrate. It has been claimed that the hypolipidemic activity of Tiafibrate in the rat was more pronounced, while its toxicity was much lower than that of Clofibrate (27).

Gemcadiol, 2,2,9,9-tetramethyl-1,10-decanediol has been developed by Parke & Davis Co. Daily doses between 1.2 and 2 g lowered serum cholesterol levels by an average of 24% in patients with Type II, and 51% in patients with Type IV hyperlipoproteinemia, respectively (28).

The two diterpenoids, Totarol and Abietic acid inhibit the intestinal absorption of cholesterol in rats when

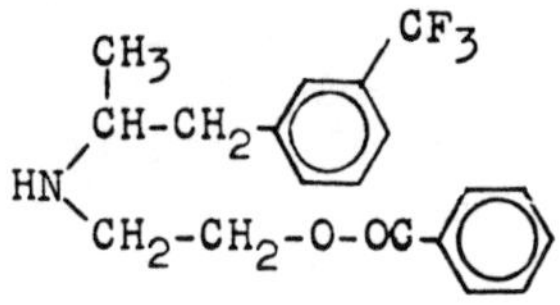

780-SE

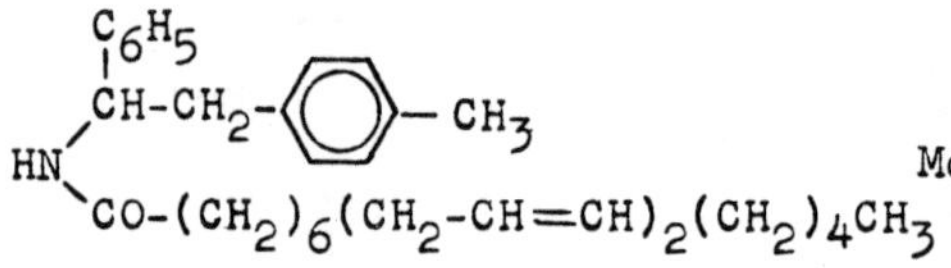

Moctamide

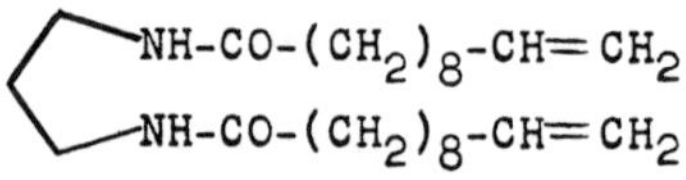

Di-undecenoyl-propylenediamine

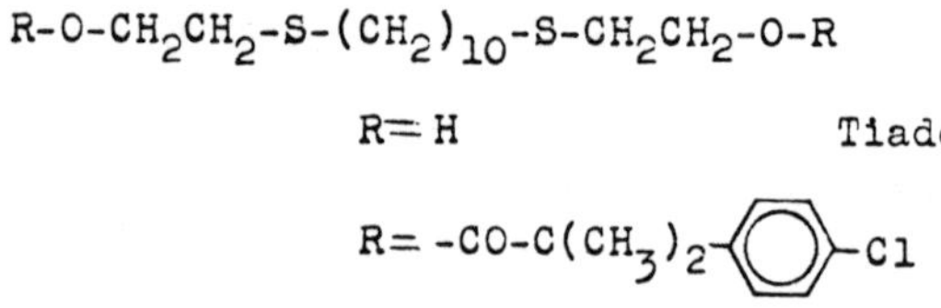

R-O-CH_2CH_2-S-$(CH_2)_{10}$-S-CH_2CH_2-O-R

R= H Tiadenol

R= -CO-C$(CH_3)_2$-C_6H_4-Cl Tiafibrate

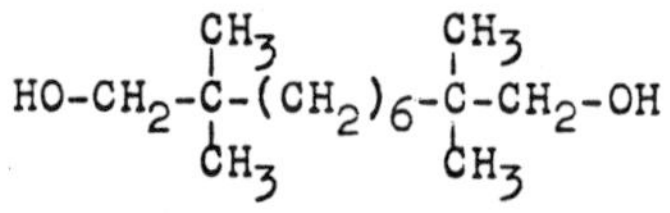

Gemcadiol

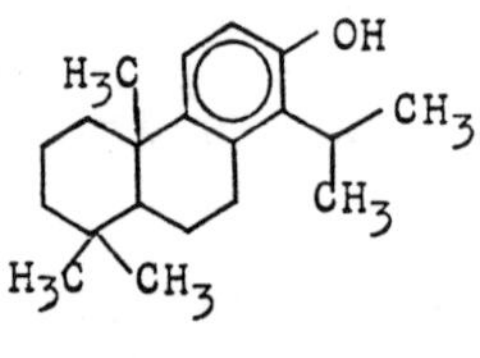

Totarol

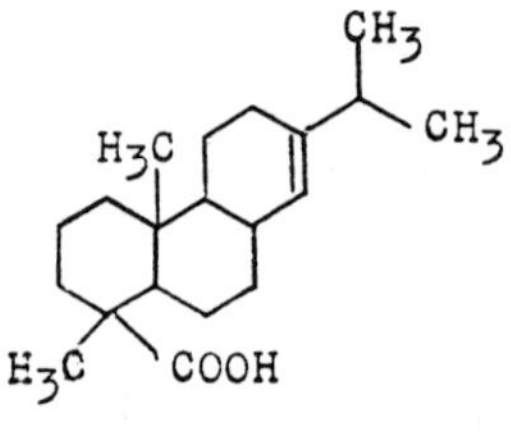

Abietic Acid

Figure 4: Inhibitors of Lipid Absorption

added to the diet at a level of 0.1-0.3% in the presence of 1% cholesterol (29).

The polymer anionic surface active agent, Tetronic 701 from Beecham Laboratories, inhibited cholesterol absorption in rats, chickens and rabbits fed an atherogenic diet (30).

METABOLIC REGULATORS

Levorotatory hydroxycitrate is the principal acid constitutent of the fruit rinds of *Garcinia cambogia*. The sodium salt of (-)-hydroxycitrate diminished lipogenesis in the rat by competitive inhibition of the cytoplasmic enzyme citrate lyase, EC 4.1.13.8. This enzyme is thought to furnish the acetyl-CoA units for lipid synthesis, particularly in the fed state after high carbohydrate intake. Of the four possible isomers, only the (-)-threo-isomer proved to be an active inhibitor of fatty acid and cholesterol biosynthesis (31). Upon prolonged administration of (-)-hydroxycitrate, citrate lyase enzyme was stimulated rather than inhibited, though the rats still kept losing weight. It appeared that (-)-hydroxycitrate turned into an anorexic agent (32).

It has been suggested that long-chain fatty-acyl-CoA derivatives are physiological regulators of fatty acid synthesis in the liver. RMI-14,514, like palmitoyl-CoA, inhibited translocation of tricarboxylate anion across the mitochondrial membrane at low concentration. Hepatic synthesis of fatty acids was reduced to one-third that of controls in rats treated with RMI-14,514. The compound was more active than clofibrate in reducing plasma cholesterol levels in the rat (33,34). Parker et al described the synthesis and biological screening of 104 analogs of RMI-14,514 (35).

The diarylether of dihydroxyacetone, 1,3-bis(p-methylphenoxy)-2-propanone at a dose of 10 mg/kg p.o. lowered serum triglyceride levels in the rat by inhibition of hepatic and intestinal microsomal glycerolipid biosynthesis (36,37).

COMPOUNDS DERIVED FROM SYNTHETIC ESTROGENS

Open-chain aliphatic analogs of 2,8-dibenzylcyclooctanone (DBCO, see Figure 3) have been prepared by Hall

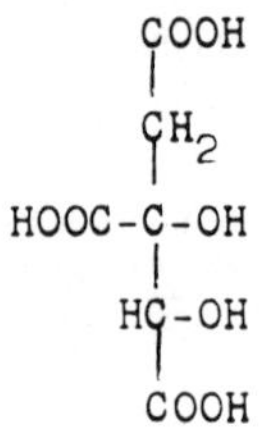

$$HOOC-C(OH)(CH_2COOH)-CH(OH)-COOH$$

(-)-threo-hydroxy-citric acid

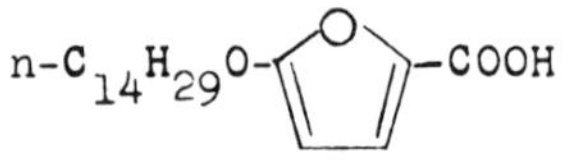

$n-C_{14}H_{29}O$-(furan)-COOH

RMI-14,514

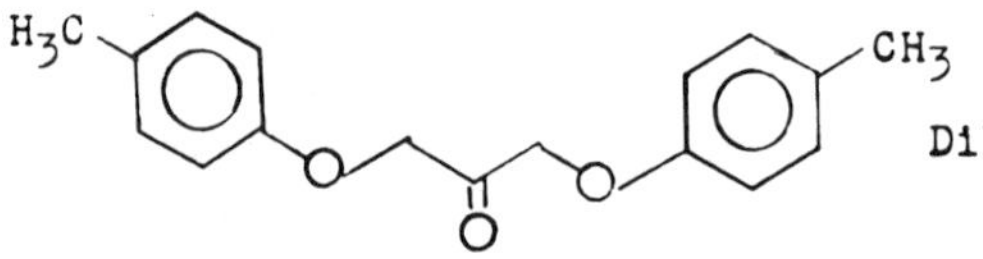

Dihydroxyacetone diarylether

Figure 5: Metabolic Regulators

and Carlson (38). 2-Octanone significantly lowered serum cholesterol, triglyceride and glycerol levels in Holtzman male rats at 10 mg/kg/day administered by oral intubation.

2-Hexadecanone reduced serum cholesterol levels significantly without altering serum triglyceride concentration. In contrast to dibenzylcyclooctanone 2-hexadecanone was not estrogenic. It reduced serum cholesterol levels in the rat by 42% at 10 mg/kg p.o. (39).

Watthey et al prepared a series of N-aryl derivatives of the known Diels-Alder adduct of maleimide and hydroxyquinone. CGS-2111 exhibited hypocholesterolemic activity in the rat and had antifertility activity even in the hamster. The bridged isoindoline derivative lacking the carbonyl group on the bridge anti to the five membered ring had no antifertility activity but did cause hypocholesterolemic effects in the rat (40).

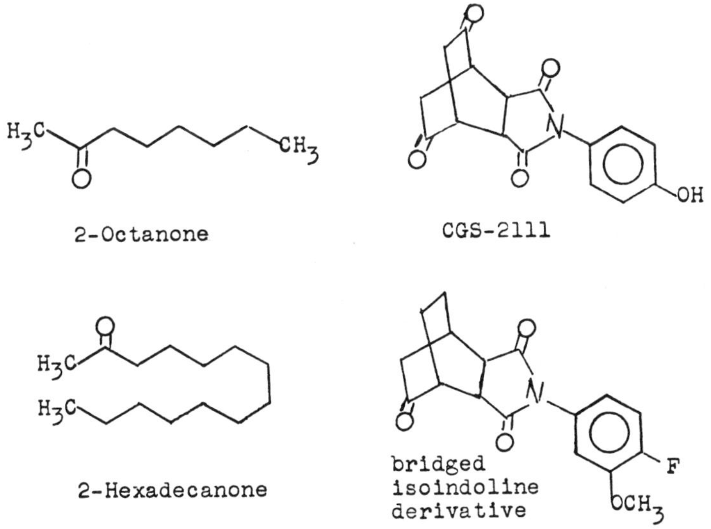

2-Octanone

CGS-2111

2-Hexadecanone

bridged isoindoline derivative

<u>Figure 6</u>: Compounds derived from synthetic estrogens

SYNTHETIC ANTIOXIDANTS

Butylated hydroxytoluene (BHT) is an antioxidant commonly added to foods, especially cooking oils, to prevent rancidity. BHT has been reported to reduce chemical carcinogenesis and retard aging in mice. Recently, BHT has been claimed to inactivate lipid-containing viruses (41).

The structural element ofBHT, the 3,4-di-tert.butyl-4-hydroxyphenyl radical has been built into a few hypolipidemic agents.

After 13 years of development by Dow Chemical Co., Probucol became an approved hypocholesterolemic agent. It appears to be a safe cholesterol lowering drug. In humans the compound causes an increase in fecal bile acids and a reduction of cholesterol synthesis and absorption. Serum triglyceride levels, in general, are not affected by probucol (42).

In contrast to probucol, the analog DH-990 does reduce serum triglyceride levels. Moreover, Renzi <u>et al</u> claimed, that DH-990 decreased the incidence of atherosclerotic lesions in the aorta of cholesterol-fed rabbits (43).

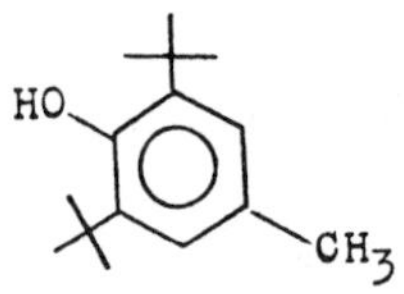

BHT 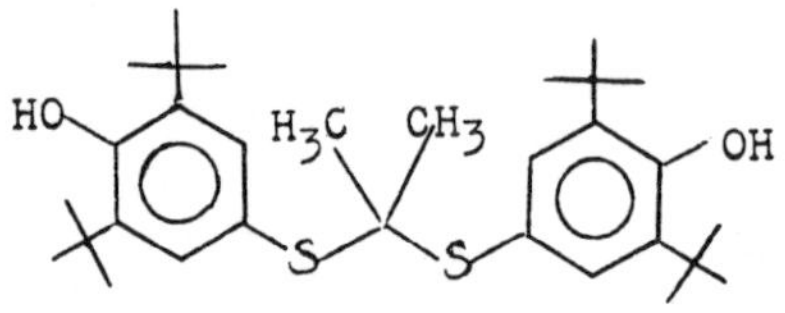 Probucol

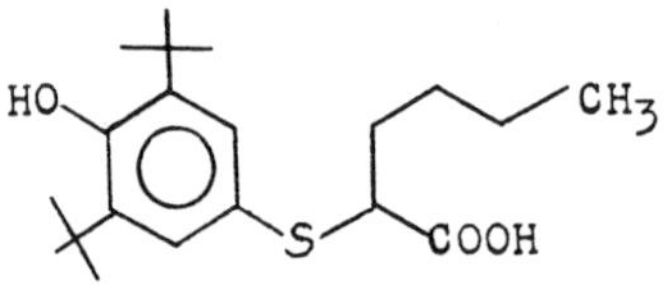

DH-990 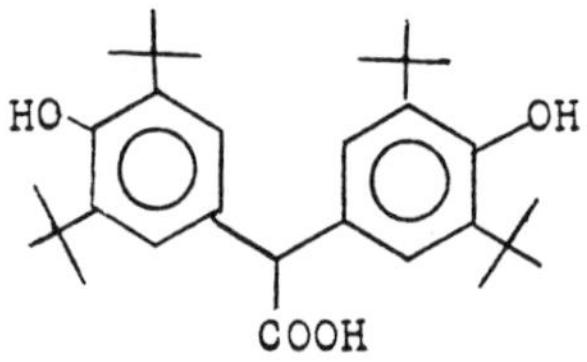 HCG-380

Figure 7: Synthetic Antioxidants

Another synthetic antioxidant HCG-380 has been claimed to be more potent than clofibrate in lowering serum cholesterol and triglyceride levels in the rat (44).

SUBSTITUTED BENZOIC ACIDS

Reddy and Krishnakanta suggested that all known hepatic peroxisome proliferators possess hypolipidemic properties, including acetylsalicylic acid which produces a moderate increase in the liver cell peroxisome population (45). Even if aspirin may never be listed in the tables of hypolipidemic agents, according to a number of clinicians it has a good chance to become an effective antiatherosclerotic drug.

A little more can be said about the hypolipidemic activity of a close relative of acetylsalicylic acid. The antitubercular drug, p-aminosalicylic acid (p-ASA) was administered in large doses (6-8 g/day) to patients with Type IIa and IIb hyperlipoproteinemia. Serum cholesterol concentration was reduced by 15-19% and triglycerides by 28% (46). Malloy _et al_ treated 20 children with familial hyperlipoproteinemia with p-ASA for 6 months. A moderate hypocholesterolemic and hypotrigly-

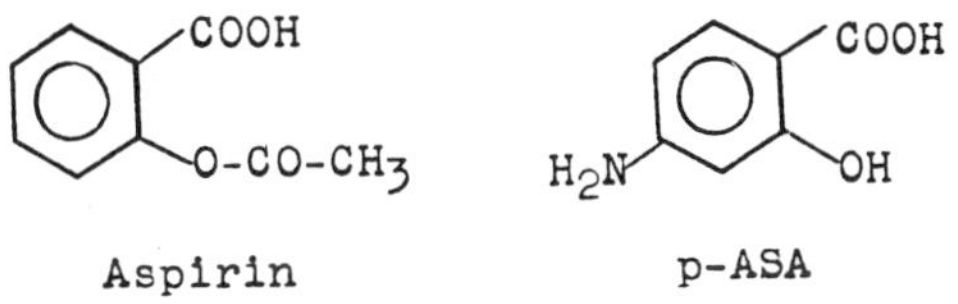

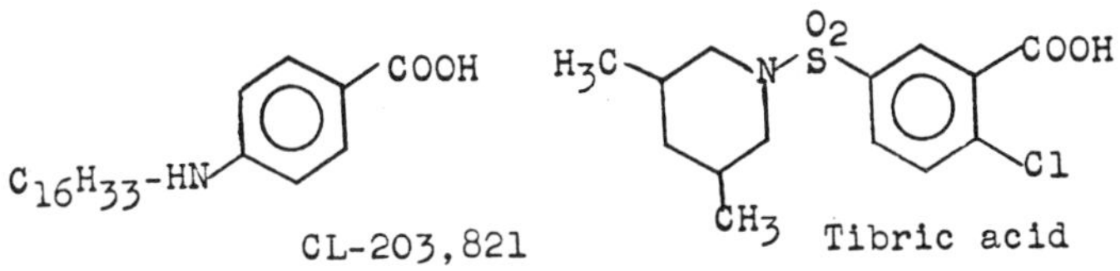

Figure 8: Substituted Benzoic Acids

ceridemic response was observed (47).

In the Lederle Laboratories a series of N-alkyl-substituted p-aminobenzoic acid derivatives have been prepared and tested for potential antiatherogenic activity in cholesterol-fed rabbits. Compound CL-203,821, p-hexadecylaminobenzoic acid, caused a significant reduction of aortic lesions and cholesterol deposition at doses of 27 and 60 mg/kg/day. A reduction of plasma esterified cholesterol levels was observed at a dose of 113 mg/kg/day (48).

Another benzoic acid derivative, tibric acid, has been developed by Pfizer. Bielman *et al* compared the hypotriglyceridemic effect of tibric acid with that of clofibrate in Type IV hyperlipidemic patients. Both drugs reduced serum triglyceride concentration but had no effect on esterified cholesterol, phospholipids and free fatty acids (49). Kritchevsky *et al* compared the influence of tibric acid on lipid metabolism in rats with three other hypolipidemic agents. Tibric acid was found to elicit hepatomegaly and a hypotriglyceridemic response (50).

NATURAL COMPOUNDS

Several hypocholesterolemic agents have been tried in the past to eliminate gallstones by dissolving the cholesterol in them. Cholesterol gallstone disease occurs in epidemic proportions. It is estimated that 10 to 15% of Europeans and 80 to 90% of the female members of certain groups of North American Indians have gallstones (51).

Chenodeoxycholic acid treatment resulted in complete dissolution of gallstones in about 20% of the treated patients. A further 50% showed a reduction in the size of the stones. Only radiolucent gallstones respond to chenodeoxycholic acid. The radioopaque stones will not dissolve upon treatment with this drug. In the responding patients small stones dissolve in 3 to 12 months. Gallstones over 10 mm in diameter may need up to 3 years of treatment (52). Fasting serum triglycerides were moderately reduced while serum cholesterol concentration was not changed during the therapy with chenodeoxycholic acid (53). However, in patients with Type II hyperlipoproteinemia chenodeoxycholic acid treatment resulted in a lowering of serum triglyceride levels by 25-54% and cholesterol by 14-28% (54).

The Coronary Drug Project Research Group reported that the incidence of gallstone formation was approximately doubled in the clofibrate and estrogen treatment groups. It was concluded that gallstone formation is a risk whenever clofibrate or estrogen is prescribed (55).

Cynarin, the 1,4-dicaffeyl ester of quinic acid, is the active constituent of the artichoke (*Cynara scolymus*). Heckers *et al* (56) treated 17 patients with familial Type IIa or IIb hyperlipoproteinemia patients with cynarin. Neither serum cholesterol nor triglyceride levels responded to the treatment. The authors refer, however, to 7 other clinical trials in which cynarin treatment elicited a hypolipidemic response.

It has been jocularly rumored that Italian men are less prone to atherosclerosis because their food is generously seasoned with garlic. Bordia *et al* (57) administered 100 g of butter with and without the freshly extracted juice of 50 g of garlic or onion to healthy subjects. The alimentary hyperlipemia induced by the butter was prevented by the essential oil of garlic and blood fibrinolytic activity was increased. Kritchevsky reported that garlic oil reduced the serum cholesterol level by about 10% and the atheromata were graded to be less severe in rabbits fed an atherogenic diet (58). Augusti and Mathew (59) administered allicin, diallyl

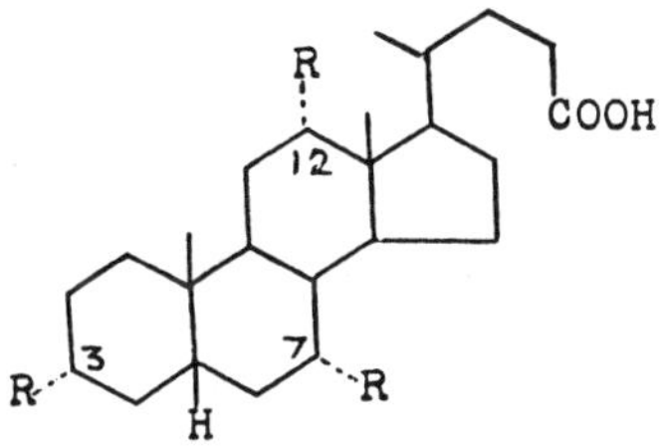

	R in position		
	3α	7α	12α
Litocholic acid	OH	H	H
Chenodeoxycholic acid	OH	OH	H
Deoxycholic acid	OH	H	OH
Cholic acid	OH	OH	OH

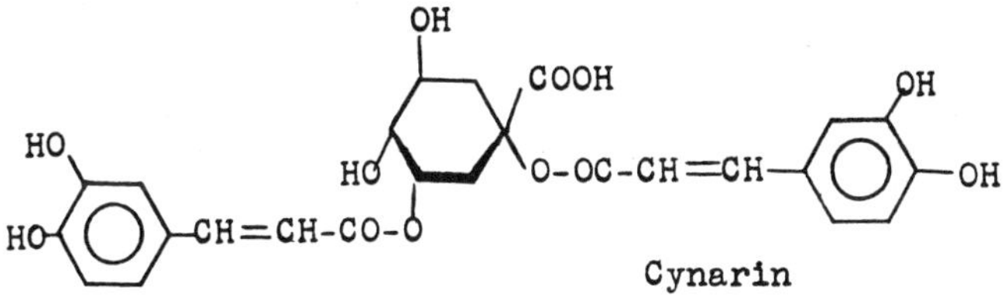

Cynarin

$CH_2{=}CH{-}CH_2{-}\overset{O\uparrow}{S}{-}S{-}CH_2{-}CH{=}CH_2$

Allicin

Figure 9: Natural Compounds

disulfide oxide, a component of the essential oil of garlic, orally to rats for a period of 2 months. A significant reduction of all types of serum lipid levels occurred as a result of the treatment.

It is proper to end this short survey of hypolipidemic agents with an optimistic note.

Regression of atherosclerotic lesions, as a consequence of hypolipidemic treatment have been observed in the rabbit, swine and Rhesus monkey. Recently, Barndt *et al* (60) reported that regression of atheromatous plaques in the femoral artery of 9 patients could be demonstrated. The regression appeared to correlate with the correction of hyperlipidemia by medical treatment. In the opinion of an editorial in the Brit. Med. J. (61): "The message seems abundantly clear."

REFERENCES

1. Finkel, M.J.
   Lipids 12: 64 (1977)
2. Sornay, R., J. Gurrieri, C. Tourne, F.J. Renson, B. Majoie and E. Wulfert
   Arneimittel-Forschung 26: 885 (1976)
3. Wulfert, E., B. Majoie and A. de Ceurriz
   Arzneimittel-Forschung 26: 906 (1976)
4. Olsson, A.G., S. Rossner, G. Walldius, L.A. Carlson, and P.D. Lang
   Atherosclerosis 27: 279 (1977)
5. Metz, G., M. Specker, W. Sterner, E. Heisler and G. Grahwit
   Arzneimittel-Forschung 27: 1173 (1977)
6. USAN Council
   J. Am. Med. Assoc. 236: 1992 (1976)
7. Okerholm, R.A., F.J. Keeley, F.E. Peterson and A.J. Glazko
   Fed. Proc. 35: 327 (1976) (abstract)
8. Newman, H.A.I., W.P. Heilman and D.T. Witiak
   Lipids 8: 378 (1973)
9. Witiak, D.T., E. Kuwano, D.R. Feller, J.R. Baldwin, H.A. Newman and S.K. Sankarappa
   J. Med. Chem. 19: 1214 (1976)
10. Witiak, D.T., G.K. Poochikian, D.R. Feller, N.A. Kenfield and H.A.I. Newman
    J. Med. Chem. 18: 992 (1975)
11. Witiak, D.T., W.P. Heilman, S.K. Sankarappa, R.C. Cavestri and H.A.I. Newman
    J. Med. Chem. 18: 934 (1975)
12. Witiak, D.T., H.A.I. Newman, G.K. Poochikian, W. Loh and S.K. Sankarappa
    Lipids 11: 384 (1976)
13. Goldberg, A.P., W.S. Mellon, D.T. Witiak and D.R. Feller
    Atherosclerosis 27: 15 (1977)
14. Miller, N.E., O.H. Forde, D.S. Thelle and O.D. Mjoes
    Lancet 1: 965 (1977)

15. Pichardo, R., L. Boulet and J. Davignon
Atherosclerosis 26: 573 (1977)
16. Schurr, P.E. and C.E. Day
Lipids 12: 22 (1976)
17. Day, C.E., P.E. Schurr, D.E. Emmert, R.E. TenBrink and D. Lednicer
J. Med. Chem. 18: 1065 (1975)
18. Sirtori, C.R., E. Tremoli, M. Sirtori, F. Conti and R. Paoletti
Atherosclerosis 26: 583 (1977)
19. Cayen, M.N., J. Dubuc and D. Dvornik
Biochem. Pharmacol. 25: 1537 (1976)
20. Chait, A., J.D. Brunzell, J.J. Albers and W.R. Hazzard
Lancet 1: 1176 (1977)
21. Danneburg, W.N., M.S. Kearney and R.T. Ruckart
Fed. Proc. 36: 1104 (1977) (abstract)
22. Duhault, J., M. Boulanger, L. Beregi, N. Sicot and F. Bouvier
Atherosclerosis 23: 63 (1976)
23. Takeuchi, N. and Y. Yamamura
Clin. Pharmacol. Therap. 16: 368 (1974)
24. Kritchevsky, D., S.A. Tepper and J.A. Story
Lipids 12: 16 (1977)
25. Linke, S. and R. Sitt
Chem. Abs. 86: P71947a (1977)
26. DeGennes, J.L., J. Truffert and J.M. LeQuere
Therapie 31: 455 (1976)
27. Martin, J.L.
Drugs of the Future 2: 138 (1977)
28. Blumenthal, H.P., J.R. Ryan, A.K. Jain and F.G. McMahon
Lipids 12: 44 (1977)
29. Enomoto, H., Y. Yoshikuni, Y. Yasutomi, K. Ohata, K. Sempuku, K. Kitaguchi, Y. Fujita and F. Mori
Chem. Pharm. Bull. (Japan) 25: 507 (1977)
30. Green, J., M.Heald, K.H. Baggaley, R.M. Hindley and B. Morgan
Atherosclerosis 23: 549 (1976)
31. Sullivan, A.C., J. Triscari, J.G. Hamilton, O.N, Miller and V.R. Wheatley
Lipids 9: 121 (1974)
32. Sullivan, A.C., J. Triscari and J.G. Hamilton
Lipids 12: 1 (1977)
33. Kariya, T., R.A. Parker, J.M. Grisar, J. Martin and L.J. Wille
Fed. Proc. 34: 789 (1975) (abstract)
34. Ribereau-Gayon, G.
FEBS Letters 62: 309 (1976)

35. Parker, R.A., T. Kariya, J.M. Grisar and V. Petrow J. Med. Chem. 20: 781 (1977)
36. Piantadosi, C., I.H. Hall, S.D. Wyrick and K.S. Ishaq J. Med. Chem. 19: 222 (1976)
37. Lamb, R.G., S.D. Wyrick and C. Piantadosi Atherosclerosis 27: 147 (1977)
38. Hall, I.H. and G.L. Carlson J. Med. Chem. 19: 1257 (1976)
39. Wyrick, S.D., I.H. Hall, C. Piantadosi and C.R. Fenske J. Med. Chem. 19: 219 (1976)
40. Watthey, J.W.H., B.J. Henrici, S. Lausten and M. Miller Abst. Papers 173rd Am.Chem. Soc.Mtg. MEDI 12 (1977)
41. Snipes, W., S. Person, A. Keith and J. Cupp Science 188: 64 (1977)
42. Barnhart, J.W., D.J. Rytter and J.A. Molello Lipids 12: 29 (1977)
43. Renzi, A.A., D.J. Rytter, E.R. Wagner and H.K. Goersch In: Lipids, Lipoproteins, and Drugs, Volume 63, Advances in Experimental Biology and Medicine, Plenum Press, New York, 1975, p. 477
44. Mauz, O. and E. Granzer Chem. Abstr. 80: P95532p (1974)
45. Reddy, J.K. and T.P. Krishnakanta Science 190: 787 (1975)
46. Barter, P.J., W.E. Connor, A.A. Spector, M. Armstrong, S.L. Connor and H.A. Newman Ann. Int. Med. 81: 619 (1974)
47. Malloy, M.J., J.P. Kane and J.S. Rowe Clin. Res. 22: 235A (1974)
48. Katocs, A.S. Jr., and S.A. Schaffer Fed. Proc. 36: 1160 (1977) (abstract)
49. Bielman, P., D. Brun, S. Moorjani, M.A. Gagnon, L. Tereault and P.J. Lupien. Int. J. Clin. Pharmacol. Biopharm. 15: 166 (1977)
50. Kritchevsky, D., S.A. Tepper and J.A. Story Arzneimittel-Forschung 26: 862 (1976)
51. Watts, J. McK., P. Jablonski and J. Toouli Drugs 10: 342 (1975)
52. Editorial. Brit. Med. J. 1: 1119 (1977)
53. Iser, J.H., R.H. Dowling, H.Y.I. Mok and G.D. Bell New Engl. J. Med. 293: 378 (1975)
54. Miller, M.E. and P.J. Nestel Lancet 2: 929 (1974)

55. Coronary Drug Project Research Group
New Engl. J. Med. 296: 1185 (1977)
56. Heckers, H., K. Dittmar, F.W. Schmahl and K. Huth
Atherosclerosis 26: 249 (1977)
57. Bordia, A., H.C. Bansal, S.K. Arora and S.V. Singh
Atherosclerosis 21: 15 (1975)
58. Kritchevsky, D.
Artery 1: 319 (1975)
59. Augusti, K.T. and P.T. Mathew
Experientia 30: 468 (1974)
60. Barndt, R., Jr., D.H. Blankenhorn, D.W. Crawford and S.H. Brooks
Ann. Int. Med. 86: 139 (1977)
61. Editorial
Brit. Med. J. 2: 1 (1977)

Metabolism: Arterial and Tissue Culture

PROPERTIES OF LIPOPROTEINS RESPONSIBLE FOR HIGH AFFINITY BINDING TO CELL SURFACE RECEPTORS OF FIBROBLASTS AND SMOOTH MUSCLE CELLS

Robert W. Mahley and Thomas L. Innerarity

Comparative Atherosclerosis and Arterial Metabolism Section, National Heart, Lung, and Blood Institute, Bethesda, Maryland, U.S.A.

INTRODUCTION

Our studies of cholesterol-induced hyperlipoproteinemia in various animal models have led to the identification of several unique lipoproteins. This discovery has provided an opportunity to explore the properties responsible for the binding of certain lipoproteins to cell surface receptors of cultured fibroblasts and arterial smooth muscle cells. After a brief description of the types of plasma lipoproteins used in these studies, we will present data to support the following conclusions: a) that specificity for lipoprotein binding to the high affinity receptor sites resides with the apoproteins; b) that either the B or the arginine-rich apoprotein (ARP) is responsible for this binding; c) that a similar stereospecific charged region or recognition site may be shared in common by the B and ARP; and d) that theARP-containing lipoproteins are more avidly bound to the receptor than are the apo-B-containing lipoproteins.

CANINE AND SWINE LIPOPROTEINS

The plasma lipoproteins from the dog and swine with their unique chemical properties have served as useful probes in examining the properties responsible for

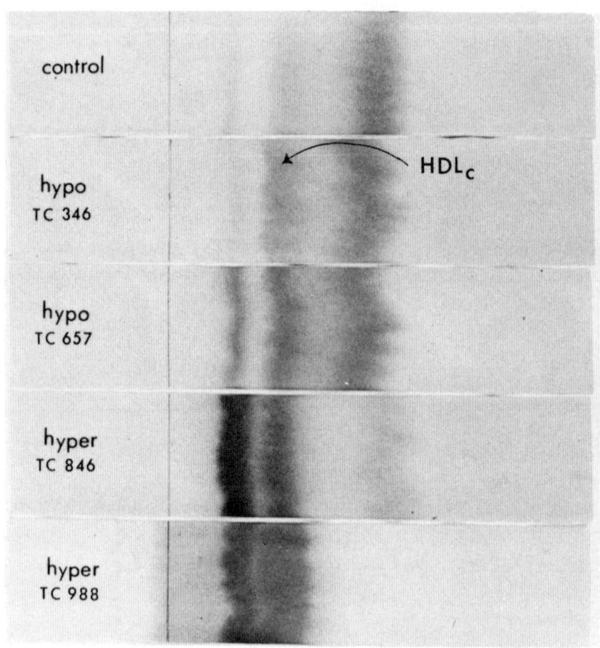

Figure 1: Electrophoretograms of canine plasma lipoproteins from a control dog (top pattern) and four hypercholesterolemic dogs. The levels of the plasma cholesterol are indicated on each pattern. Reproduced with permission (2).

specific binding. The lipoproteins of a dog on a control chow diet are compared to those induced by cholesterol feeding in Figure 1. In the control dog (top pattern), the lipoproteins routinely seen are the low density lipoproteins (LDL) and two α-migrating lipoproteins referred to as HDL_1 and HDL_2. The two α-migrating lipoproteins have been classified as high density lipoproteins (HDL) because they contain the A-I apoprotein indicative of HDL and lack the B apoprotein. The HDL_2 are the main plasma lipoproteins of control dogs and are equivalent to the typical high density lipoproteins of man.

In the cholesterol-fed dogs, as the plasma cholesterol begins to increase, the principal lipoprotein to carry the cholesterol is one having α_2-mobility similar to the HDL_1. We have called these cholesterol carrying lipoproteins HDL_c, the subscript c indicating that they

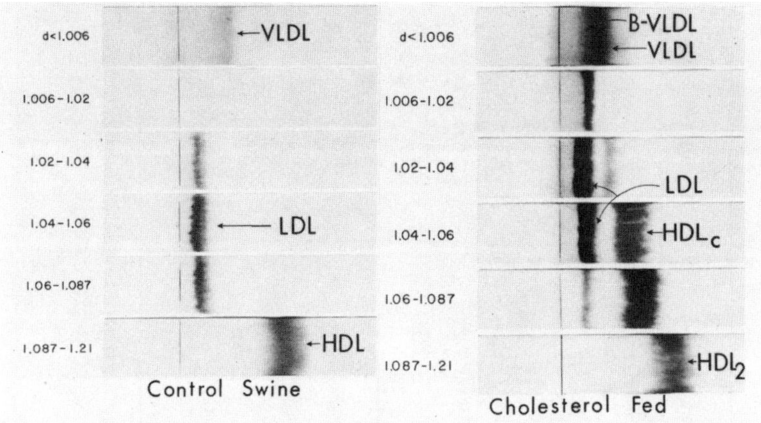

Figure 2: Electrophoretograms of lipoproteins in the various ultracentrifugal density fractions of control and cholesterol-fed swine. Reproduced with permission (5).

are cholesterol induced. The HDL_c of the cholesterol-fed dog appear to be HDL_1 which become loaded with cholesterol. As the plasma cholesterol increases further, the HDL_c increase in concentration. Furthermore, an increase in the β-migrating lipoproteins represented by B-VLDL and LDL and a decrease in the typical HDL_2 accompany the increase in plasma cholesterol.

The HDL_c and LDL are both cholesterol rich with similar composition and particle size (200 Å in diameter). However, they are dissimilar with respect to their apoprotein content. Canine LDL, like human LDL, contain primarily the B apoprotein. The HDL_c lack the B apoprotein and contain either the ARP as the exclusive apoprotein or the ARP and A-I apoproteins (for a review of canine lipoproteins see ref. 1-4).

Miniature swine fed a control chow diet have lipoproteins which are equivalent to human VLDL, LDL, and HDL (Fig. 2). When a high cholesterol diet is fed, the plasma lipoproteins are markedly altered (Fig. 2). The β-migrating lipoproteins including B-VLDL and LDL increase and HDL_c occur. The HDL_c and LDL of the swine are similar to those lipoproteins described in the dog (for review see ref. 4 and 5). Similar lipoproteins have been described in other species (6-8).

Table 1

CHARACTERISTICS OF THE PLASMA LIPOPROTEINS

	Human Lipoproteins		Dog and Swine Lipoproteins		
	LDL	HDL	LDL	HDL_c	HDL_2
Electrophoretic Mobility	β	α_1	β	α_2	α_1
Density	1.02-1.05	1.125-1.21	1.02-1.06[a]	1.02-1.06[a]	1.10-1.21
Composition[b]	CE-rich	Protein, PL	CE-rich	CE-rich	Protein, PL
Size (Å)	170-220	70-100	160-240	150-260	80-100
Major Apoproteins	B	A-I, A-II	B	ARP, A-I	A-I
Heparin Precipitable	+	-	+	+	-
HMG-CoA Reductase Regulation	+	-	+	+	-
High Affinity Receptor Binding	+	-[c]	+	+	-[c]

[a]The LDL and HDL_c are isolated at d=1.02-1.06 by ultracentrifugation and purified by Geon-Pevikon block electrophoresis (13). In some cases a different density fraction is used as noted.

[b]Cholesteryl ester, CE; phospholipid, PL.

[c]High affinity binding of HDL occurs to a limited extent when added to the tissue culture media at high protein concentrations (discussed below).

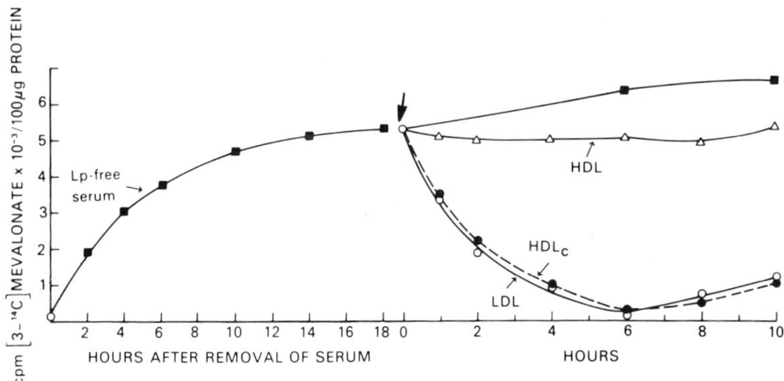

Figure 3: Time course of induction and suppression of 3-hydroxy-3-methylglutaryl coenzyme A (HMG CoA) reductase activity by serum lipoproteins . Modified from (10).

Our studies designed to determine the properties of the specific lipoproteins responsible for binding to the cell surface receptors are based on comparisons of the binding activities of canine and swine LDL, HDL_c, and HDL_2 and human LDL and HDL. The characteristics of the canine and swine lipoproteins are summarized in Table I. The LDL and HDL_c are cholesteryl ester rich lipoproteins, whereas the HDL_2 are rich in protein and phospholipid. The LDL and HDL_c are 200 Å and HDL_2 are 100 Å in diameter. The LDL contain the B apoprotein; HDL_c lack the B apoprotein and contain exclusively the ARP or the ARP and A-I apoproteins; HDL_2 contain primarily the A-I apoprotein. LDL and HDL_c are both precipitated by heparin/Mn. Finally, of great importance particularly to these studies is the ability of both HDL_c and LDL to be bound, internalized, and degraded by fibroblasts and smooth muscle cells and to suppress cholesterol synthesis by regulation of HMG-CoA reductase (3,9-12).

LIPOPROTEIN BINDING TO THE CELL SURFACE RECEPTORS OF FIBROBLASTS AND SMOOTH MUSCLE CELLS

Lipoprotein research has realized a major advance in the recognition by Goldstein, Brown and coworkers (14,15) that cell surface receptors on fibroblasts bind plasma lipoproteins and initiate a series of events which regulate cholesterol synthesis and lead to the accumulation of cholesterol esters within the cells. Their observation that LDL and VLDL, which contain the B apoprotein,

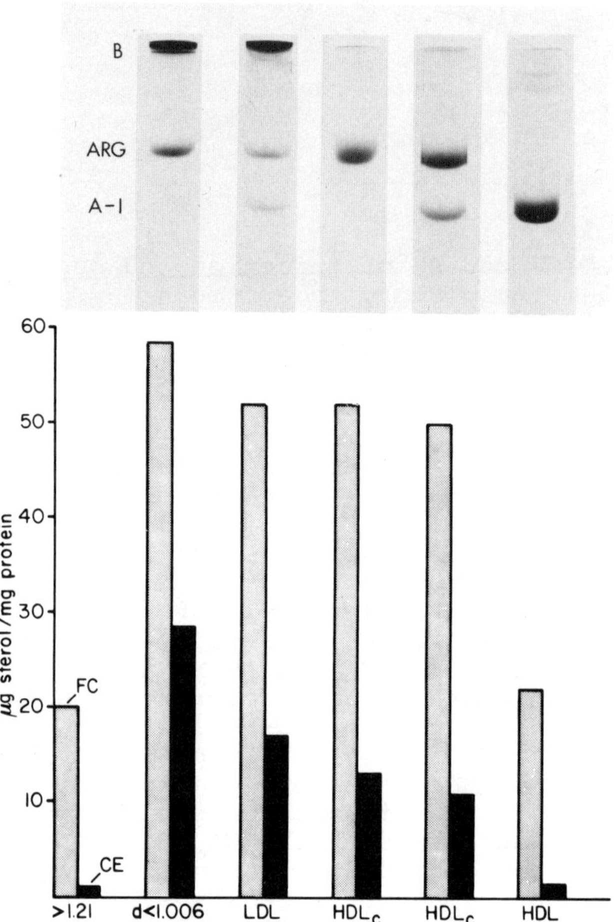

Figure 4: Sterol accumulation by canine aortic smooth muscle cells in culture in response to 24-hr incubation with lipoproteins (200 μg/ml cholesterol) from a cholesterol-fed dog. The apoprotein patterns of the lipoproteins used are shown at the top of the figure. FC, free cholesterol. CE, cholesteryl ester. d>1.21, lipoprotein deficient sera. ARG, arginine-rich apoprotein. Reproduced with permission (3).

are bound to the cell surface receptors, while HDL, which lack apo-B, do not bind significantly led initially to the postulate that the receptor might be specific for the B apoprotein. However, we have found that HDL_c bind to the same receptor as LDL, although HDL_c lack the B apoprotein and in some cases contain only the arginine-rich apoprotein.

Our initial studies suggest that swine LDL and HDL_c can both interact with cells and regulate cholesterol metabolism by processes similar to those observed with human LDL. When smooth muscle cells are incubated with lipoprotein-deficient serum, HMG-CoA reductase activity increases (Fig. 3). The addition of LDL or HDL_c results in a similar nearly complete suppression of cholesterol synthesis within six hours, whereas typical HDL_2 have little effect (10). Similar results have been obtained with human fibroblasts; furthermore swine LDL and HDL_c (11), like human LDL (14), are incapable of suppressing reductase activity in the receptor-negative homozygous Type II fibroblasts. These studies suggest that cholesterol from both LDL and HDL_c enters the smooth muscle cells and normal fibroblasts and regulates cholesterol synthesis.

In fact, we have demonstrated that both swine and canine LDL and HDL_c can cause accumulation of cholesterol and cholesteryl esters within these cells (3,11). The response of canine smooth muscle cells to canine LDL which contain primarily the B apoprotein, two HDL_c fractions which lack the B apoprotein and contain primarily or exclusively the ARP, and typical HDL_2 which contain primarily the A=I apoprotein are compared (Fig. 4). The lipoproteins are added at a concentration of 200 μg/ml of cholesterol in the media and cellular free and esterified cholesterol are measured after 24 hours. The basal (control) sterol content of the cells is determined by incubation of the cells in lipoprotein-deficient sera. The LDL and HDL_c cause a marked and similar increase in sterol content. However, typical HDL_2 containing primarily the A-I apoprotein do not increase the cellular cholesterol. Thus, both LDL and HDL_c cause an accumulation of cellular cholesterol (3). It should be pointed out that canine smooth muscle cells accumulate sterol to a greater extent than occurs with smooth muscle cells of swine (Table 2). Furthermore, swine smooth muscle cells accumulate esterified cholesterol at levels similar to those described for human fibroblasts (16) and rhesus monkey smooth muscle cells (17). The extent to which

Table 2

ACCUMULATION OF FREE AND ESTERIFIED CHOLESTEROL BY CANINE AND SWINE SMOOTH MUSCLE CELLS

	CANINE		SWINE	
Lipoproteins[b]	Free[c]	Esterified	Free	Esterified
Canine d<1.006	58±4	29 ±4	42±2	9 ±1
HDL	52±4	17 ±3	45±2	4.5±0.3
HDL_c	52±5	13 ±2	44±1	4.4±0.4
HDL_2	22±1	1.3±0.2	29±2	1.8±0.4
d>1.21	20±1	1.1±0.1		
Swine d>1.21			32±3	1.4±0.2
Swine LDL	48±6	28 ±2	47±4	4.4±0.4
HDL_2	23±3	3 ±0.6	32±2	1.3±0.2
d>1.21	23±2	2.7±0.5	30±2	1.2±0.2
Canine LDL	47±2	35 ±3		
HDL_2	20±2	3.6±0.4		
d>1.21	23±3	2.8±0.5		

[a]Results presented at the top and bottom of the table were performed with different cell lines to confirm the observation at different times and with different cells.

[b]Cholesterol concentration in the media was 220 μg/ml. The swine lipoproteins were from animals on a normal diet. The swine LDL were obtained at d=1.02-1.063 and the HDL_2 at d=1.10-1.21. The d>1.21 was the lipoprotein deficient sera to compare the response of added lipoproteins.

[c]Free and esterified cholesterol expressed as μg of sterol/mg cell protein±S.D. All determinations were performed in triplicate or quadruplicate. Table reproduced with permission (3).

sterol accumulates in canine smooth muscle cells is only observed in rat smooth muscle cells and fibroblasts after treatment of these cells with chloroquine, a known inhibitor of lysosomal hydrolases (18). The enhanced cholesterol accumulation by canine smooth muscle cells in response to canine or swine LDL may be of physiologic significance in that the atherosclerosis of dogs is characterized by massive deposition of lipid within the smooth

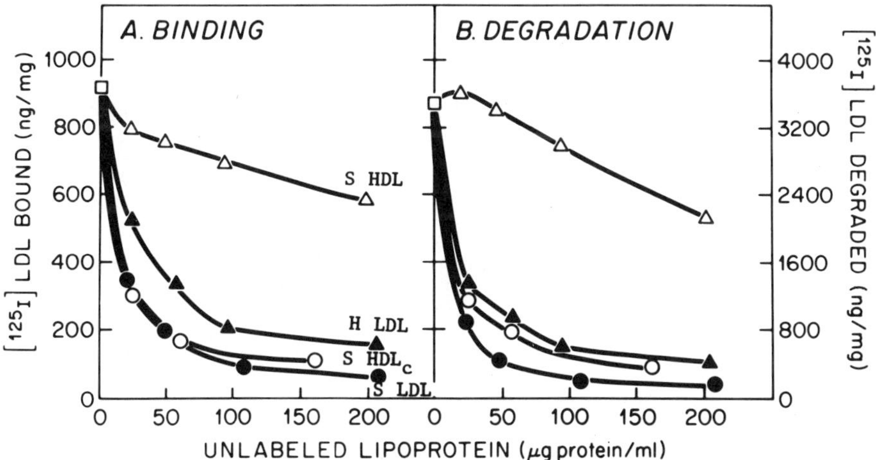

Figure 5: Ability of human LDL (▲), swine LDL (o), swine HDL_c (∘) or swine HDL_2 (△) to compete with human ^{125}I-LDL for binding and degradation in normal human fibroblasts. Modified from (11).

muscle cells of the media of the artery and less of the proliferative intimal response characteristic of swine or human atherosclerosis (3,19).

In order to determine whether LDL and HDL_c interact with the same or different cell surface receptors, we have undertaken competitive binding and degradation studies using the various swine lipoproteins and cultured human fibroblasts. Goldstein and Brown (15) have shown that when ^{125}I-labeled LDL are incubated with human fibroblasts, the LDL are bound to the cell surface receptors, internalized, and degraded. The ability of the various lipoproteins to compete with human ^{125}I-LDL for binding to the cell surface receptor is shown in Fig.5 (11). Swine LDL and HDL_c (bottom two curves) are seen to be as effective as human LDL in competing with iodinated LDL for the high-affinity binding sites. Swine HDL_2 are much less effective in displacing the iodinated LDL from the receptors, as previously described for human HDL (20). These data suggest that the LDL and HDL_c are bound at the same cell surface receptor sites. At this point it is reasonable to postulate that the cell surface receptors might recognize both the B apoprotein of LDL and the arginine-rich apoprotein of the HDL_c through a similar structural sequence common to both apolipoproteins.

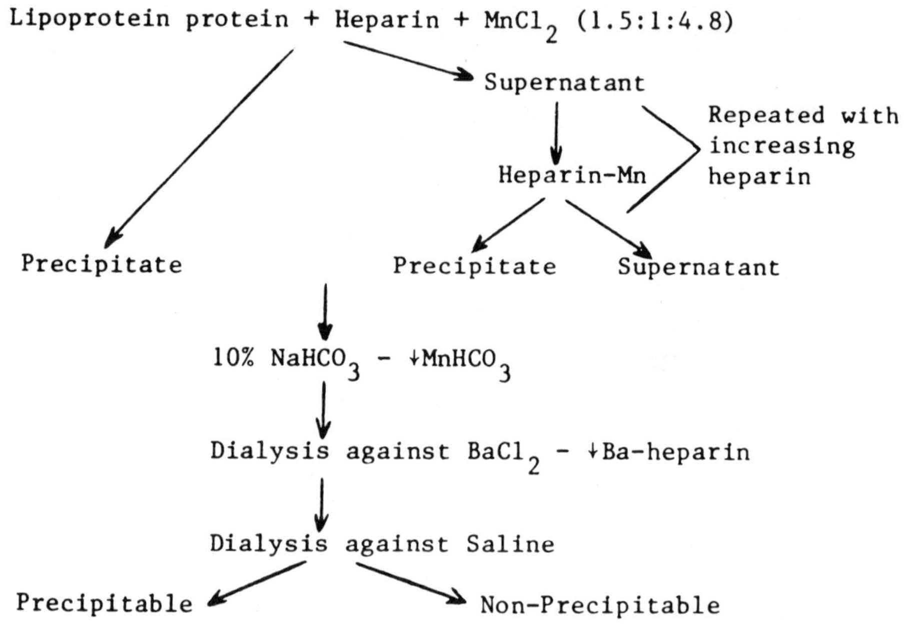

Figure 6: Schematic drawing of the heparin/Mn precipitation procedure.

To gain a further understanding of the properties of lipoproteins which might account for receptor binding of certain classes of lipoproteins, and not others, we have compared the activity of various dog lipoproteins in tissue culture (9). One of the properties of HDL_1 of the control dog and HDL_c of the cholesterol fed dog which we studied was heparin/manganese (Mn) precipitation. The HDL_1 and HDL_c are variably precipitated by heparin/Mn, and the most readily precipitable HDL_1 and HDL_c are those which contain the largest concentration of arginine-rich apoprotein. Thus, by use of the heparin/Mn precipitation, subfractions of HDL_1 or HDL_c which have different apoprotein contents, particularly with respect to the ARP, are isolated.

Using the scheme shown in Figure 6, precipitate and supernatant fractions are obtained upon addition of heparin/Mn. A single addition of heparin precipitates 95-99% of the canine LDL, whereas the typical dog HDL_2 are less than 10% precipitable. HDL_1 and HDL_c are 50 to

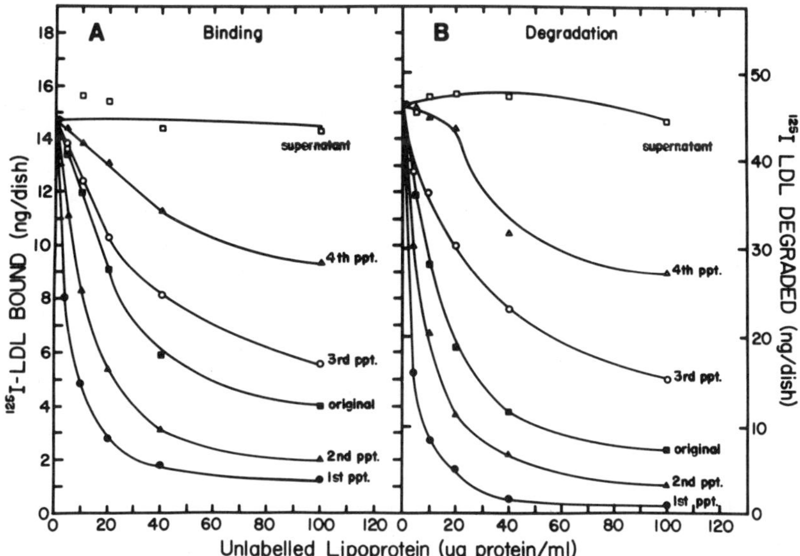

Figure 7: Ability of canine HDL_1, the four precipitated HDL_1 fractions, and supernatant HDL_1 to compete with canine ^{125}I-LDL for binding and degradation in normal human fibroblasts. Reproduced with permission (9).

80% precipitable by a single addition of heparin/Mn. Further precipitates of HDL_1 and HDL_c can be obtained by adding increasing amounts of heparin/Mn to the original supernatant. Thus, by multiple additions of heparin, several precipitates and a final supernatant are obtained. A comparison of the effectiveness of the precipitable and nonprecipitable HDL_1 and HDL_c fractions with respect to binding and degradation by human fibroblasts has been undertaken.

Competitive binding and degradation studies have been performed using canine ^{125}I-LDL in normal human fibroblasts (Fig.7). Increasing concentrations of the various subfractions of the unlabeled HDL_1 are added to the cells along with the ^{125}I-LDL. The most readily precipitable HDL_1 (the first precipitate which occurs at the lowest concentration of heparin/Mn) is the most effective in competing with the ^{125}I-LDL for binding and degradation. Displacement of the ^{125}I-LDL is progressively less with each successive precipitate and the least with the HDL_1 which remain in the supernatant following the fourth precipitation. Note that the

Table 3

CHARACTERIZATION OF HDL_1, PRECIPITATED HDL_1, AND SUPERNATANT HDL_1

	Ppt I[b]	Ppt II	Ppt III	Ppt IV	Super-natant	Original
Apoproteins[a]						
B	0	0	0	0	0	0
ARP	++++	+++	++	+	0	++
A-I	+	++	++	+++	++++	++
C's	++	++	++	+	+	++
% Composition						
T. Cholesterol[c]	43.8	38.8	38.1	34.9	28.5	37.4
Phospholipid	44.4	47.1	45.4	45.5	44.5	45.6
Protein	11.8	14.1	16.5	19.6	27.0	17.1
TC/PL	1.0	0.82	0.84	0.77	0.64	0.82
TC/Protein	3.7	2.8	2.3	1.8	1.1	2.2
Diameter, Å[d]						
Mean	256	259	223	221	218	252
Range	180-360	160-340	180-300	160-320	180-300	160-380

[a]Prominence of apoproteins as assessed qualitatively by SDS polyacrylamide gel electrophoresis.

[b]Ppt I was the HDL_1 fraction which precipitated at the lowest concentration of heparin-Mn (4:1:4.8). Ppt IV precipitated at the highest concentration of heparin and the supernatant HDL_1 remained nonprecipitable.

[c]The % esterified cholesterol was not different among the fractions (range: 65-68% of total).

[d]200 particles measured.

Table modified from (9).

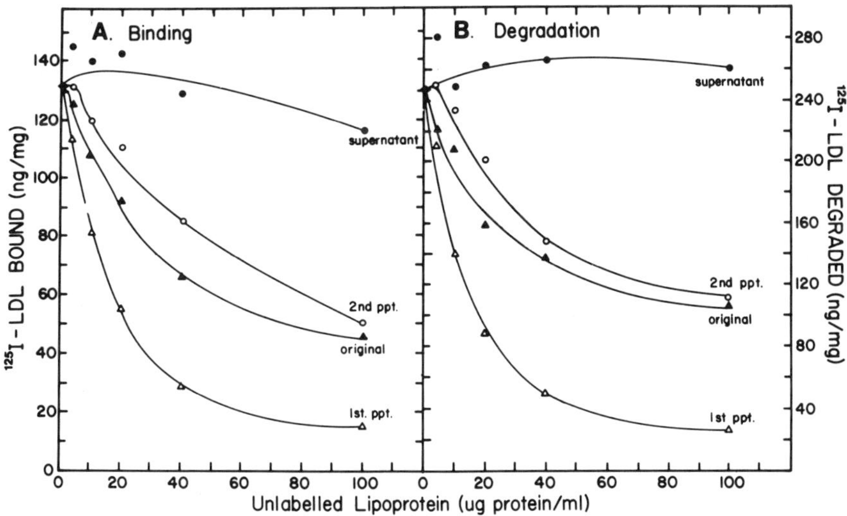

Figure 8: Ability of swine HDL_c (▲), the two heparin/manganese precipitable fractions (△, first fraction precipitated; o, second precipitate) and the supernatant (●) of the HDL_c to compete with swine ^{125}I-LDL for binding and degradation in normal human fibroblasts. Reproduced with permission (9).

original untreated HDL_1 give intermediate results. Thus, the most readily bound lipoproteins are those which are most readily precipitated by heparin (9). It is now possible to compare the properties of the subfractions (Table 3).

The HDL_1 subfraction which is most active and precipitates at the lowest concentration of heparin is the first precipitate, and it is found to contain more ARP than any other fraction including the original HDL_1. Progressively less ARP is present in each of the successive precipitates (II-IV), and no ARP is seen in the supernatant HDL_1 by polyacrylamide gel electrophoresis. The chemical composition of the subfractions reveals that the first precipitate contains more cholesterol and less protein than do the other precipitates or the supernatant (Table 3). Also, the mean particle size decreases as one compares the first through the fourth precipitates and supernatant. However, the change in particle size is only 40 Å, and the supernatant HDL_1, which are very ineffective in displacing the ^{125}I-LDL from the binding

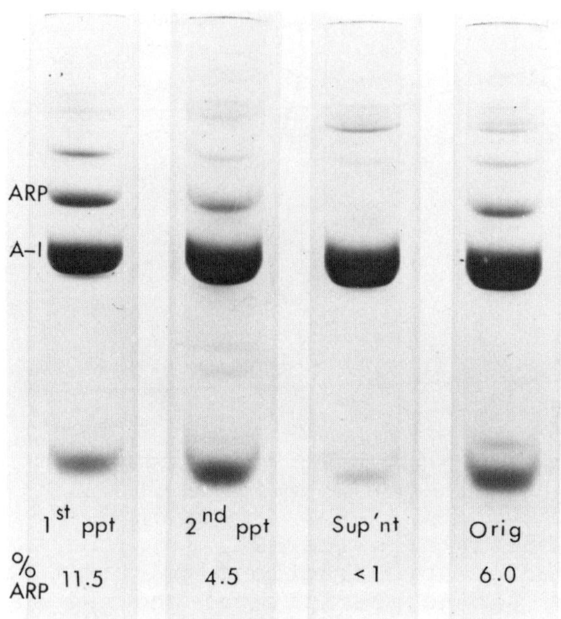

Figure 9: Sodium dodecyl sulfate polyacrylamide gel electrophoresis of the original swine HDL_c (Orig.), the two heparin/manganese precipitable fractions (1st Ppt and 2nd Ppt) and the HDL_c which remain in the supernatant (Sup'nt). The per cent of the total lipoprotein protein represented by the arginine-rich apoprotein is shown for each fraction. Modified from (9).

sites, are 218 Å in diameter (approximately the size of LDL). Particle size in the 200-300 Å range does not appear to be an important determinant for cell surface receptor binding under these conditions (9).

Swine HDL_c have also been subfractionated by heparin/Mn precipitation. Two precipitates and a supernatant fraction are obtained. As shown in Fig. 8, the first precipitate is most effective in displacing the ^{125}I-LDL. The second precipitate and the original HDL_c give similar results and the supernatant is very ineffective in displacing the ^{125}I-LDL from the receptor of the human fibroblasts. The properties of the two precipitated subfractions and the final supernatant fraction are similar with respect to chemical composition and size but are quite different with respect to apoprotein content. The first precipitate, which is most active in displacing the ^{125}I-LDL, contains more ARP than the original or the other fractions (Fig. 9). The per cent of the total lipoprotein protein represented by the ARP for each lipoprotein fraction is indicated in Fig. 9. The supernatant HDL_c fraction contains $< 1\%$ ARP as determined by quantitative two-dimensional immunelectrophoresis and is the least active subfraction (9). The HDL_c fraction which precipitated at the lowest concentration of heparin/Mn is at least as active as LDL in displacing the ^{125}I-LDL from the binding sites and yet the ARP content of this fraction represents only 11.5% of the total apoproteins.

These studies further suggest that the ARP of HDL_1 or HDL_c might play an important role in binding and internalizing these lipoproteins. The subfractions which are most readily precipitated by heparin are the most efficient in competing with LDL for binding and degradation. The most striking consistent characteristic of the precipitated HDL_1 and HDL_c which are most efficiently bound is the occurrence of the arginine-rich apoprotein. It is reasonable to speculate that the property of the lipoproteins responsible for binding to heparin and to the cell surface receptor is the same and might represent a positively charged region on the lipoprotein surface shared in common with both B and ARP. Surface charge has been suggested by previous studies to be important since heparin competes with the receptor on fibroblasts for binding with human LDL (21).

Since one of the components of a lipoprotein which is positively charged at physiologic pH is the amino acid arginine, studies have been undertaken to modify selectively the arginyl residue of the various apolipoproteins (12). A reagent which reacts specifically with arginine or the arginyl residues of proteins under very mild conditions is 1,2-cyclohexanedione (CHD). It has been demonstrated that CHD reacts only with the guanido groups of arginine and with no other residues (22,23). We have found that the product of the reaction of CHD with LDL is stable, but that the reaction can be quantitatively reversed by incubation of the lipoprotein with hydroxylamine (12). Previous studies with CHD have shown it is possible to block selectively the reactions of certain enzymes, such as pancreatic ribonuclease A, which have arginine in the active site of the molecule, and then to regenerate most of the enzymatic activity following the removal of the 1,2-cyclohexanedione (24). Based on these observations, we wanted to know what effect CHD modification of the arginyl residues of the various

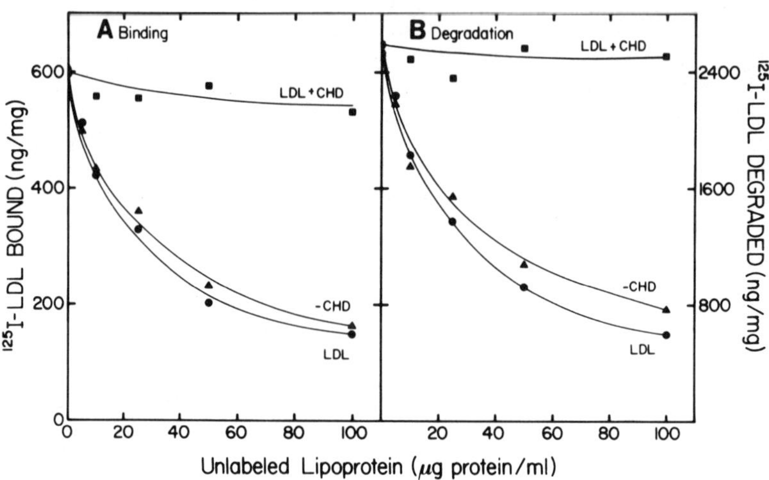

Figure 10: Ability of native LDL (●), LDL modified with 1,2-cyclohexanedione (■) and LDL from which cyclohecanedione has been removed (▲) to compete with human ^{125}I-LDL for binding (A) and proteolytic degradation (B) in normal human fibroblasts at 37°. On day 7 the media was replaced by 10% human lipoprotein deficient serum, 5 μg/ml of human ^{125}I-LDL protein (67 cpm/ng), and the unlabeled lipoproteins as indicated. The experiment was performed for 5 hr. LDL was allowed to react with 0.1 M CHD in 0.166 M borate buffer, pH 8.1, for 2 hr at 35°. The CHD was removed from the LDL by incubation at 35° for 16 hr in 0.5 M hydroxylamine and 0.15 M mannitol. Reproduced with permission (12).

apolipoproteins might have on competitive binding, internalization, and degradation. As shown in Fig. 10, the treatment of human LDL with 0.1 M CHD for two hours markedly inhibits the ability of this lipoprotein to compete with the ^{125}I-LDL for binding, internalization, and degradation by human fibroblasts at 37°. Untreated LDL give the typical competitive displacement curve for binding and degradation. The effects of the CHD are reversed by the removal of the CHD from the LDL by incubation with hydroxylamine (Fig. 10) (12).

Likewise, in studies performed at 4°, in which binding occurs but internalization does not, the CHD-modified LDL (top line) are incapable of displacing the ^{125}I-LDL from the high affinity receptor sites (Fig. 11). The

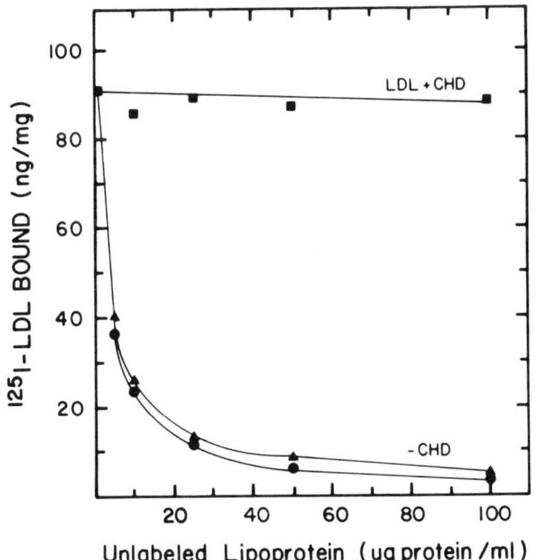

Figure 11: Ability of untreated human LDL (●), LDL modified with 1,2-cyclohexanedione (■), and LDL from which the cyclohexanedione had been removed (▲) to compete with human ^{125}I-LDL for binding at 4° to normal human fibroblasts. On day 7, 2.5 μg/ml of ^{125}I-LDL (210 cpm/ng of protein) and unlabeled LDL were added. Incubation was for 2 hr. Reproduced with permission (12).

untreated LDL and the regenerated LDL give very similar results in displacing the ^{125}I-LDL from the receptors. In other experiments CHD modification of iodinated LDL has demonstrated a direct effect of CHD on the inhibition of binding.

It is important to determine that the reaction of human LDL with CHD and the subsequent release of the CHD do not alter the physical or chemical properties of the lipoproteins. We can show by negative staining electron microscopy that the original LDL, CHD-treated LDL, and regenerated LDL (CHD treatment followed by CHD removal) are the same size (200 Å) and have the same morphologic appearance (individual spherical particles). The chemical composition is likewise unchanged when the original, CHD-treated, and regenerated LDL are compared. By paper electrophoresis, the CHD-LDL are relatively more negative and migrate further than the original or regenerated LDL. However, the original and regenerated LDL migrate as a

Table 4

AMINO ACID COMPOSITION OF HUMAN LDL

Amino Acids	Untreated	CHD Treated	Regenerated
Aspartic Acid	27.1 (27)[a]	27.4 (27)	27.2 (27)
Threonine	14.0 (14)	14.9 (15)	13.4 (13)
Serine	20.9 (21)	20.5 (21)	20.5 (21)
Glutamic Acid	30.8 (31)	31.4 (31)	31.0 (31)
Proline	10.1 (10)	10.6 (11)	10.5 (11)
Glycine	12.1 (12)	12.3 (12)	11.9 (12)
Alanine	15.3 (15)	15.9 (16)	15.6 (16)
Valine	13.6 (14)	14.0 (14)	14.0 (14)
Methionine	3.9 (4)	3.7 (4)	3.8 (4)
Isoleucine	14.4 (14)	14.5 (15)	14.5 (15)
Leucine	30.6 (31)	30.6 (31)	30.4 (30)
Tyrosine	8.4 (8)	8.4 (8)	8.3 (8)
Phenylalanine	12.4 (12)	12.4 (12)	12.3 (12)
Lysine	21.2 (21)	20.0 (20)	20.8 (21)
Histidine	6.3 (6)	6.2 (6)	6.1 (6)
Arginine	8.6 (9)	5.2 (5)	8.1 (8)

[a]Amino acid residues calculated per mole assuming 250 residues per mole. Value in parentheses is rounded off to nearest whole number. Conditions for the modification and regeneration were as described in Fig. 10. Table reproduced with permission (12).

sharp β band. These results in combination with the competitive binding and degradation studies indicate that the reaction is mild and does not irreversibly alter the physical or chemical properties (12).

We have synthesized ^{14}C-labeled cyclohexanedione and shown that 98% of the activity is associated with the protein and less than 2% appears in the lipid extract. The CHD in the lipid extract appears to be free CHD; none of it is detected in association with the phospholipid classes separated by two-dimensional thin-layer chromatography.

To determine the extent of the modification of the protein by the CHD treatment, the amino acid compositions of the lipoproteins are compared before and after reaction with CHD and after release of CHD by hydroxylamine

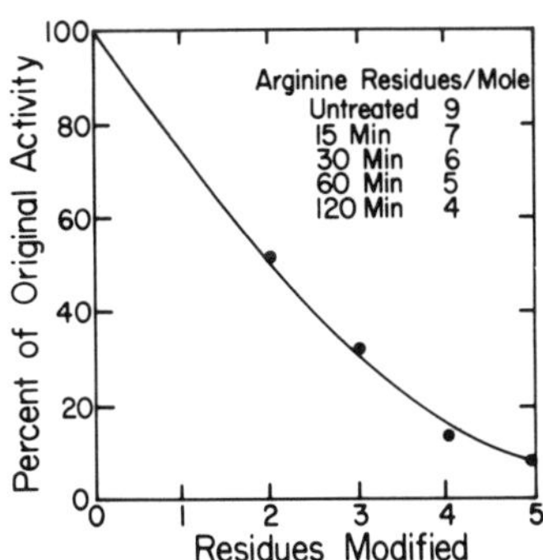

Figure 12: Changes in the binding activity of human LDL as a function of the number of arginyl residues modified by cyclohexanedione. Reproduced with permission (12).

treatment. It is possible to determine the number of amino acid residues which react with CHD by difference amino acid analysis, since the modified residues are not detected on the analyzer. The analyses of the LDL reveal that only the arginyl residues are modified (Table 4). The untreated LDL contain nine residues of arginine per mole as compared with five residues in the CHD-treated LDL (i.e., four of the nine residues are modified). After the release of CHD with hydroxylamine, eight residues of arginine are detected by amino acid analysis.

It is possible to demonstrate a direct correlation between the number of arginyl residues modified and the ability of the LDL to inhibit ^{125}I-LDL binding and degradation. When CHD is allowed to react with LDL for 15,30,60, and 120 minutes, the number of arginyl residues determined by amino acid analysis decreases with time (Fig. 12). A modification of two arginine residues results in a 50% decrease in the capacity of the modified LDL to inhibit degradation of the ^{125}I-LDL as compared with untreated LDL. Modification of four or five out of a total of nine residues results in the abolishment of greater than 85% of the activity of the LDL (Fig. 12). Thus, CHD treatment, as well as being mild and reversible, is specific for arginine, and binding activity is abolished by modification of approximately half of the arginyl residues of LDL (12).

CHD modification of canine LDL likewise eliminates their binding activity. Release of CHD from canine LDL restores most of the activity to the LDL. It appears

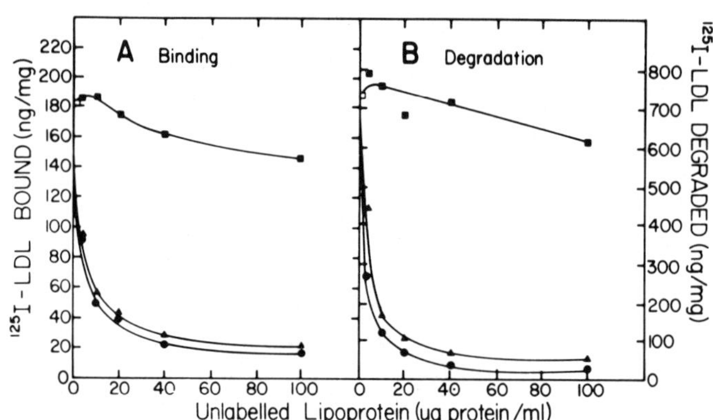

Figure 13: Ability of canine HDL_1 (●), HDL_1 modified with 1,2-cyclohexanedione (■) and HDL_1 regenerated by the removal of cyclohexanedione (▲) to compete with canine ^{125}I-LDL for normal human fibroblasts at 37°. Reproduced with permission (12).

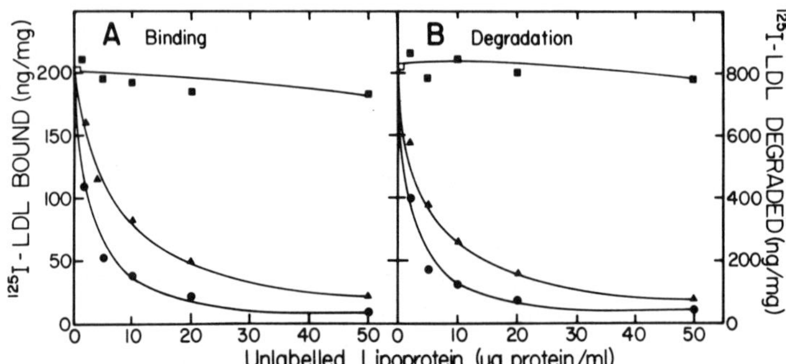

Figure 14: Ability of canine HDL_c (●), HDL_c modified with cyclohexanedione (■) and HDL_c regenerated by removal of cyclohexanedione (▲) to compete with canine ^{125}I-LDL for binding, internalization, and degradation in normal human fibroblasts at 37°. Reproduced with permission (12).

that modification of the B apoprotein of human and canine LDL prevents binding.

It is of interest to determine whether CHD treatment of canine HDL_1 and HDL_c which lack the B apoprotein and contain the arginine-rich apoprotein will prevent their binding. This would obviously suggest a common property through which the reactive lipoproteins bind to the receptor. Indeed, CHD modification of HDL_1 has been shown to abolish the ability of the HDL_1 to displace the ^{125}I-LDL from the receptors (Fig. 13). The same is true for the HDL_c. As shown in Fig. 14, the modification of HDL_c markedly reduces their ability to displace the ^{125}I-LDL. Most of the original activity of the HDL_c is restored after removal of the CHD. The HDL_c used in the experiment shown in Fig. 14 contain the arginine-rich apoprotein as the only detectable protein. Amino acid analysis of this apolipoprotein reveals that the untreated HDL_c contain 30 residues of arginine per mole, assuming 290 residues/mole of protein. The HDL_c treated with CHD for two hours retain 13 arginine residues; i.e., the modification of slightly more than half of the arginyl residues abolishes the binding activity. Following the regeneration of HDL_c by removal of CHD, 28 arginyl residues are determined by amino acid analysis. The other amino acid residues are unchanged by the CHD treatment, as is true for the LDL (12).

It appears that the recognition site on the LDL and HDL_c which react with the cell surface receptor resides with the apoprotein constituents and that the B and arginine-rich apoproteins are involved. It also appears that a similar positively charged region of the B and ARP on the lipoprotein surface is involved and that arginyl residues are functionally significant residues in the lipoprotein recognition site. However, the precise mechanism by which the CHD modification of the B or ARP prevents binding awaits more information on the nature of lipoprotein-cell receptor interactions and more detailed structural characterization of the recognition site.

Data thus far obtained indicate that the B and ARP interact with the same cell surface receptors and initiate similar intracellular events. However, as is evident from a comparison of the data in Fig. 13 and 14, the ARP-containing lipoproteins (HDL_1, HDL_c) are much more active in displacing the ^{125}I-LDL from the high affinity cell surface receptors of human fibroblasts than the B-containing LDL (Fig. 10). Competitive binding

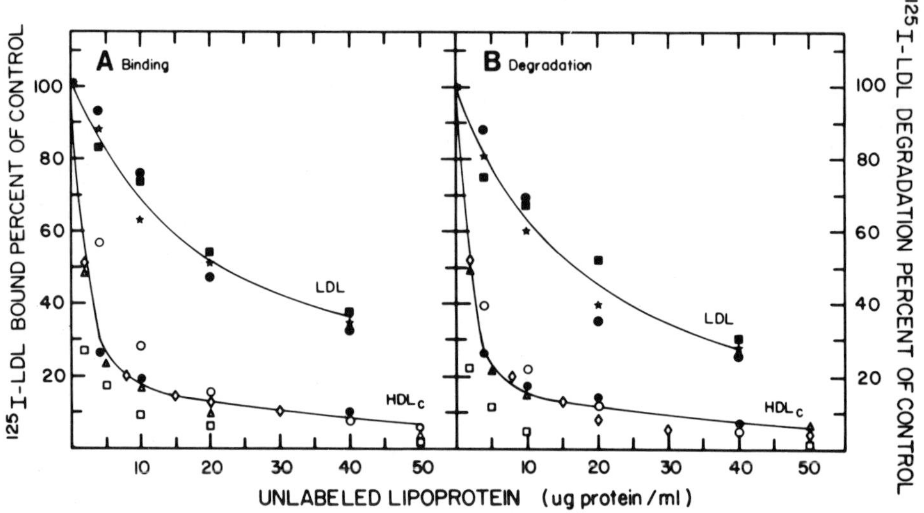

Figure 15: Ability of canine LDL (top curve) and canine HDL_C which contained only the arginine-rich apoprotein (bottom curve) to compete with 5 μg of canine ^{125}I-LDL for binding and degradation in normal human fibroblasts at 37°. Incubation performed for 5 hr.

and degradation studies performed at 37° using canine ^{125}I-LDL (5 μg/ml of protein) reveal that LDL displace approximately 50% of the labeled LDL at a concentration of 25 μg/ml of protein as compared with a 50% displacement by HDL_C at a concentration of 2-2.5 μg/ml of protein (Fig. 15). As shown in Fig. 16, a competitive binding assay performed at 4° reveals the canine HDL_C which contain only the ARP to be 100-fold more active than LDL which contain the B apoprotein (25). The LDL and HDL_C used in this experiment had similar lipid and protein compositions by weight and were approximately the same size but differed with respect to their apoprotein content. The enhanced binding activity of ARP may be related to a greater number of recognition sites (more arginyl residues or active sites per mole of protein) available on the ARP-containing lipoproteins than on LDL (I, Fig. 17). An increased number of recognition sites would increase the likelihood of ARP interacting with the receptors as compared with the B apoprotein. Another possibility (II) is that the receptor binding or affinity constant for ARP is greater than for the B apoprotein due to a "positive cooperativity" by which adjacent recognition sites on the ARP may enhance the

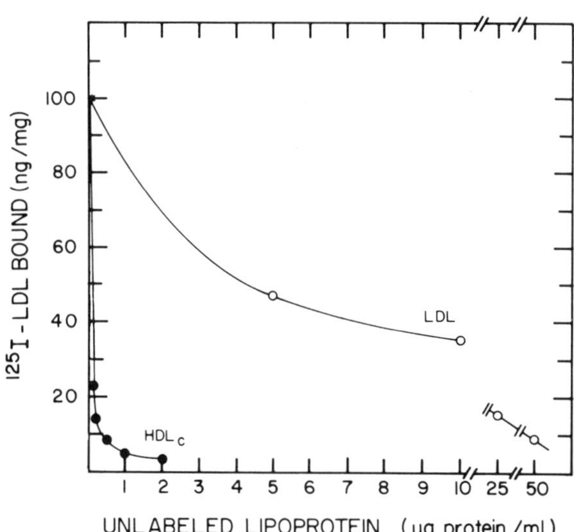

Figure 16: Ability of canine HDL_c which contained only the arginine-rich apoprotein (●) and human LDL (o) to compete with human ^{125}I-LDL for binding in normal human fibroblasts at 4°. Incubation performed for 2 hr.

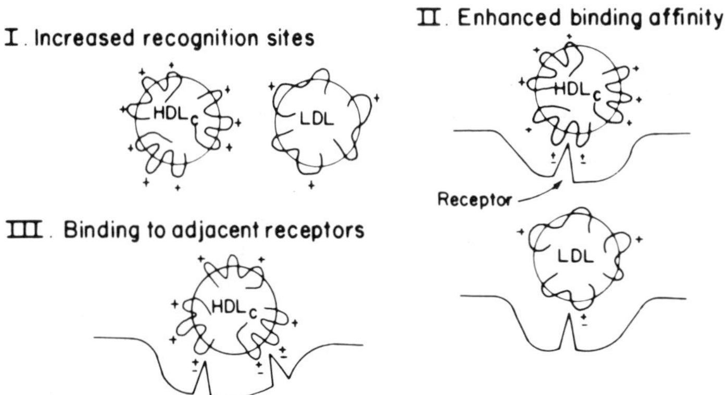

Figure 17: Possible mechanisms to explain the enhanced binding activity of the arginine-rich apoprotein containing lipoproteins.

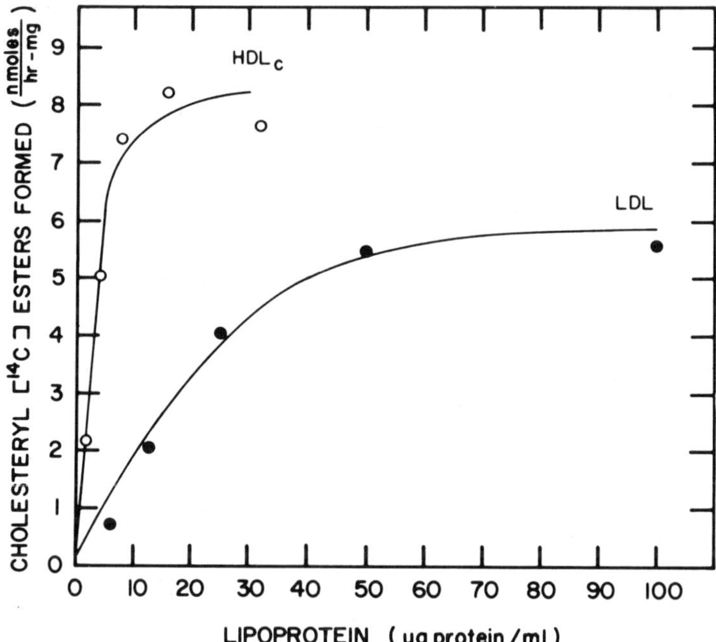

Figure 18: Incorporation of ^{14}C-oleate into cholesteryl esters as a function of LDL (●) and HDL$_c$ (o) concentration. Normal human fibroblasts were incubated with the indicated amount of lipoproteins for 15 hr and then pulsed with ^{14}C-oleate (0.1 mM, 40,000 cpm/nmol for 2 hr. The cells were harvested and the cholesteryl ^{14}C-esters determined.

binding of these lipoproteins to a single receptor. On the other hand, a single ARP-containing lipoprotein particle might bind to two adjacent receptor sites (III, Fig. 17). At the present time it is impossible to distinguish among these or alternate mechanisms.

In addition to the enhanced binding activity of the ARP-containing lipoproteins, the intracellular events mediated by these lipoproteins are likewise affected as reflected by an increased esterification of intracellular cholesteryl esters. Previously, an enhancement in the rate of incorporation of ^{14}C-oleate into cholesteryl esters as a consequence of internalization and degradation of human LDL by fibroblasts has been described (14, 15). When canine HDL$_c$ which contain only the ARP are

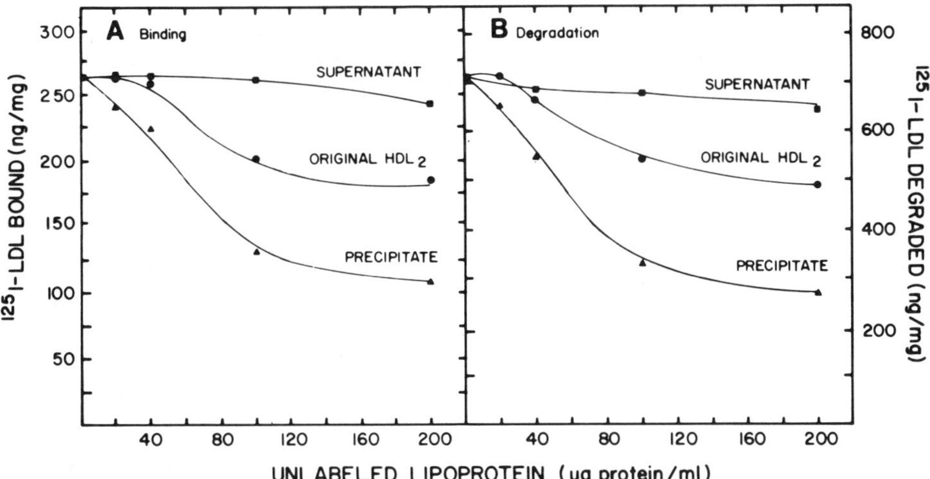

Figure 19: Ability of swine HDL (d=1.09-1.21) (●), heparin/manganese precipitated HDL (▲) and the HDL that remained in the supernatant (■) to compete with swine ^{125}I-LDL for binding and degradation in normal human fibroblasts. Five μg/ml swine ^{125}I-LDL (274 cpm/ng) and the unlabeled HDL fractions were added to the cells after 7 days in culture. Experiment performed for 5 hr at 37°.

incubated with fibroblasts for 15 hr and then pulsed for 2 hr with ^{14}C-oleate, the incorporation of ^{14}C-oleate into cellular cholesteryl esters is greatly enhanced as compared to the results obtained with human LDL (Fig. 18). The concentration of LDL which stimulated half-maximal incorporation of ^{14}C-oleate into cholesteryl esters is 18 μg/ml of protein. The HDL_c give a half-maximal incorporation at a much lower concentration (3 μg/ml of HDL_c protein) and achieve a higher absolute level of cholesteryl ester synthesis (25).

Because of the enhanced binding activity of ARP, a small quantity of ARP in a minor, but potent, subfraction of the typical HDL (d=1.09-1.21) of swine and man could account for the observed binding activity. Previously, Carew et al.(26) and Miller et al.(27) have shown that typical HDL from swine and from normal man bind to the cell receptor of smooth muscle cells and fibroblasts to a significant extent only at high HDL concentrations in the culture media. As shown in Fig. 19, swine HDL (d=1.09-1.21) can displace up to 30% of the ^{125}I-LDL (5 μg/ml of protein) at a concentration of 200 μg/ml of HDL protein in the media. To determine if this activity is associated with an active subfraction, swine HDL are subjected to the heparin/Mn precipitation procedure and the binding activities of the precipitable and non-precipitable (supernatant) fractions are compared. The precipitable fraction of the HDL, which accounts for 15% of the total HDL, contains a detectable amount of ARP (no apo-B) and possesses all the binding activity of the fraction (Fig. 19). The supernatant fraction, representing 85% of the total HDL protein, has little or no capacity to displace the ^{125}I-LDL from the receptor sites on human fibroblasts and lacks detectable ARP. Except for the presence of ARP in the precipitable HDL, no other physical or chemical properties are notably different when the precipitate and supernatant fractions are compared. It is suggested that the presence of small amounts of the highly reactive ARP could account for most, if not all, of the high-affinity receptor binding activity of HDL.

SUMMARY

The uniqueness of the apoprotein content and chemical composition of certain canine and swine lipoproteins has proved to be useful in examining the properties responsible for the specificity of lipoprotein binding to the high affinity receptors of cultured fibroblasts and arterial smooth muscle cells. The conclusions based on observations derived from studies with canine, swine, and human lipoproteins are as follows:

1. The apoproteins appear to be the constituents responsible for the specificity of binding certain lipoproteins (e.g. LDL and HDL_c) to the cell surface receptors.

2. Either the B or the arginine-rich apoprotein can interact with the receptor.

3. There appears to be a similar structural sequence or positively charged region associated in common with both the B and arginine-rich apoproteins which interacts with the receptor site.

4. The amino acid arginine in the B and arginine-rich apoproteins is associated with the recognition site on the lipoprotein surface responsible for binding to the cell receptors. Modification of approximately half of the arginyl residues of either the B or arginine-rich

apoprotein containing lipoproteins with 1,2-cyclohexanedione totally abolishes their ability to bind to the cell receptors. Only the arginyl residues are modified by this procedure, and removal of the cyclohexanedione from the lipoprotein restores most of the original binding activity.

5. Heparin precipitability within a given class of lipoproteins is directly correlated with the ability of the lipoproteins to bind to the receptor. With the canine, swine, and human lipoproteins studied, either the B or arginine-rich apoproteins are necessary for both precipitability and binding.

6. The arginine-rich apoprotein containing lipoproteins (HDL_c and certain HDL) are more readily bound, internalized and degraded than are the apo-B containing LDL. The binding activity is 25- to 100-fold greater for the arginine-rich than for the apo-B containing lipoproteins.

7. The high affinity binding of typical HDL (d-1.09-1.21) of man and swine appears to correlate with the presence of a variable amount of a highly reactive subfraction of the HDL which contains the arginine-rich apoprotein. The fraction which binds to the receptor is precipitated by heparin/Mn and usually represents less than 15% of the HDL fraction. The HDL_c production induced by cholesterol feeding in animals may occur by overloading an HDL subfraction with cholesterol and the arginine-rich apoprotein. The effects of dietary cholesterol in altering the HDL of man is an important unanswered question.

In summary, some of the parameters of lipoprotein structure which may be important in the regulation of cellular cholesterol metabolism have been identified. However, the metabolic role of the B versus arginine-rich apoprotein in regulating cellular cholesterol content and the plasma cholesterol level _in vivo_ remains to be determined.

ACKNOWLEDGEMENTS

The authors gratefully acknowledge the collaboration of the coworkers who have contributed to this review: K.S. Arnold, T.B. Bersot, M.L. Broderick, D.L. Fry, K.S. Holcombe, B.L. Kahler, S. Oh, R.E. Pitas, and K.H. Weisgraber. We thank Mrs. Exa Murray and Ms. Patricia Hartman for typing the manuscript. Portions of this work were performed under contract with Meloy Laboratories.

REFERENCES

1. Mahley, R.W. and Weisgraber, K.H.
Circ. Res. 35: 713 (1974)
2. Mahley, R.W., Weisgraber, K.H. and Innerarity, T.L.
Circ. Res. 35: 722 (1974)
3. Mahley, R.W., Innerarity, T.L., Weisgraber, K.H. and Fry, D.L.
Am. J. Path. 87: 205 (1977)
4. Mahley, R.W.
In: The Physiology of Lipids and Lipoproteins in Health and in Disease, J.M. Dietschy, editor, in press
5. Mahley, R.W., Weisgraber, K.H., Innerarity, T.L. Brewer, H.B., Jr., and Assmann, G.
Biochemistry 14: 2817 (1975)
6. Mahley, R.W. and Holcombe, K.S.
J. Lipid Res. 18: 314 (1977)
7. Mahley, R.W., Weisgraber, K.H., and Innerarity, T.L.
Biochemistry 15: 2979 (1976)
8. Weisgraber, K.H., Mahley, R.W. and Assmann, G.
Atherosclerosis, in press
9. Mahley, R.W. and Innerarity, T.L.
J. Biol. Chem. 252: 3980 (1977)
10. Assmann, G., Brown, B.G., and Mahley, R.W.
Biochemistry 14: 3996 (1975)
11. Bersot, T.P., Mahley, R.W., Brown, M.S. and Goldstein, J.L.
J. Biol. Chem. 251: 2395 (1976)
12. Mahley, R.W., Innerarity, T.L., Pitas, R.E., Weisgraber, K.H., Brown, J.H., and Gross, E.
J. Biol. Chem., in press
13. Mahley, R.W. and Weisgraber, K.H
Biochemistry 13: 1964 (1974)
14. Brown, M.S., Ho, Y., and Goldstein, J.L.
Ann. N.Y. Acad. Sci. 275: 244 (1976)
15. Goldstein, J.L. and Brown, M.S.
Ann. Rev. Biochem. 46: 897 (1977)
16. Brown, M.S., Faust, J.R., and Goldstein, J.L.
J. Clin. Invest. 55: 783 (1975)
17. St. Clair, R.W.
In: Atherosclerosis Reviews, Vol. 1, edited by R. Paoletti and A.M. Gotto, Jr., New York, Raven Press, 1976, p. 61-117
18. Stein, O., Vanderhoek, J. and Stein, Y.
Atherosclerosis 26: 465 (1977)

19. Mahley, R.W., Nelson, A.W., Ferrans, V.J. and Fry, D.L.
Science 192: 1139 (1976)
20. Brown, M.S. and Goldstein, J.L.
Proc. Natl. Acad. Sci. USA 71: 788 (1974)
21. Goldstein, J.L., Basu, S.K., Brunschede, G.Y. and Brown, M.S.
Cell 7: 85 (1976)
22. Patthy, L. and Smith, E.L.
J. Biol. Chem. 250: 557 (1975)
23. Dietl, T. and Tschesche, H.
Hoppe-Seyler's Z. Physiol. Chem. 357: 657 (1976)
24. Patthy, L. and Smith, E.L.
J. Biol. Chem. 250: 565 (1975)
25. Innerarity, T.L. and Mahley, R.W., in preparation
26. Carew, T.E., Koschinsky, T., Hayes, S.B. and Steinberg, D.
Lancet I: 1315 (1976)
27. Miller, N.E., Weinstein, D.B., and Steinberg, D.
J. Lipid Res. 18: 438 (1977)

THE LIPIDS IN HUMAN ATHEROSCLEROSIS - MORPHOLOGICAL DEMONSTRATIONS OF FIVE FORMS OF ATHEROMA LIPIDS

Yoshiya Hata and Toshiharu Ishii

Department of Medicine and Pathology, Keio University School of Medicine, Tokyo, Japan

INTRODUCTION

In the development of atherosclerosis in mammals including man, arterial tissue undergoes three fundamental changes: proliferation of smooth muscle cells, deposition of intra- and extracellular lipids, and accumulation of extracellular matrix of collagen, elastin and proteoglycans (1). Among these processes, the accumulation of lipids in atherosclerosis is featured by accretion of cholesteryl esters, particularly oleate in the early lesions of fatty streak (2-6), while cholesteryl linoleate accumulates in addition to oleate with a marked increase in free cholesterol and phospholipids in the intermediate lesions of fibrous plaque and in the advanced lesion of complicated lesions (2,3, 4,6-9).

These accumulations of lipids in tissue seem to play a crucial role in genesis and development of atherosclerosis for five reasons: a) there is no atherosclerosis without accumulation of lipids in arterial tissues (10), b) arterial lipid contents are closely related to both the serum lipid levels and the severity of lesions (11), c) atherosclerosis is more common and severe in the population taking high fat diet (12), d) in experimental animals atherosclerosis can be induced by cholesterol feeding (13), and e) it regresses when serum cholesterol is lowered (14,15). However, the exact mechanism of how the lipids accumulate in arterial tissues to initiate and develop the lesion or how they are absorbed to induce regression of the lesion is not yet fully known.

This lack of knowledge seems to arise in part from the intrinsic limitations in methods, both morphological and biochemical, employed so far for studies on lipids in normal and atherosclerotic lesions. Since chemical method deals only with the lipids extracted from the homogenized tissue, then dissolved in organic solvents in an amorphous form regardless of their original configuration in tissue site, and morphological method deals with the lipids exposed to dehydrating organic solvents which may dissolve and even extract lipids during tissue preparations. Due to these intrinsic limitations in methods and artifacts involved in prepared specimens, we have only scanty information on macromolecular organization of lipids in the environment of biological tissues, where all the physiological components are integrated in unity and even foreign bodies are organized in certain sites of certain cells.

To elucidate the nature of lipids accumulating in human atherosclerotic lesions of fatty streak, fibrous plaque and complicated lesions as close as possible to *in vivo* state avoiding both extraction with solvents and distortion due to dehydrating agents or embedding materials, we have employed a combined use of ordinary and polarizing light microscopy (16), together with silver nitrate staining (17) and immunofluorescence method (18), for demonstration of five forms of lipids in atherosclerotic lesions. They are recognized as structure-bound lipids, lipoprotein lipids, anisotropic lipid inclusions, isotropic lipid inclusions and solid crystals. In this paper they are morphologically demonstrated and the relationship between the proportions of each type of lipid and the developmental stage of atherosclerosis is discussed.

MATERIAL AND METHODS

Human aortas were used for demonstration of lipids in normal and atherosclerotic tissues. They were obtained at autopsy and opened along the anterior margin. The cleaned intimal surface was examined by the naked eye for differentiation of type of lesions.

The grossly normal intima was defined as pinkish white, smooth surface covered by a fine transparent membrane without any damage or deterioration. The lesions were identified by visual inspection according to the WHO classification (19) as fatty streaks, fibrous plaque and complicated lesions. Fatty streak lesions were defined as yellowish, slightly raised areas of opaque spots or streaks covered by a delicate translucent membrane, whose underlying internal elastic lamina and media appeared apparently normal in color, texture and consistency. Fibrous plaque lesions were recognized as pearly whitish, raised areas of opaque firm tissue covering a pale yellow core of lipids in the intima which often extended in the media. Complicated lesions were noted as hard roughened surface either with ulceration, haemorrhage, thrombosis or calcareous deposits.

A portion of endothelial surface of normal intima from a 59 year-old male, who died of gastric cancer, was immersed with 0.25% silver nitrate for 1 minute and rinsed in 0.9% saline solution, then exposed to a mercury vapor UV lamp with a filter of 70% transmittance at the 25-37 line for 7 minutes (17). The stained specimen was freeze-sectioned in Cryostat at -10°C as thin as possible along the endothelial surface, and stained further with haematoxylin-eosin for nuclei and cytosols.

A piece of unfixed fatty streak lesions from a 43-year-old male who died of a myocardial infarction was teased in 0.9% saline solution under a dissecting microscope and immersed in 80% glycerol to demonstrate anisotropic and isotropic lipid inclusions in clusters of foam cells under a polarizing light microscope with a polarizer and an analyser crossed at 90° (20).

The anisotropic and isotropic lipid inclusions were isolated by mincing five to ten fatty streak lesions with fine dissecting scissors in 2 ml of 0.9% saline solution until the tissue fragments were about 0.7-1.0 mm cubes and a turbid suspension was produced. An aliquot of 0.2 ml of the suspension was crudely isolated by aspiration with a Pasteur pipet. The aliquot was mixed with four volumes of glycerol to stabilize the inclusions and reduce their Brownian movement under the polarizing microscope (20).

An area of fibrous plaque lesions of a 73 year-old male who died of thyroid tumor was frozen and sectioned to obtain specimens with a thickness of six to ten microns. The sectioned specimens were reacted with anti-human LDL rabbit sera labelled with fluorecein isothiocyanate (FITC) at 37°C for 60 minutes, then viewed under a fluorescent microscope with BV excitation-1 and Ratten 2B-1 filters (18).

A portion of complicated lesions from the same patient was dissected with sharp needles in 0.9% saline solution into fine pieces to show solid crystals in tissue under a polarizing light microscope.

RESULTS

Figures 1 to 5 present the results of the observations. Figure 1 illustrates the enface-view of the endothelium of the human aorta stained with silver nitrate and hematoxylin eosin. Dark stained were the spindle-shaped boundaries of elongated endothelial cells, whose longer axis was oriented longitudinally, parallel to the

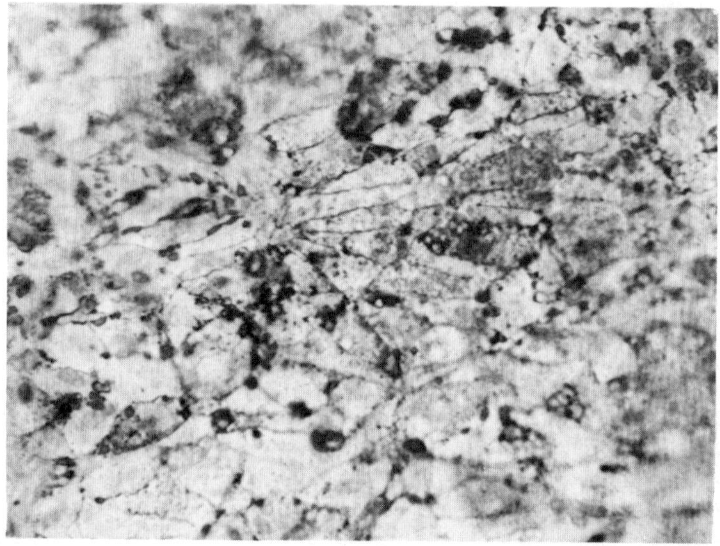

Figure 1: Endothelial cell boundaries visualized by silver nitrate staining for a Häutchen preparation of the aorta from a 59 year-old male subject. The cell boundaries are of irregular spindle-shape and the endothelial cells aligned with their longer axis parallel to the direction of blood stream.

blood stream. In normal intima the size and shape of cells appeared homogeneous, and their linings trim and regular.

Figure 2 shows the presence of LDL in atherosclerotic tissue by immunofluorescence technique. The bright fluorescent areas in intima and partly in media indicated the locations where the anti-LDL area were specifically bound to LDL in tissue, and made luminous by the fluorescence due to FITC bound to anti-LDL serum. The fluorescent areas in lesions differed in size from granular spots to insular clusters.

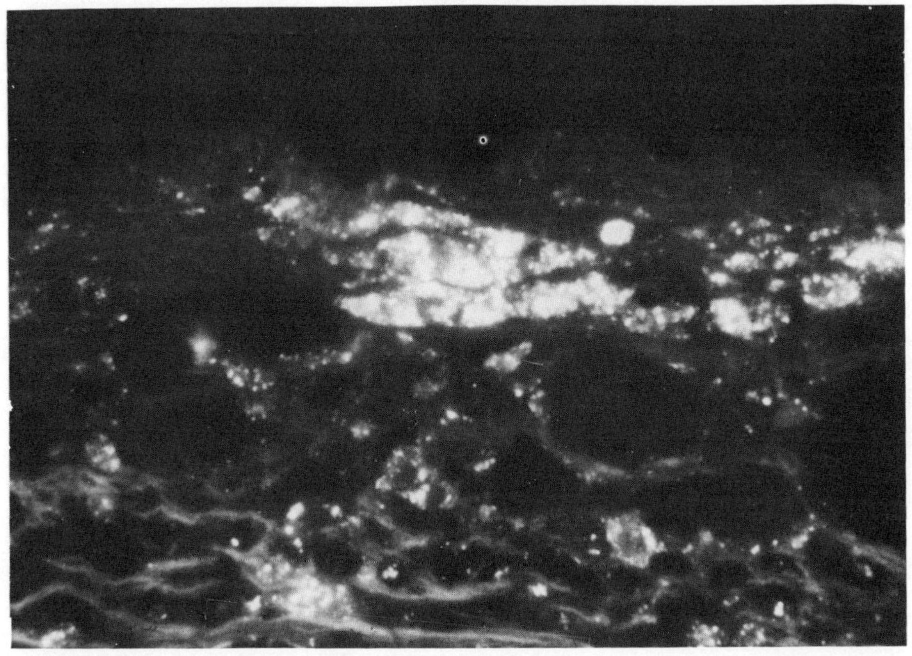

Figure 2: Immunofluorescence of LDL in fibrous plaque lesion from the thoracic aorta of a 73 year-old male. Bright areas in the intima and partly in the media represent immunofluorescence due to anti-human LDL rabbit serum labelled with FITC (x40).

Figure 3 demonstrates the lipid inclusions *in situ* in thin-layer of unfixed fatty streak lesions examined by polarizing light microscopy. The light areas of birefringence represent anisotropic lipid inclusions clustered in spindle-shaped intimal cells. Diffuse areas of brightness indicate similar clusters of double refractile material above and beneath the plane of focus of the microscope.

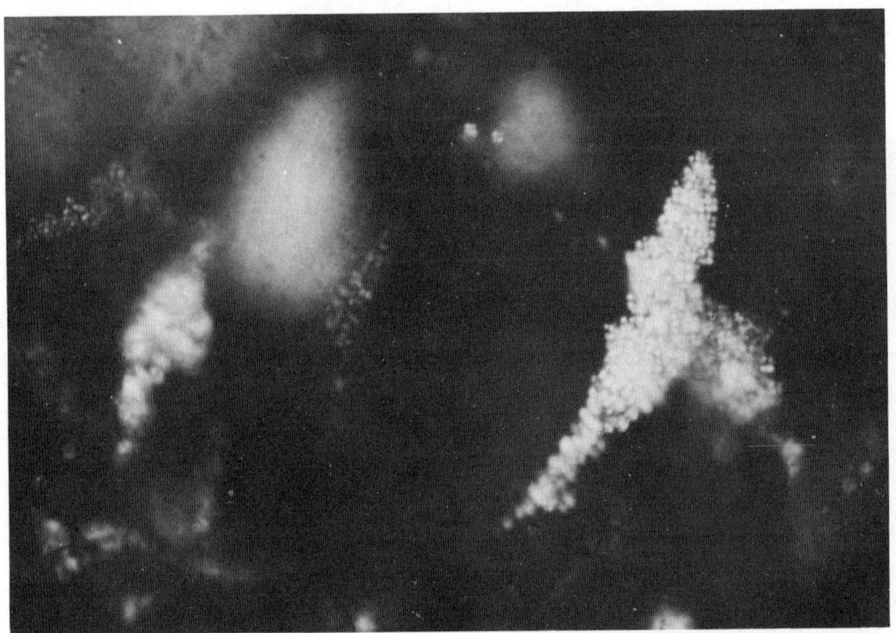

Figure 3: Anisotropic lipid inclusions *in situ* in thin preparation of unfixed fatty streak lesion from the thoracic aorta of a 43 year-old male examined with a polarizing light microscope. The bright area of birefringence represents anisotropic lipid inclusions clustered in spindle-shaped intimal cells (x20).

Figure 4 is the photograph of preparation of isolated lipid inclusions from unfixed fatty streak lesions suspended in 80% glycerol, and examined under a polarizing light microscope with the analyser rotated slightly off the 90° cross with the polarizer to visualize isotropic lipid inclusions as homogenous grey bodies. Anisotropic lipid inclusions show divisions into quadrants by sharp Formee cross image. All anisotropic inclusions demonstrated similar orientation of the cross image and interference colors under a tint plate. Their size varied from 0.6 to 3μ.

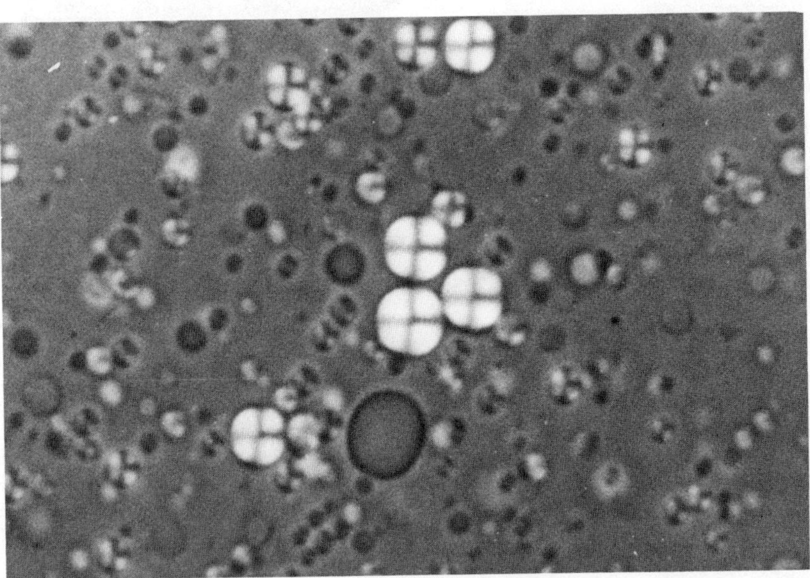

Figure 4: Isolated lipid inclusions from unfixed fatty streak lesions of a 43 year-old male examined under a polarizing light microscope which resolved into mixtures of anisotropic and isotropic inclusions: the former spheres were divided into equal quadrants by a black cross image whose arm directions coincided with those of polarizer and analyser crossed at 90°, while isotropic inclusions appeared as homogenous dark grey spheres (x40).

Figure 5 shows the crystal pieces in the advanced lesion of complicated lesions unfixed and teased in 0.9% saline solution, and viewed under a polarizing light microscope. The crystal pieces were mostly in thin plate of tetragonal shape with an approximate dimension of 10 to 20μ. Upon rotating the microscope stage, they demonstrated interference colors of first order yellow and second order blue.

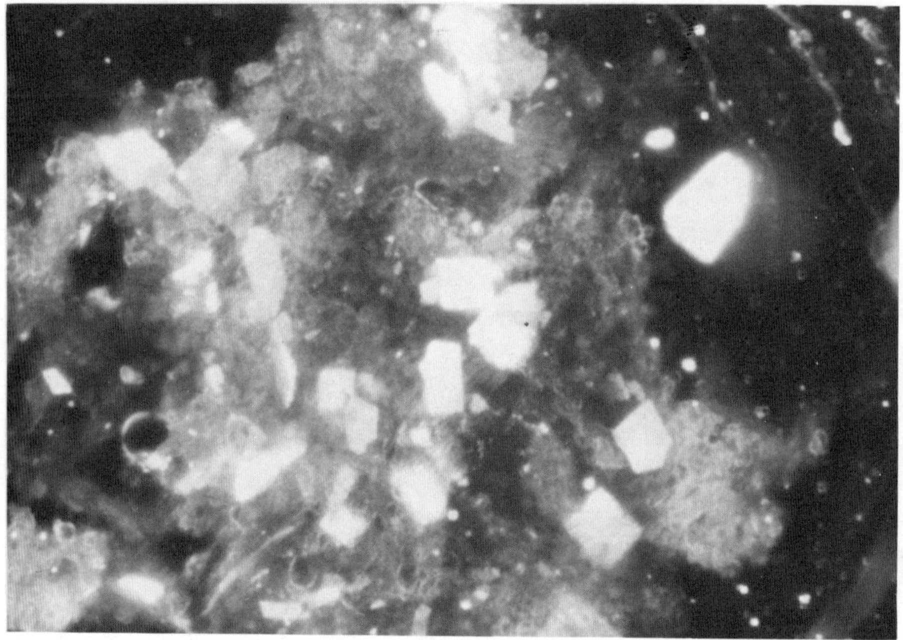

Figure 5: Crystal pieces in unfixed complicated lesions from the thoracic aorta of a 73 year-old male. Under polarizing microscope, crystals appeared birefringent thin plate in tetragonal shape (x10).

DISCUSSION

Lipids in normal and atherosclerotic lesions have been studied by several methods in which the aortic specimens are neither exposed to organic solvents for dehydration nor embedded in resin materials except for frozen-section performed in preparation for Figures 1 and 2. Thus minimizing possible source of artifacts, we have demonstrated the atheromatous lipids in a form as close as possible to *in vivo* state of tissues.

Firstly, there are lipids in the form of membrane matrix or those bound to intercellular substances in arterial tissues. They are visualized by silver nitrate staining of the Häutchen preparation of endothelial cells (17,21,22) as in Fig. 1. Since silver nitrate is readily reduced to metallic silver under such oxidative conditions as involving double bonds and ultraviolet lights, the silver grains formed along the cell boundaries indicate that such lipids containing double bonds as cholesterol and phospholipids are present in arterial tissue either in the form of membrane matrix (23). or in the form of lipids bound to interstitial substances. Such interstitial cement substances as collagen, elastin and proteoglycans tend to trap and accumulate the lipoprotein lipids into their macromolecular organization (24,25).

Secondly, there are lipids in the form of lipoproteins incorporated into arterial tissue. The immunofluorescence detected in the intima and media indicates that there exist LDL's in the tissue (11,26,27), since the LDL antibody is specifically prepared for human serum LDL, and the LDL is known to be incorporated into endothelial and smooth muscle cells via the LDL pathway (28,29) of arterial tissue. Therefore, the immunofluorescence observed in Figure 2 reveals the presence of lipoproteins probably in a particulate form solubilized in cytosols and intercellular space of the tissue.

Thirdly, there are lipids in the form of anisotropic and isotropic lipid inclusions. The inclusions from fatty streak have 85% anisotropy, while those from fibrous plaque lesions have 68% isotropy (20). Chemical analysis has revealed the inclusions of 85% anisotropy consisted of cholesteryl esters 94.9%, free cholesterol 1.7%, phospholipids 1.0% and triglycerides 2.4% (30), while those of 68% isotropy had cholesteryl esters 59.6%, free cholesterol 12.9%, phospholipid 17.6% and triglycerides 9.9% (9). Crystallographic examinations show that the main constituent molecules of cholesteryl esters are oriented in radial symmetry, forming a concentric lamellar structure incorporating water molecules between layers. Because of this molecular alignment, the cholesteryl ester-rich inclusions are defined as liquid crystal named lyotropic smectic mesophase (20,31).

Finally, there are lipids in the form of solid crystals. They are often found in fibrous plaque lesions (20), and invariably exist in complicated lesions. Mostly there are thin plates in tetragonal shape (32,33), rather than in needle-shape, of 10 to 20μ in dimensions. Under polarizing light microscope, they are double-refractile and, upon rotating microscope stage with a tint plate, show interference colors of first order yellow and second order blue which are similar to those from pure authentic crystals.

These five forms of lipids in human atheromatous lesions are tentatively designated as (I) structure-bound lipids, (II), lipoprotein lipids, (III) anisotropic lipid inclusions, (IV) isotropic lipid inclusions and (V) solid crystals. This classification features also the physical states of lipids in biological environments; the structure-bound lipids represent membrane lipid in bilayers (23), the lipoprotein lipids a pseudomicellar state (34), anisotropic inclusions a liquid crystalline state (20,31), isotropic inclusions a liquid state (20), and solid crystals a solidified form of regular molecular orientation.

Although it is shown that the amount of tissue lipid content is to some extent proportional to serum cholesterol levels (10,11) and that 60 to 80% of the total cholesterol in lesion comes from serum cholesterol (35, 36), while 90% of phospholipids in lesion is synthesized *in situ* (37), the exact origin and precise mechanism of formation and transformation of these five forms of lipids remain to be investigated. However, it is likely that each type of lipid plays a different role in genesis and progression of atherosclerosis, since, as in Table 1, the major lipid accumulated in atherosclerotic tissue characterizes the lesion types, and the proportions of each type of lipid differ in the amount from lesion to lesion. For instance, in normal arterial tissue, we usually find only the structure-bound lipids and the lipoprotein lipids in arterial tissue. In contrast to the normal, once the lesion of fatty streak develops,

Table 1

RELATION OF ACCUMULATION FORM OF LIPIDS TO ARTERIAL TISSUE TYPES

Form of Lipid	Tissue Type				
	Normal	Aged	Fatty Streak	Fibrous Plaque	Complicated Lesion
I. Structure-Bound Lipids	+	++	+	++	++
II. Lipoproteins in Cytosol	±	+	++	+	+
III. Anisotropic Lipid Inclusions	-	-	++	+	+
IV. Isotropic Lipid Inclusions	-	-	+	++	++
V. Crystal Lipids	-	-	-	+	++

the lipids in the form of anisotropic inclusions appear in addition to the structure-bound lipids and the lipoprotein lipids, and become the major type of lipids in intimal cells to form foam cells. As the lesion advances from fatty streak to fibrous plaque, the lipids in the form of isotropic inclusions increase in the amount in the tissue space, besides the former three forms of lipids. In complicated lesions, the lipids in the form of solid crystal turn into the major lipids in the tissue.

Thus the major type of lipid in the arterial tissue seems not only to characterize the stage of development of atherogenesis, and determine the type of atherosclerotic lesions, but also to play a different role in the development of atherosclerosis. The structure-bound lipids may be related to the membrane fluidity of endothelial and smooth muscle cells, which regulates the permeability and activities of enzymes bound to the membrane (38). When serum lipoproteins, particularly LDL, are incorporated into arterial cells, their constituent lipids will be the precursor for the formation of lipid inclusions (39). Once anisotropic spherical inclusions are formed within cytosol, they remain unchanged within the homeostatic medium of cytosol for a long period of time because of their stable inner structure having molecular organization in radial symmetry. The increase of the inclusions in number within cells may do harm to the metabolism of intimal cells, and the changes in size and shape of inclusions by swelling or phase transition (40) from anisotropic to isotropic inclusions or to solid crystals will also be damaging and destructive to tissue. Based on the identification of these five forms of lipids in human atherosclerosis, we can view the entire process of atherosclerosis with comprehension and analyze the specific role of each type of lipid in atherosclerosis and probably in regression of atherosclerosis.

ACKNOWLEDGEMENTS

The authors express their sincere thanks to Dr. T. Taketomi, Department of Biochemistry, Institute of Adaptation Medicine, Shinshu University School of Medicine, for providing us with anti-human LDL rabbit serum, and to Mm K. Ogawa, K. Miyazaki and K. Takakura for their help given to this work. This study is supported by the grants-in-aid for scientific research C-57301, C-157244, and C-257206, Ministry of Education, Science and Culture, Japan, the 6th Kanae Scientific Award for Medical Research (1975), a grant-in-aid for research provided by the University Funds for Educational Promotion, Keio University, Tokyo (1976) and the grants in-aid for medical research from Keio Health Counselling Center, Tokyo (1976 and 1977).

REFERENCES

1. Ross, R. and J.A. Glomset
Science 180: 1332 (1973)
2. Böttcher, C.J.F.
In: Drugs Affecting Lipid Metabolism, S. Garattini and R. Paoletti, editors, Elsevier, Amsterdam, 1961, pp. 54-63
3. Mead, J.F. and M.L. Gouze
Proc. Soc. Exp. Biol. Med. 106: 4 (1961)
4. Smith, E.B.
J. Atheroscler. Res. 5: 224 (1965)
5. Insull, W., Jr. and G.E. Bartsch
J. Clin. Invest. 45: 513 (1966)
6. Panganamala, R.V., J.C. Geer, H.M. Sharma and D.G. Cornwell
Atherosclerosis 20: 93 (1974)

7. Buck, R.C. and R.J. Rossiter
Arch. Path. 51: 224 (1951)
8. Myer, B.J., A.C. Meyer, W.J. Pepler and J.J. Theron
Am. Heart J. 71: 68 (1966)
9. Insull, W.
In: Atherosclerosis III, G. Schettler and A. Weizel, editors, Springer-Verlag, Heidelberg, 1974, p. 11-14
10. Hirsch, E.F. and S. Weinhouse
Physiol. Rev. 23: 185 (1943)
11. Smith, E.B. and R.S. Slater.
In: Atherogenesis: Initiating Factors, R. Porter and J. Knight, Associated Scientific Publishers, Amsterdam, 1973, p. 39-52
12. Keys, A.
In: Atherosclerosis and Its Origin, M. Sandler and G.H. Bourne, Academic Press, New York, 1963, p. 263-299
13. Anitschkow, N.N.
In: Cowdry's Arteriosclerosis 2nd Edition, H.T. Blumenthal, editor, Charles C. Thomas, Springfield, 1967, pp. 21-44
14. Lofland, H.B., Jr., R.W. St. Clair and T.B. Clarkson
In: Pharmacological Control of Lipid Metabolism, Advances in Experimental Medicine and Biology Volume 26, W.L. Holmes, D. Kritchevsky and R. Paoletti, editors, Plenum, New York, 1972, p. 91
15. Armstrong, M.L.
Atherosclerosis Rev. 1: 137 (1976)
16. Bloss, F.D.
An Introduction to the Methods of Optical Crystallography, Holt Rinehart and Winston, New York, 1961, p. 47-213
17. Duff, G.L., G.C. McMillan and A.C. Ritchie
Am. J. Pathol. 33: 845 (1957)
18. Coons, A.H. and M.H. Kaplan
J. Exp. Med. 91: 1 (1950)
19. WHO Technical Report Series: Classification of Atherosclerotic Lesion. No. 143: 3-20 (1958)
20. Hata, Y., J. Hower and W. Insull, Jr.
Am. J. Pathol. 75: 423 (1974)
21. Lautsch, E.V., G.C. McMillan and G.L. Duff
Lab. Invest. 2: 397 (1953)
22. Florey, H.W., J.C.F. Poole and G.A. Meek
J. Path. Bact. 77: 625 (1959)
23. Singer, S.H. and G.K. Nicolson
Science 175: 720 (1972)

24. Berenson, G.S., S.R. Srinivasan, B. Radhakrishnamurthy, and E.R. Dalferes
In: Arterial Mesenchyme and Arteriosclerosis, W.D. Wagner and T.B. Clarkson, editors, Advances in Experimental Medicine and Biology Vol. 43, Plenum, New York, 1974, p. 141-159
25. Kramsch, D.M., C. Franzblau and W. Hollander
In: Arterial Mesenchyme and Arteriosclerosis, W.D. Wagner and T.B. Clarkson, editors, Advances in Experimental Medicine and Biology, Vol. 43, Plenum, New York, 1974, p. 193-210
26. Watts, H.F.
In: Evaluation of the Atherosclerotic Plaque, R.J. Jones, editor, University of Chicago Press, Chicago, 1963, p. 117-132
27. Walton, K.W.
In: Atherosclerosis III, G. Schettler and A. Weizel, editors, Springer-Verlag, Heidelberg, 1974, p. 93-99
28. Brown, M.S. and J.L. Goldstein
Science 191: 150 (1976)
29. Goldstein, J.L. and M.S. Brown
In: Current Topics in Cellular Regulation Vol. 11, B.L. Horecker and E.R. Stadtman, Academic, New York, 1976, p. 147-181
30. Lang, P.D. and W. Insull
J. Clin. Invest. 49: 1479 (1970)
31. Hata, Y. and W. Insull, Jr.
Jap. Circulation J. 37: 269 (1973)
32. Servelle, M., C. Hiltenbrand, H.M. Antoine, L. Vavvon, J. Meunier, F. Bacour, P. Levitcharon and B. Andrieux
Sem. Hop. 48: 3483 (1972)
33. Adams, C.W.M. and O.B. Bayliss
Atherosclerosis 22: 629 (1975)
34. Havel, R.J.
In: Lipids, Lipoproteins, and Drugs, D. Kritchevsky, R. Paoletti and W.L. Holmes, editors, Advances in Experimental Medicine and Biology Vol. 63, Plenum, New York, 1975, p. 37-55
35. Swell, L. and C.R. Treadwell
In: Atherosclerosis and Its Origin, M. Sandler and G.H. Bourne, Academic, New York, 1963, p. 301-347
36. Dayton, S. and S. Hashimoto
Exp. Mol. Pathol. 13: 253 (1970)
37. Newman, H.A.I. and D.B. Zilversmit
J. Atheroscler. Res. 4: 261 (1964)
38. Jackson, R.L. and A.M. Gotto
Atheroscler. Rev. 1: 1 (1976)

39. Rothblat, G.H., L. Arbogast, D. Kritchevsky, and M. Naftulin
Lipids 11: 97 (1976)
40. Small, D.M.
In: Surface Chemistry of Biological Systems, M. Black, editor, Plenum, New York, 1971, p. 55-82

APPLICATION OF IMMUNOLOGICAL TECHNIQUES TO THE INVESTIGATION OF ATHEROGENESIS

Kenneth W. Walton

Department of Experimental Pathology
University of Birmingham, England

PREVIOUS APPLICATIONS OF IMMUNOLOGICAL TECHNIQUES TO THE STUDY OF ATHEROGENESIS

It is now coming to be widely agreed that the formation of atherosclerotic lesions is associated with the movement of intact serum lipoproteins (rather than of the simple serum lipids in their free state) into the arterial wall at segregated areas of altered vascular permeability (1). Some of the evidence in support of this view has been obtained using immunological techniques. For example, it has been shown by immunofluorescence that the apolipoprotein B (apo-Lp B) which is common to very low density, intermediate density, and low density lipoproteins (or VLDL, IDL and LDL respectively) is present in atherosclerotic plaques at all stages of their development (2). However, in addition, apolipoprotein C, which is characteristic of lipoproteins larger in molecular size than LDL, is also demonstrable in these lesions while, in some individuals, the antigen characteristic of the variant lipoprotein known as LP(a) lipoprotein is also detectable (3,4).

On applying the immunohistological method and conventional histological staining sequentially to the same tissue sections, it has been found that the topographic distribution of the above-mentioned apolipoproteins has corresponded precisely with that of extracellular lipid shown by conventional fat "stains." The latter are simply pigments preferentially soluble in fat but unreactive with proteins. On the other hand, antilipoprotein antibodies react mainly or exclusively with the protein part of lipoprotein molecules (5). The correspondence of distribution found by the two techniques thus formed the basis for the inference that intact lipoprotein molecules were present in the lesions.

Similar observations have been made in relation to certain lipid-containing extravascular lesions found in association with hyperlipidemia and severe atherosclerosis in humans, such as lipid deposits in heart valves (6); xanthomata (7); and the corneal arcus (8). Very similar findings were obtained at corresponding sites in lipid-fed rabbits with experimental atherosclerosis (9-11).

Another immunochemical technique has been used to show that there is not a selective movement of low density lipoproteins alone into the arterial wall but rather an "insudation" of plasma into the intima with apparently selective binding of apoLp B-containing lipoproteins. This was demonstrated by comparing two-dimensional electrophoresis of plasma, or of the tissue-fluid contained in samples of arterial intima, into antiserum-containing gels. This established that almost all the proteins of plasma enter the intimal connective tissue. But if intimal samples from areas affected by atherosclerosis were electrophoresed in this manner until no further plasma protein emerged and the same intimal sample was then examined by immunofluorescence, it was possible to demonstrate a residual firmly-bound fraction of apo-Lp-B-containing-lipoprotein still present in the tissue (12,13).

These observations seemed to indicate that the evolution of atherosclerotic lesions depends not merely upon the entry of plasma proteins into the arterial wall but upon the selective binding and/or uptake at such sites of the lipoproteins by connective tissue components. However, for technical reasons previously discussed elsewhere (1,5) the immunological methods so far described were inadequate to define precisely the upper limit of molecular size of lipoproteins showing atherogenic potential. Also, in relation to immuno-histology, the methods could only be applied in the light microscope. Recent developments in technique have overcome these limitations.

THE IMMUNOPEROXIDASE TECHNIQUE AND ITS APPLICATIONS

This technique is similar in principle to immunofluorescence except that the antibody is conjugated to a plant enzyme (horse-radish peroxidase is most frequently used) instead of to a fluorochrome (14). After purification the conjugate is allowed to react with a tissue section so that immunospecific interaction occurs at sites where antigen is present in the tissue. Following washing to remove unbound conjugate, the sites at which bound labelled-antibody is present are revealed by incubation of the tissue with di-aminobenzidine and hydrogen peroxide. This gives a dark-brown reaction product at these sites. The reaction product is visible in the light microscope but can also be visualized, after treatment with osmic acid, in the electron microscope. A modification of the technique consists in conjugation of the enzyme to a peptide subcomponent of the antibody globulin containing the antigen-combining site - either the Fab fragment obtained by papain digestion of the $(Fab')_2$ fragment after pepsin treatment of immunoglobin G. This gives a labelled-reagent of smaller molecular size than the intact labelled immunoglobin so that more effective penetration of the tissue by diffusion occurs and, in practice, equal specificity but reduced "background" staining is obtained.

The immunoperoxidase technique has been applied to the study of atherosclerosis in cerebral arteries (15) and also in the aorta, basilar, coeliac axis and splenic arteries and to lipid depositions in heart valves (16) using labelled antisera to apo-Lp B. The appearances seen have varied with the sites at which and with the forms in which lipid has been present in lesions.

For example, where lipid has been identified by conventional fat stains as being present as pools of amorphous lipid in the interstitial matrix of the intima, a brown reaction product was present in corresponding sections treated with peroxidase labelled anti-apo Lp B and examined in the electron microscope. The same areas, similarly treated and examined in the electron microscope, resolved into large numbers of electron-dense spherical particles of varying size. The electron opacity was seen to be due to a coating with the immuno-specific reaction product, which identified the material as containing apo-Lp B. In some instances, the plane of section was such as to show granules of reaction product arranged in circles, as though surrounding a hollow sphere (Figure 1).

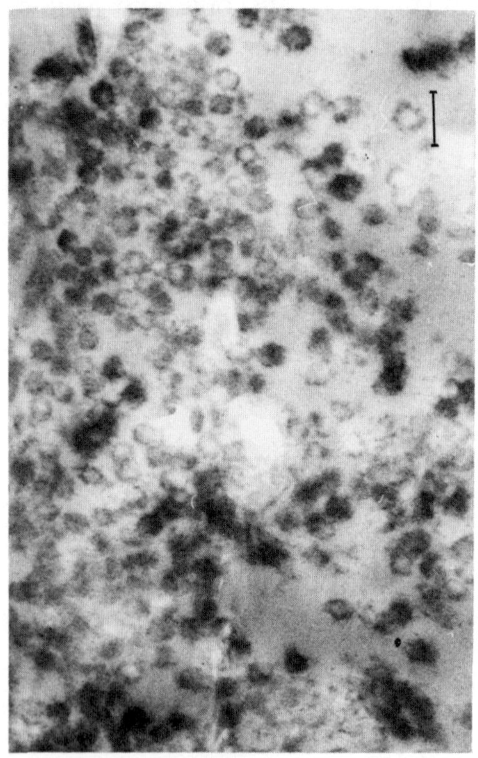

Figure 1: Small area of lipid pool in interstitial matrix of intima from fatty aortic plaque in man aged 74. Tissue treated with peroxidase-labelled anti-apo B and examined in electron microscope. Note circular structures of varying size, some uniformly coated and others surrounded by rings of electron-dense reaction product (compare with Figure 2).

Scale marker = 100nm x 75,000

internal diameters of such structures varied between about 22 and 48nm. This corresponds to the range of molecular diameters found for individual lipoprotein molecules (e.g. see Figure 2) when isolated and purified fractions of LDL, IDL and VLDL are examined in the electron microscope (17). In addition larger spherical lipid particles, some bearing partial or complete coatings of reaction product were seen. It was not possible to decide

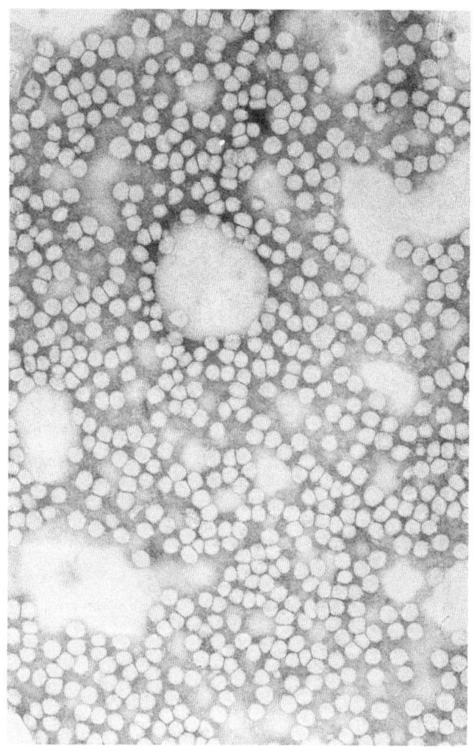

Figure 2: Ultracentrifugally isolated and purified human LDL after negative-staining with sodium phosphotungstate. For comparison with Figure 1.

x 75,000

whether these were aggregates of LDL or VLDL or whether some were chylomicra.

On the other hand, lipid (lipoprotein) deposition also occurs in association with collagen fibres and bundles as "peri-fibrous lipid" (18). Areas showing this appearance (in the light microscope) after treatment of the tissue by the immunoperoxidase method and when examined in the electron microscope reveal a heavy deposit of electron-dense reaction product enclosing spherical particles on the outer surface of bundles of collagen fibrils in the intima. When collagen bundles are cut transversely or tangentially, reaction product

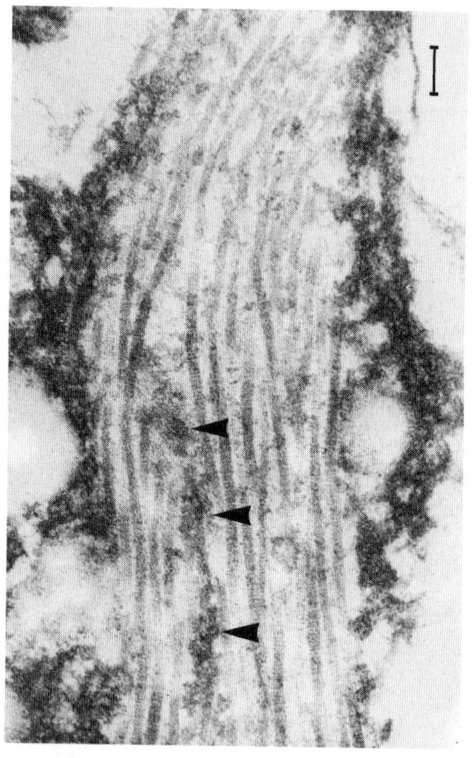

Figure 3: Collagen bundle consisting of longitudinally disposed fibrils of native collagen. Tissue treated with peroxidase-labelled anti-apo Lp B. Note electron-dense reaction product surrounding spheres of varying size which are applied to outer aspect of collagen bundle. But note similar structures in peri-fibrillar distribution along course of individual fibrils within bundle (arrows).

Scale marker = 100nm x 60,000

can also be seen surrounding individual fibrils (Figure 3) which have the (normal) appearance of 64-67nm-banded native collagen.

In occasional instances lipid (identified as lipoprotein by its reactivity with immunoperoxidase-labelled anti apoLp B) is found in association with polymorphic

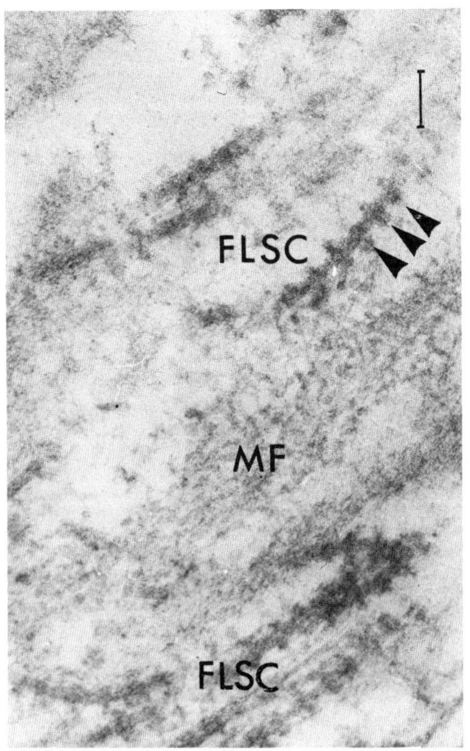

Figure 4: Polymorphic forms of collagen in atherosclerotic plaque. Tissue treated with peroxidase-labelled anti-apo Lp B. Note randomly disposed mesh-work of microfibrils (MF) and fibrous-long-spacing collagen (FLSC) with electron-dense reaction product applied at regular periodicity (arrows).

Scale marker = 200nm x 37,500

forms of collagen in both the superficial and deeper regions of plaques and at the intimal/medial junction. These appear as disorganised collections of microfibrils lying in a structureless matrix; and also as bundles of fine fibrils in parallel array and with marked transverse striations traversing the bundles at regular intervals (fibrous long-spacing collagen). In this latter instance the electron-dense reaction product is also disposed at regular intervals being bound at the transverse bands at intervals of about 120nm along the bundles (Figure 4).

The peroxidase-labelled anti-apoLp B also allows identification of binding of the lipoprotein to elastin, and upon the cytoplasmic membrane or to intracytoplasmic structures in smooth-muscle cells (16).

DISCUSSION

The results obtained with the immunoperoxidase technique support the inferences drawn from previous studies using immunofluorescence. The latter, which showed apolipoproteins C and Lp(a) to be identifiable in plaques in addition to apo-Lp B, led to the conclusion that lipoproteins larger in molecular size than LDL participate in atherogenesis. This conclusion is confirmed visually by the immunoperoxidase technique used as described. This is because apo-Lp B is known to be present in the whole spectrum of lipoproteins from LDL through IDL to VLDL and peroxidase labelled antibody to this apolipoprotein reacts with spherical particles (molecules) in plaques with particle diameters corresponding to those of this range of lipoproteins.

The combination of two-dimensional electro-immunodiffusion, applied to the interstitial fluid of arterial intima, with subsequent examination of the same tissue by immunofluorescence demonstrates a "firmly-bound" fraction of apo-Lp B-containing-lipoproteins in the tissue (12,13). It has been suggested by many authors (for references see Ref.1) that this binding of lipoproteins occurs by their interaction with sulphated glycosaminoglycans or proteoglycans of the connective tissues of the arterial wall. The ultrastructural distribution of the lipoprotein found by the immunoperoxidase technique in relation to native collagen, elastin and in the interstitial matrix of the intima is compatible with a molecular mechanism of binding of this kind.

Such a mechanism is even more likely in the case of the binding of lipoprotein to fibrous long-spacing collagen (FLSC). This "abnormal" polymorphic form of collagen is known to be formed in altered microenvironments in connective tissues in a variety of pathological conditions (19,20) although its occurrence in atherosclerotic plaques has only recently been described (16,21). Structural studies on FLSC have suggested that its characteristic morphology arises from the occurrence of unpaired positively-charged side chains which recur with a regular periodicity becoming aligned in parallel in adjoining fibres by intermolecular bridging by glycosaminoglycans (GAG's) interacting with these side-chains (20). The finding of LDL at precisely the same periodicities suggests that the GAG's also bind lipoprotein.

In relation to the structural organization of the arterial wall, the occurrence of FLSC in plaques may be of significance since the tensile strength of this abnormal form of collagen is likely to be less than normally cross-linked native collagen. Its occurrence may thus be conducive to arterial dilatation and other complications associated with reduced tensile strength of the arterial wall.

ACKNOWLEDGEMENTS

Figures 1-4 are reproduced from Walton, K.W. and Morris, C.J. (reference No. 16) with the permission of the Editor and publishers of Prog. Biochem. Pharmacol.

REFERENCES

1. Walton, K.W.
   Amer. J. Cardiol. 35: 542 (1975)
2. Walton, K.W. and Williamson, N.
   J. Atheroscler. Res. 8: 599 (1968)
3. Walton, K.W.
   In: Atherosclerosis III: Proceedings of the Third International Symposium, G. Schettler and A. Weizel, editors. Springer-Verlag, Berlin, 1974, p. 93.
4. Walton, K.W., Hitchens, J., Magnani, H.N. and Kahn, M.
   Atherosclerosis 20: 323 (1974)
5. Walton, K.W.
   In: Lipids, Lipoproteins and Drugs, D. Kritchevsky, R. Paoletti and W.L. Holmes, editors. Adv. Exp. Med. Biol., Plenum, New York, 1975, Vol. 63, p. 85
6. Walton, K.W., Williamson, N. and Johnson, A.G.
   J. Pathol. 101: 205 (1970)
7. Walton, K.W., Thomas, C. and Dunkerley, D.J.
   J. Pathol. 109: 271 (1973)
8. Walton, K.W.
   J. Pathol. 111: 263 (1973)

9. Walton, K.W.
In: Lipids, Lipoproteins and Drugs, D. Kritchevsky, R. Paoletti, and W.L. Holmes, editors. Adv. Exp. Med. Biol., Plenum, New York, 1975, p. 371
10. Walton, K.W. and Dunkerley, D.J.
J. Pathol. 114: 217 (1974)
11. Walton, K.W.
Nutr. Metabol. 15: 59 (1973)
12. Walton, K.W. and Bradby, G.V.H.
In: Atherosclerosis: Metabolic, Morphologic and Clinical Aspects. G.W. Manning and M.D. Haust, editors, Adv. Exp. Med. Biol., Plenum, New York, 1977, p. 888
13. Bradby, G.V.H. and Walton, K.W., in preparation
14. Nakane, P.K. and Kawaoi, A.
J. Histochem. Cytochem. 22: 1084 (1974)
15. Hoff, H.F. and Gaubatz, J.W.
Virchow's Arch. Path. Anat. Histol. 369: 111, 1975
16. Walton, K.W. and Morris, C.J.
In: Atherosclerosis: International Conference, Wien, April 1977, H. Sinzinger, editor. Prog. Biochem. Pharmacol., Karger, Basel, 1977, Vol. 14, in press
17. Forte, G.M., Nichols, A.V. and Glaser, R.M.
Chem. Phys. Lipids 2: 326 (1968)
18. Smith, E.B., Evans, P.H. and Downham, M.D.
J. Atheroscler. Res. 7: 171 (1967)
19. Banfield, W.G., Lee, C.K. and Lee, C.W.
Arch. Pathol. 95: 262 (1973)
20. Doyle, B.B., Hukins, D.W.L., Hulmes, D.J.S., Miller, A. and Woodhead-Galloway, J.
J. Molec. Biol. 91: 79 (1975)
21. Veress, B.
In: Atherosclerosis: International Conference, Wien, April 1977, H. Sinzinger, editor, Prog. Biochem. Pharmacol., Karger, Basel, 1977, Vol. 14, in press

THE ROLE OF CONNECTIVE TISSUE IN ATHEROSCLEROSIS

Dieter M. Kramsch, M.D.

Cardiovascular Institute, Boston University
Medical Center, Boston, Massachusetts, U.S.A.

INTRODUCTION

In man atherosclerosis generally involves the large and medium sized arteries in which connective tissue proteins comprise more than half the dry weight. Connective tissue contributes to some of the most important alterations in the significant human lesion, the fibrous plaque. It is this lesion which poses the most serious threat to health and life. As recently reviewed by Smith and Smith (1), it is still open to debate whether or not fibrous plaques, or at least some of them, develop from fatty streaks. We, therefore, will restrict our discussion to fibrous lesions. Fibrous lesions begin to develop in the second to third decade of life in almost all individuals of our type of society. However, it takes decades of slow growth before they produce clinical symptoms.

MORPHOLOGICAL ASPECTS

Let us briefly review some of the morphological features of fibrous lesions.

The raised intima of the fully developed fibrous plaque (Fig. 1) consists of fibro-cellular cap with or without an underlying lipid-rich necrotic core. The cap contains massive depositions of collagen, cells (sometimes filled with lipid), and frequently some fine elastic elements. The intimo-medial elastica of most

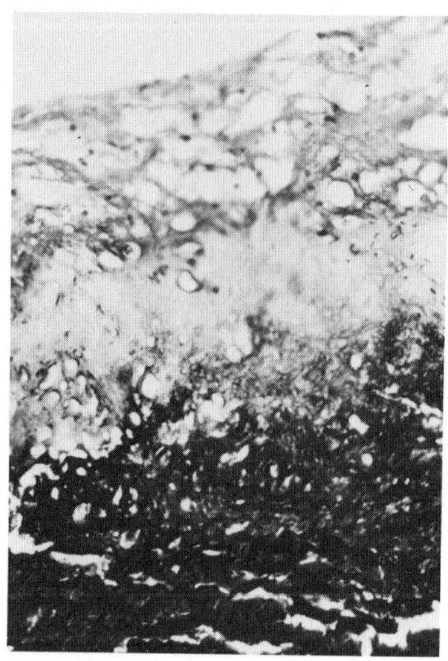

Figure 1: Human fibrous plaque of aorta. Note fibrous cap (top) with some lipid-filled "foam cells" overlying a necrotic core (middle). The intimo-medial elastica (bottom, black) was fragmented and deranged. Verhoeff's-Van Gieson, x102. (Reduced 50% for purposes of reproduction.)

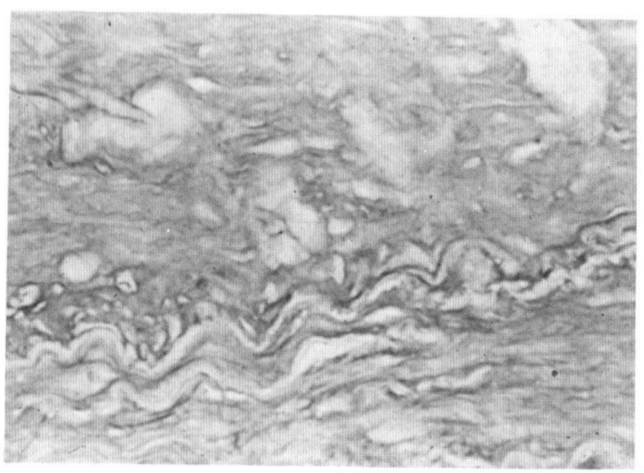

Figure 2: Sequential section of the same plaque as in fig. 1. Alcian Blue staining material indicating glycosaminoglycans (dark grey) on the deranged elastica (light undulating bands) and in "lakes" in the raised intima. There also was PAS-staining material (light grey) in close association with the duplicated elastica and in the overlying intima (top half). PAS-Alcian Blue, x200. (Reduced 50% for purposes of reproduction.)

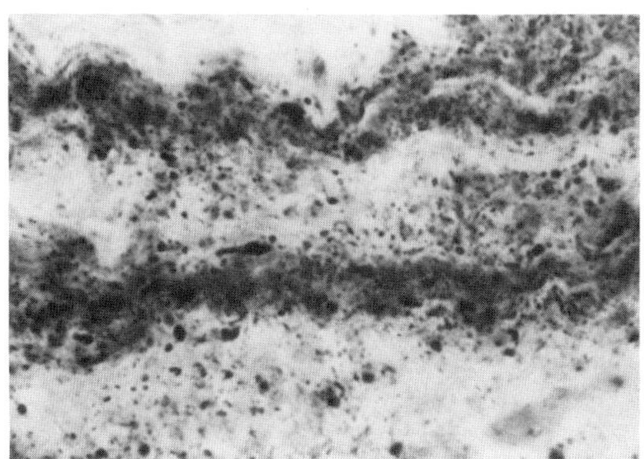

Figure 3: Sequential section of the same plaque as in figure 1. Lipid droplets (black, red in the original) were on and around the duplicated internal elastica and in cells (top). Oil Red O, x256. (Reduced 50% for purposes of reproduction.)

plaques is fragmented and deranged often deep into the media. Accumulations of glycosaminoglycans (acid mucopolysaccharides) (Fig. 2) frequently can be demonstrated enveloping the deranged or duplicated elastica and in "lakes" over the collagenous part of the cap. PAS-staining material, perhaps glycoproteins, also may be seen deposited in close association with duplicated elastica and with what appears to be collagen of the fibrous cap. Depositions of stainable lipids, if present, often are associated (Fig.3) with duplicated and/or fragmented elastic laminae, their coat of glycosaminoglycans or with collagenous areas of the cap. Finally, calcium can be deposited in fibrous lesions. In mild plaques (Fig. 4), the calcium is deposited predominantly on the deranged elastica. In advanced lesions, collagen areas or the entire plaque can calcify rendering it impossible to differentiate with which structural plaque elements the calcium minerals are associated. Calcification of advanced plaques often can be so massive as to be grossly recognizable as a stone-hard plate.

The connective tissue alterations sometimes may involve only the elastica. Figure 5 shows a split internal elastica with deposition of stainable lipids in an otherwise normal human coronary artery. Lillie _et al_ (2) recently also have observed selective lipid staining of human arterial elastica, apparently preceeding the

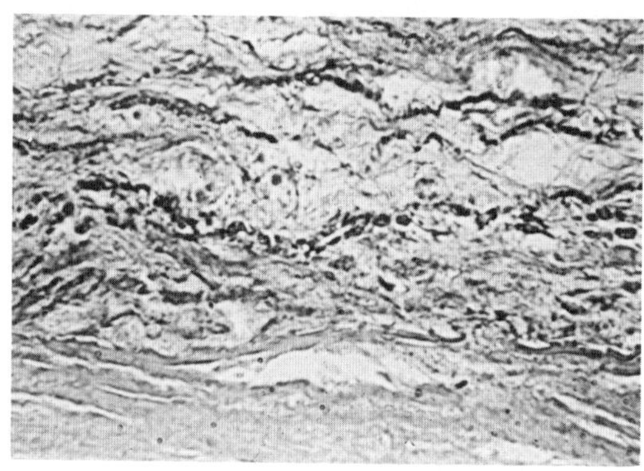

Figure 4: Mild human fibrous plaque of aorta without necrotic core. Calcium (black) was deposited on the fragmented and deranged intimo-medial elastica (top two-thirds). Alizarin Red-Light Green, x 128. (Reduced 50% for purposes of reproduction.)

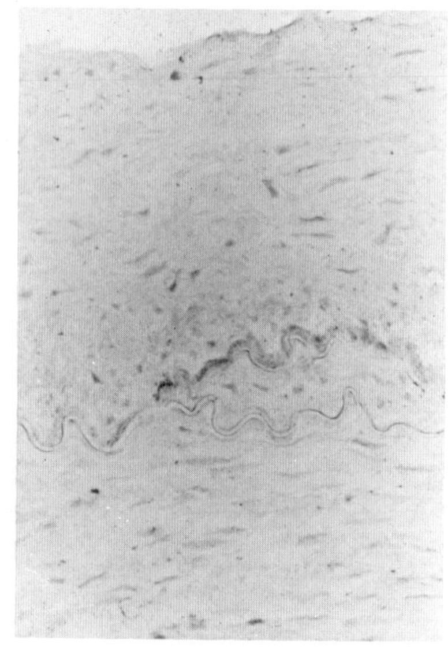

Figure 5: Grossly normal human coronary artery showing splitting (or reduplication) of the internal elastica (undulating bands) with lipid droplets (black) on the upper strand of the duplicated elastica. Note the paucity of lipid deposition in cells of the intima and media. Oil Red O, x102. (Reduced 50% for purposes of reproduction.)

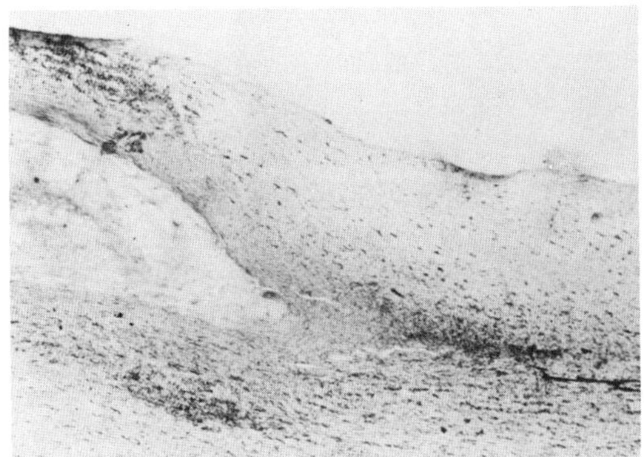

Figure 6: Autoradiograph of an advanced encapsulated fibrous plaque of human aorta. The intravenously injected tritiated cholesterol radioactivity (black dots) was seen deposited over collagen areas of the plaque capsule and on duplicated intimo-medial elastica (black bands) at the border of the plaque. Note the virtual absence of cholesterol radioactivity over the encapsulated necrotic (lipid-rich) core. Hematoxylin-Van Gieson, x102. (Reduced 50% for purposes of reproduction.)

appearance of fibrous plaques by some years. These and other authors (3-11) have advanced that elastica changes may be the earliest alterations in atherosclerosis.

Figure 6 shows an autoradiograph of an advanced encapsulated plaque of aorta from a moribund patient, who had been intravenously injected with a tracer dose of tritiated cholesterol 4 months prior to death. It is of interest that the injected radioactive cholesterol was mainly deposited in the plaque capsule: in cells, over collagen and especially over the elastica at the border of the plaque. It is also noteworthy that very little, if any, cholesterol radioactivity was found over the lipid-rich core of the plaque. This finding suggests that the cholesterol contained in the necrotic core of encapsulated plaques may not easily exchange with the cholesterol circulating in the blood stream.

Figure 7a shows a micrograph of a fibrous plaque of femoral artery from the same patient. Although no lipid was detectable in this lesion by Oil Red O staining of a sequential section from this lesion, the radioautograph of another sequential section (Fig. 7b) revealed marked

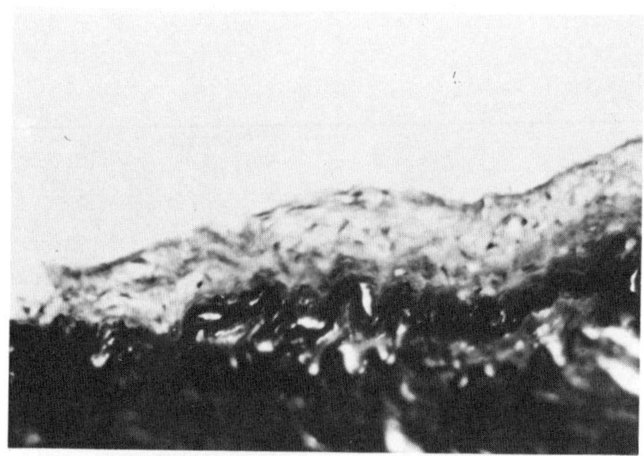

Figure 7a

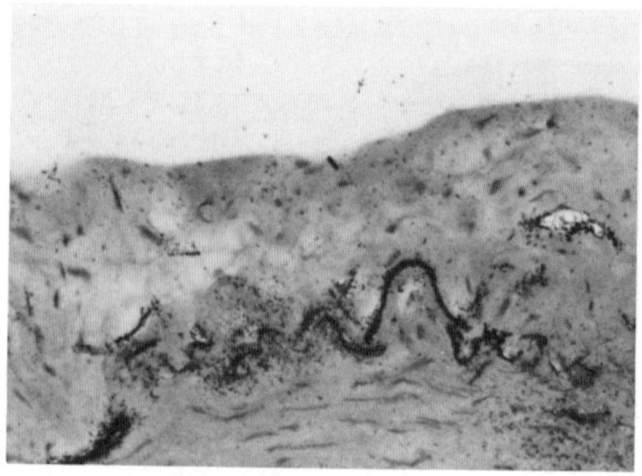

Figure 7b

Figure 7: Sequential sections through a small fibrous plaque of human femoral artery. a. The intima is mildly raised by an accumulation of collagen and proliferation of cells; the internal elastica was duplicated. Verhoeff's-Van Gieson, x102. (Reduced 50% for purposes of reproduction.) Oil Red O staining of a sequential section did not reveal the presence of lipids in the lesion. b. Autoradiograph showing the presence of intravenously injected tritiated cholesterol on and around the split elastica as well as in areas of collagen deposition but not in intimal cells, Hematoxylin-Eosin, x128. (Reduced 50% for purposes of reproduction.)

deposition of radioactive cholesterol on the fragmented elastica and in areas of collagen accumulation. The finding indicates that if no lipid is detectable by staining - as in many fibrous plaques - it does not necessarily mean that none is present. It may be masked, for example, by other proteins or proteoglycans that are associated with the connective tissue proteins.

These observations indicate that fibrous plaques appear to have several pools of lipid deposition: small amounts contained in cells and larger amounts associated with the connective tissue or contained in the necrotic core and in the extracellular cholesterol clefts. It appears that the cholesterol contained in several of these lipid pools may not freely exchange with the circulating cholesterol, at least that contained in the necrotic core and - as we shall see below - the cholesterol bound to plaque elastin and possibly collagen.

BIOCHEMICAL ASPECTS

Classes of Arterial Connective Tissue and their Alterations in Plaques

Fibrous plaques are biochemically characterized by focal accumulations of four classes of extracellular macromolecules: collagen, elastin, glycosaminoglycans and glycoproteins.

Collagen. The largest component of these accumulated macromolecules obviously is collagen, which is known to increase with the increasing severity of atherosclerosis, with maximal per cent increases in calcified plaques (12). The composition of plaque collagen appears to be altered. There are 3 distinct species of collagen contained in arteries: type I, III and IV (13). In normal arteries, type III appears to predominate. In plaques, however, type I appears to be the predominant collagen (14) while changes in type IV (the basement membrane collagen) have as yet not been reported to occur in lesions. But it is of great interest that immuno-histochemical studies have shown that the subendothelial layer of the fibrous cap appears to contain predominantly type III collagen (15). Type III collagen is, at least *in vitro*, the most potent stimulator of platelet aggregation and, potentially, thrombosis (16).

Collagen already normally has a marked affinity for

lipids which may be structural components of the protein (17). In atherosclerosis, this association appears to be increased with about 8-10% of the total cholesterol of human fibrous plaques being contained in the insoluble plaque collagen (18,19). Furthermore, collagen from plaques but not from adjacent normal intima appears to have especially pronounced antigenic properties which could represent autoantigenicity (19). Immunoglobulins G (IgG) and A (IgA) as well as complement were extractable with the acid soluble tissue-bound collagen fractions, as well as by collagenase. A small amount of collagen-bound IgG appeared to be synthesized locally in plaques.

Elastin. Elastin appears to be quantitatively the second major extracellular macromolecule of fibrous plaques. Although no exact data on the content of elastin in human fibrous lesions are available, there is no question from many animal experiments (20-22) that arteries with induced fibrous-type atherosclerosis have an increased content of elastin (as well as of collagen) if expressed in absolute amounts per length-defined artery.

In atherosclerotic lesions, elastin, the backbone protein of elastic lamellae, is qualitatively altered in man (23-26) as well as in rabbits and monkeys (26). The amino acid composition of normal elastin from normal arteries or normal areas of diseased arteries was remarkably similar in adult animals and humans and did not appear to change markedly with increasing age. However, the alkali-isolated elastin fraction from atherosclerotic lesions had a markedly greater content in polar amino acids (Table I), an abnormality which increased with increasing severity of the disease. Similar increases in polar amino acids of alkali-isolated elastin have been found in atherosclertic arteries of monkeys and rabbits (Table I). There were no significant changes in the remaining amino acids of these elastin fractions. The compositional abnormality of plaque elastin may have been due to a close binding of one or more other proteins to the original elastin, such as the normally closely associated microfibrillar glycoprotein (27) or the likewise normally closely associated proteoglycans (28-30), as well as elastase or lysyl oxydase, both of which are known to bind to elastin (31, 32). Robert et al. (33) have shown that solubilized peptides of arterial elastin are antigenic and that the microfibrillar glycoprotein of elastic tissue has one of the most powerful antigenic properties. It therefore is possible that antimicrofibrillar and/or antielastin immunoglobulins may have become tightly bound to the elastin. Still another possibility is that at least part of these

Table I

CHANGES IN THE AMINO ACID COMPOSITION OF ALKALI-INSOLUBLE AORTIC "ELASTINS" IN HUMAN AND EXPERIMENTAL ATHEROSCLEROSIS
(Residues/1000 residues; Means ± S.D.)

HUMAN ATHEROSCLEROSIS					ANIMALS ON ATHEROGENIC DIETS	
Amino Acid	Normal Aorta[a]	Fatty Streak	Moderate Fibrous Plaque	Severe Fibrous Plaque	Macaca Fascicularis[b] No Drugs	Rabbit[c] Without Drugs
OH-PRO	10.5±1.5	13.2±4.0	14.5±4.6	15.2±0.6	13.0±2.5	13.5±2.5
ASP	5.6±1.6	14.6±4.7*	21.5±2.7*	22.7±3.9*	13.1±4.2*	8.2±2.0*
THR	12.5±2.4	16.8±2.2	16.9±1.6**	18.0±1.8*	10.2±2.8	9.9±3.4
SER	9.5±1.1	14.8±3.1*	16.9±2.6*	18.1±1.8*	13.6±1.4*	12.6±2.3
GLU	21.2±2.3	33.1±5.2*	39.2±6.2*	40.7±2.7*	31.0±6.9*	27.3±2.8*
LYS	6.0±1.2	12.2±2.3*	14.9±2.2*	12.4±1.2*	9.3±1.6**	8.3±1.0**
HIS	1.9±1.1	4.4±1.1*	5.4±0.9*	5.0±0.6*	2.3±1.3	1.0±0.8
ARG	4.9±0.9	11.5±3.6*	14.7±1.1*	14.2±1.2*	8.9±2.1*	7.9±1.4*

[a]Normal elastin [b]Cholesterol and butter [c]Cholesterol and peanut oil

*$P < 0.01$ from normal values **$P < 0.05$ from normal values

secondary proteins may be derived from low density and very low density lipoproteins, both of which have been shown by immunohistochemical techniques to associate with plaque elastica (and collagen) (34,35). A small portion of these secondary proteins of plaque elastin could be collagen (25).

On the other hand, it cannot be excluded that newly synthesized elastin already has an altered composition, possibly by close association with one or more of the above listed proteins (especially the microfibrillar proteins and proteoglycans) that cannot be removed by hot alkali. It is of interest in this context that Dr. Franzblau's laboratory has shown (36) that newly synthesized alkali-isolated elastin at certain stages of arterial smooth muscle cell cultures also is rich in acidic (polar) amino acids, reminiscent of the abnormal elastin from lesions.

As reported by our laboratory and by others (23,26, 37-40), normal arterial elastin as well as elastin from plaques appears to be a protein-lipid complex with the lipids presumably bound by hydrophobic stacking to hydrophobic sites of the elastin molecule (41). While the lipid moiety of normal elastin was small, it increased markedly, especially ester cholesterol, in the abnormal elastin from plaques in man (23) as well as in atherosclerotic arteries from monkeys and rabbits (26). In uncomplicated fibrous plaques of man, about 30% of the total cholesterol was contained in the altered plaque elastin (18). Whether the fatty acid composition of the cholesterol esters associated with this abnormal protein complex is similar to that reported for "perifibrous" lipids (42) is not known. The prerequisite for the increased lipid binding appears to be the altered amino acid composition of the plaque elastin protein and the mechanism of binding appears to be a transfer, predominantly of ester cholesterol, from serum and/or arterial LDL and VLDL but not from HDL and chylomicrons to the abnormal protein - at least as shown *in vitro* (18). *In vivo* binding of radioactive cholesterol to arterial elastin also was demonstrated in man (18) and rats (43). The ester cholesterol transferred *in vitro* from lipoproteins to plaque elastin protein was firmly bound to the elastin and could not be removed by subsequent incubations with apo-LDL, apo-VLDL, apo-HDL, intact HDL or treatment with trypsin and hot alkali (18). These findings suggest that the lipid pool associated with plaque elastica may be rather stagnant and not easily removed. Wagner and

Clarkson (39) arrived at a similar conclusion from regression experiments in animals with induced atherosclerosis.

Glycosaminoglycans. A third major component of the extracellular matrix of arteries is the glycosaminoglycans (GAGs). Stevens and his co-workers at Dr. Karl Schmid's laboratory (44) have unequivocally shown that the glycosaminoglycans also increase in human lesions with increasing severity of atherosclerosis when their content was expressed per cm^2 of intima instead of in gram per dry defatted tissue. There was approximately a 10-fold increase of these macromolecules in advanced fibrous plaques. This increase was mainly due to large increases in dermatan sulfate while heparin sulfate decreased slightly and classical chondroitin-4-sulfate (chondroitin sulfate A) was not detectable in diseased or normal aortic intima. However, hyaluronic acid was present in the intima of lesions and non-lesions in agreement with the small amounts required for the aggregation of proteoglycans. The increase of dermatan sulfate in lesions is of great interest since it is this GAG which has been shown *in vitro* to bind most avidly but reversibly LDL and VLDL.

Except for hyaluronic acid, all GAGs are bound to proteins of various composition to form proteoglycans. It is noteworthy that the protein moieties of all arterial proteoglycans contained large amounts of the polar amino acids, glutamic acid and aspartic acid, according to a recent report of Radhakrishnamurty *et al.* (45). These authors also reported that in normal bovine aorta a fairly large amount of proteoglycans are soluble and can be extracted with 0.15 M NaCl. These proteoglycans contained about 50% of the total aortic content of chondroitin-4 and 6-sulfates and almost all chondroitin. About 75% of hyaluronic acid also was extractable by saline solutions. These soluble proteoglycans and hyaluronic acid presumably constitute the major portion of the so-called "ground substance" as well as proteoglycans bound to soluble collagen. Most of the remaining proteoglycans and glycosaminoglycans not extractable by saline appeared to be bound to the arterial connective tissue proteins elastin (which *per se* is an insoluble protein) and the insoluble collagen. The insoluble collagen was mainly associated with proteoglycans containing large amounts of chondroitin-6-sulfate as well as smaller amounts of chondroitin-4-sulfate, dermatan sulfate and hyaluronic acid, while the proteoglycans associated with elastin contained exclusively heparin sulfate.

However, it is of interest that elastase solutions (containing inhibitors of non-specific proteolytic activity) also solubilized large amounts of dermatan sulfate along with the elastin from the NaCl-extracted aortic tissue (45). This finding suggests that protein-free dermatan sulfate may be bound to arterial elastin and could also explain the deposition of LDL and VLDL seen on plaque elastica by immunohistochemical techniques (34,35). One could speculate that an increase in the glycosaminoglycans bound to elastin of plaques in turn facilitates an increased deposition of LDL and VLDL from which an increased transfer of cholesterol esters to plaque elastin could occur *in vivo*. Unfortunately, it was technically not possible to demonstrate any such role of glycosaminoglycans in our own studies (18,23) since the hot alkali used to isolate an elastin protein-lipid complex with a reasonably collagen-free moiety was so drastic that virtually all glycosaminoglycans also were destroyed and none were detectable in the purified elastin fraction. However, the protein moiety of the proteoglycans associated with plaque elastin may not have been destroyed completely by the alkali and may in part account for the high content of glutamic and aspartic acid in the elastin. In contrast to our lack of knowledge as to the quantity of GAGs bound to the plaque elastin fraction, is is known (19) that about 18% of the total GAGs of plaques are bound to the insoluble plaque collagen. These GAGs could play a role in the direct or indirect binding of lipoproteins and lipids to the collagen of lesions.

Glycoproteins. The fourth class of extracellular macromolecules is the glycoproteins. As opposed to proteoglycans in which the protein moiety is small and the bulk of the macromolecules consists of acidic polysaccharides, glycoproteins are predominantly proteins in nature, bearing a small number of branched oligosaccharide units. According to a recent review by Anderson (46), the presence of four distinct varieties of glycoproteins in arteries has definitely been established. They are: 1. glycoproteins that are closely associated with collagen; 2. the microfibrillar glycoproteins of elastin; 3. glycoproteins that are covalently bound to the basement membrane; and 4. glycoproteins concerned with the aggregation of proteoglycans. Many of these glycoproteins are soluble, such as those linked with NaCl-soluble collagen and proteoglycans. The glycoproteins that are tightly bound to insoluble arterial components such as elastin, insoluble collagen, basement membranes or associated with the proteoglycans bound to these insoluble structures also are insoluble in NaCl and can be broadly termed structural glycoproteins.

It has been proposed by Robert and Robert (47) that these structural intercellular matrix macromolecules direct the oriented formation of collagen fibers, elastic laminae and basement membranes. Because of this capacity, any alterations of glycoproteins in plaques would play a major role in atherosclerosis. However, little is known about quantitative of qualitative changes of glycoproteins in plaques. The only exception is the probable role of structural glycoproteins as autoantigenic factors in the formation of atherosclerotic lesions (48) and their apparent overproduction in plaques, especially their presumed increase in the elastin fraction, as a result of tissue degradation in the original lesion (49). It is of interest, however, that very acidic glycoproteins are known to be involved in the calcification of collagen (46,50).

Formation and Degradation of Connective Tissue in Plaques

The cells responsible for the synthesis of connective tissue macromolecules appear to be mainly the arterial smooth muscle cells, although cultured endothelial cells (51) also have been reported to synthesize collagen. Arterial smooth muscle cells in culture have been shown to synthesize cross-linked collagen (52), including type I and type III collagen (53), and the microfibrillar glycoprotein of elastin (52), other glycoproteins (54), as well as cross-linked elastin (36) and the GAGs dermatan sulfate, chondroitin sulfates and hyaluronic acid (55). Collagen and elastin appear to be extruded from the cells first as soluble pro-collagen and tropo-elastin via - at least in part - a system of microtubules including the Golgi apparatus as demonstrated with certainty for collagen (56); elastin possibly is extruded in a similar manner. Before extrusion, pro-collagen is hydroxylated at certain proline and lysine residues by the enzymes prolyl and lysyl hydroxylase. Unhydroxylated pro-collagen is not secreted by the cells (57). A sensitive method for detecting early increases in collagen synthesis is the determination of prolyl hydroxylase (58). Cross-linking of soluble precursors occurs extracellularly, resulting in the extracellular deposition of collagen and elastin fibers. The biochemical mechanisms for the synthesis and secretion of GAGs and glycoproteins by arterial smooth muscle cells are less well understood. Furthermore, GAGs are known to circulate in the blood stream (59) and plasma GAGs also could be a source for the GAG increase in plaques.

Little is known about factors that might trigger the sclerogenic response of arteries leading to the formation of fibrous plaques. As recently reviewed in part by Armstrong (60), morphological studies in experimental animals have implicated dietary factors such as cholesterol, saturated fats in general, peanut oil, as well as mono-unsaturated and trans-polyunsaturated cholesterol esters; diabetes, immune reactions, hypertension and various chemical and mechanical injuries to the arterial wall or just its endothelial layer also appear to be fibrogenic.

The turnover rate of arterial collagen in normal adults is believed to be slow; the half-life of normal mature elastin is considered to approximate the life span of the animal (61). And yet, as recently shown by Yu and Yoshida (62), most of the ^{14}C-labeled elastin implanted into the peritoneal cavity of normal rats was degraded between 6-15 days, probably by macrophages present in large numbers at the implantation site.

In experimental atherosclerosis, however, the turnover of arterial collagen appears to be accelerated with the synthesis outweighing degradation (63-65), leading to a net increase of collagen in advanced lesions (64). The arterial wall was found to have a marked collagenolytic activity, at least in rabbits (64); collagenases also are thought to be contained in the serum (64) in platelets and polymorphnuclear leucocytes (66) as well as in macrophages (67). Macrophages are known to be actively engaged in the resorption of tissue collagen (68,69).

No exact data are available on the turnover rate of elastin, GAGs and glycoproteins in atherosclerosis. It is of interest, however, that our laboratory in recent preliminary studies (70) was able to show that the *in vivo* synthesis of elastin appeared to be increased in atherosclerosis. It is possible that the doubling of elastica seen by microscopy in lesions may result from new formation of elastic tissue (reduplication).

On the other hand, the doubling of lesion elastica also may be caused by degradation (splitting). There is good evidence (71) that naturally occurring hydrophobic ligands such as free fatty acids bind to isolated elastin *in vitro*, presumably to hydrophobic sites, increasing elastolysis by pancreatic elastase up to 25-fold with linoleic acid being the most effective. Recent studies by Kagan and Lerch (72) revealed that approximately 70% of the potentially anionic dicarboxylic residue of elastin, glutamic and aspartic acids, are amidated, rendering the intrinsic negative charge of elastin considerably lower than previously suspected. The positively charged enzyme elastase, however, needs negative charges on elastin in order to attach to its substrate and unfold its elastolytic activity. This would explain why anionic hydrophobic ligands, such as fatty acids bound to elastin, could attract elastase and increase its elastolytic effect so dramatically. In recent studies by Dr. Kagan and ourselves (73), we have shown that in perfused intact rabbit aortae, linoleic acid also increased markedly the effect of elastase in degrading the intimo-medial elastic lamellae of normal aortae. An increased amount of free fatty acids has been observed in lesion elastin with increasing severity of atherosclerosis (74).

It has been advanced that elastase, presumably of pancreatic origin, circulates in the blood stream (75) where it is inhibited by α_1-antitrypsin and presumably α_2-macroglobulin (76). Proteases with elastolinolytic activities have been obtained from human spleen (77) and from granules of circulating granulocytes (78) and platelets (66,79). Since platelets also contain other proteolytic enzymes (such as cathepsin) and polysaccharide-degrading enzymes (66), it seems possible that proteolytic and mucolytic enzymes released from platelet thrombi forming on elastic laminae after endothelial (or other arterial) injury (80,81) can destroy the protective proteoglycan coat of elastin (82), exposing it to elastolysis by elastase. However, neutrophil elastase appears to be different from pancreatic elastase. Its effect on elastin was not increased but inhibited by unsaturated fatty acids (83).

It is of particular interest that an especially active form of elastase has been found in macrophages (84) which also are known to contain many other proteolytic and mucolytic enzymes. Glagov (85) and also Schwarz (86) recently have demonstrated that monocytes, the circulating precursors of macrophages can be found in experimental animals deep in the arterial media in areas of endothelial injury. A substantial number of monocyte-derived macrophages have recently been detected in diet-induced lesions of non-human primates (87). It is very possible that these macrophages are involved in the degradation of arterial elastica. Presumably, both processes, degradation and *de novo* synthesis of elastin also occur simultaneously in atherosclerosis with the synthesis outweighing degradation. As shown by Clark and Glagov (88) elastic branch fascicles are attached to arterial smooth muscle cells and form one functional unit. One can imagine what deleterious effect the destruction of large segments of elastica must have on the functional integrity of the arterial wall.

The Role of Calcium in the Patho-biochemistry of Connective Tissue

Calcium appears to play an important role in the patho-biochemistry of the intercellular matrix macromolecules. Calcium ions are required for the complexing of LDL and VLDL to GAGs from the serum (89) as well as to GAGs from arteries (45). At the appropriate concentration and appropriate ionic strength Ca^{++} has been shown to significantly increase elastolysis by pancreatic elastase *in vitro* (90). The calcium chelator EDTA inhibits the elastolytic activity of macrophage elastase (84). And, as we have heard at this symposium from Dr. Packham, the adherence of platelets to collagen, their aggregation and release reaction require Ca^{++}; all these phenomena could be prevented by EDTA or citrate (91).

Calcium appears to play an important part in the binding of secondary proteins to lesion elastin either through Ca^{++} bridges or simply by incrustation of the whole elastic fiber with calcium minerals (25). Proposed possible nucleation sites for calcium mineralization include: the polar microfibrillar glycoprotein associated with the elastin (27) or the likewise closely associated glycosaminoglycans (92,93) or neutral peptide groups of the elastin itself (94). Acidic phospholipids also have been shown to bind Ca^{++} (95). It is noteworthy that the phospholipid content of the elastin fraction from plaques - though small - also was increased 10-fold as compared to that of normal arterial elastin. Calcium and phosphorus have been shown to bind to arterial elastin purified with formic acid (96). Binding of Ca^{++} to normal arterial elastin *in vitro* has been shown to cause configurational changes in this protein, exposing more hydrophobic sites and giving rise to an increased absorption of other hydrophobic molecules such as cholesterol (97).

The principal target tissue for calcification of arteries in atherosclerosis and aging appears to be the elastica (25,92,98,99). Calcium mineralization of aortic elastica in preference over collagen also has been demonstrated *in vitro* (100). The main constituents of the minerals associated with elastins appears to be calcium and phosphorus (24,93) which appeared to be present - at least at later stages - in the form of hydroxyapatite crystals (92,98,101) as indicated by x-ray diffraction and electron microscopy.

Plaque collagen also can calcify presumably with associated glycoproteins serving as nucleation sites (46). But there are several examples of calcified tissues that contain proteins other than collagen indicating that collagen is not essential for calcification (46). A λ-carboxyglutamic acid-containing non-collagenous protein which binds Ca^{++} and phospholipids has been detected in calcified plaques but not in the tissue from normal areas of human aortae (102). However, it is as yet not known with what plaque components this protein is associated.

It also should not be overlooked that all processes leading to the formation of fibrous plaques, the biosynthesis of connective tissue macromolecules and their degradation, require energy in the form of Ca^{++}- (and Mg^{++})-dependent high energy phosphates.

Inhibition, Prevention, Arrest and Reversal of Connective Tissue Alterations

It is the alterations of the arterial connective tissue which render atherosclerosis so dangerous: by raising the intima to the point of stenosis, initiation of thrombosis, loss of elastica causing aneurysms, calcification of whole arterial segments leading to brittleness and rupture. It therefore is imperative to search for means to prevent, reverse or at least arrest the disease.

There has been a recent report (103) stating that morbidity and mortality from cardiovascular disease has slightly declined in the U.S. during the last decade.

However, it appears still too early to say whether this is the result of less pronounced atherosclerosis or rather due to a diminishing and/or better treatment of its sequellae, notably thrombosis and cardiac complications. With some notable exceptions (104,105), all means to lower elevated serum cholesterol levels in western man have resulted in serum cholesterol levels still above the level that would be atherogenic in non-human primates (11,60,106). Even if the serum cholesterol levels in our population can be lowered to non-atherogenic levels - which is considered by several investigators (60,106-108) to be around 150-160 mg/100 ml - regression of fibrous lesions might be extremely slow, if one can extrapolate from several pertinent experiments in non-human primates (21,106). Heavily calcified human plaques may not regress at all.

Since it still appears uncertain whether serum cholesterol levels in our society generally can be lowered to the required non-atherogenic levels, it seems reasonable to test agents that might inhibit or prevent the disease despite continued high serum cholesterol levels. Several such studies already have been performed using rabbits and pigeons on various atherogenic regimens. Wartman et al. (63) reported diminished accumulation of aortic collagen and elastin after treatment with Mg-EDTA; Hollander et al. (109) reported complete prevention of collagen and elastin accumulation by treatment with the microtubular disruptive drug colchicine and the copper chelator penicillamine; Rosenblum et al. (110) reported inhibition of lesion formation and calcium mineralization in rabbits by treatment with relatively low dosages (up to 5 mg/kg body weight/day) of ethane-1-hydroxy-1,1-diphosphonic acid (EHDP); Wagner et al. (111) very recently suppressed the usually occurring calcium mineralization of lesions during regression from induced atherosclerosis in pigeons, also with similar small doses of EHDP.

Our laboratory has been experimenting in past years to achieve these goals in rabbits and monkeys on fibrogenic atherogenic diets. The animals were treated with EHDP, an agent which is known to prevent soft tissue calcification, including in arteries (110-112). EHDP also has been shown to inhibit calcium ion transport through a membrane as well as to inhibit the proline hydroxylation of pro-collagen (113). Other animals on the atherogenic diet were treated with 2-thiophene carboxylic acid (ThCA) and its methylated derivative (Methyl-ThCA), agents which exert a thyrocalcitonin-like effect on maintaining calcium homeostasis (114); still others were treated with the microtubular disruptive drug (115) n-acetyl-n-methyl-colchicine (Colcemid), which probably, like its parent compound, colchicine, increases the biosynthesis of collagenase (116).

The fibrogenic atherogenic diets (FAD) for rabbits contained 8% peanut oil and 2% cholesterol according to a slight modification of the method of Kritchevsky et al. (117); those for monkeys contained 10% unsalted butter and 0.1% cholesterol as previously described (118). The control diets (CD) were Purina Rabbit and Monkey Chow with banana mash added to the ground monkey chow.

Six groups of 10 New Zealand White Rabbits each and 5 groups of 3 Macaca fascicularis (cynomolgus) monkeys each were fed CD or FAD: rabbits for 8 weeks, monkeys for 18 months. One group of rabbits was fed CD and one group FAD alone while 4 groups were given FAD + EHDP, Colcemid, Colcemid and EHDP or Methyl-ThCA, respectively. Likewise, one group of monkeys was fed CD and one group FAD alone, while 3 groups were given FAD + EHDP, Colcemid and Methyl-ThCA, respectively. Five additional groups of 10 rabbits and 3 groups of 3 monkeys were fed CD after their respective period on FAD: rabbits for 8 weeks, monkeys for 14 months. After cessation of FAD, 1 group of rabbits and 1 group of monkeys were given CD alone while 4 groups of rabbits received CD + EHDP, Colcemid, Colcemid and EHDP, or Methyl-ThCA, respectively; 2 groups of monkeys were given CD + EHDP or Colcemid + ThCA, respectively. The daily oral dosages of the drugs/kg body weight were: EHDP = 20 mg for rabbits and 30 mg for monkeys (active substance of the hexahydrate), ThCA and Methyl-ThCA = 280 mg, Colcemid = 0.06 mg. Due to the small number of monkeys per group, all monkey studies were regarded as pilot studies.

In all animals on the fibrogenic atherogenic diet, the serum cholesterol was markedly elevated to about the same levels regardless of whether any of the drugs were given or not (Table II). In animals on FAD alone the serum calcium levels were also significantly elevated while addition of any of the drugs normalized serum calcium levels in both species.

In rabbits during the induction period of fibrous atherosclerosis, best results were obtained with a combination of Colcemid and EHDP and with Methyl-ThCA alone (Table III). Both drug treatments completely suppressed

Table II

SERUM COMPONENTS OF ANIMALS ON CONTROL DIETS (CD) AND ON FIBROGENIC ATHEROGENIC DIETS WITH AND WITHOUT DRUGS:
RABBITS = 8 WEEKS; MONKEYS = 18 MONTHS

Experimental Groups	RABBITS Cholesterol (mg/100 ml; Mean ± S.D.)	RABBITS Calcium (mg/100 ml; Mean ± S.D.)	MONKEYS Cholesterol (mg/100 ml; average)	MONKEYS Calcium (mg/100 ml; average)
Control Diet (CD)	82± 23	13.7±0.3	139	10.5
Ath. Diet (FAD), no drugs	3,499±954*	15.8±0.6*	539	13.6
FAD + EHDP	3,535±738*	13.4±0.5	492	10.2
FAD + Colcemid	3,841±938*	13.9±0.6	583	11.5
FAD + Colcemid & EHDP	2,973±865*	13.2±0.8	---	----
FAD + Methyl-ThCA	3,324±716*	13.4±0.7	488	10.8

SERUM COMPONENTS OF ANIMALS ON FAD WITHOUT DRUGS FOLLOWED BY CD WITH AND WITHOUT DRUGS:
RABBITS = FAD 8 WEEKS CD 8 WEEKS; MONKEYS = FAD 18 MONTHS CD 14 MONTHS

Experimental Groups	RABBITS Cholesterol (mg/100 ml, mean ± S.D.)	RABBITS Calcium (mg/100 ml, mean ± S.D.)	MONKEYS Cholesterol (mg/100 ml, average	MONKEYS Calcium (mg/100 ml, average
FAD → CD, no drugs	1,380±259*	14.1±0.5	147	11.0
FAD → CD + EHDP	1,022±166*	13.9±0.4	---	----
FAD → CD + Colcemid	1,232±187*	14.3±0.8	---	----
FAD → CD + Colcemid & EHDP	1,451±193*	13.8±0.3	---	----
FAD → CD + Methyl-ThCA	994±272*	16.1±0.4*	161	9.2
FAD → CD + Colcemid & ThCA	----------	--------	157	10.4

* Highly significant increases from control values ($p < 0.01$)

Table III

COMPONENTS OF AORTIC INTIMA-MEDIA FROM ANIMALS ON CONTROL DIETS (CD) AND ON FIBROGENIC ATHEROGENIC DIETS (FAD) WITH AND WITHOUT DRUGS: RABBITS = 8 WEEKS; MONKEYS = 18 MONTHS

RABBITS	COLLAGEN	"ELASTIN"	CHOLESTEROL	CALCIUM	NON-LIPID PHOSPHORUS
	(Absolute amounts in mg/whole aorta; mean ±SD)				
Control (CD=8 weeks)	11.9±1.5	55.8±3.8	1.6±0.6	0.03±0.01[a]	0.17±0.03
Ath. Diet (FAD), no drugs	18.7±2.3[a]	82.5±4.3[a]	12.8±2.7[a]	0.12±0.04	0.34±0.05[a]
FAD + EHDP	13.6±1.0[b]	78.8±3.5[a]	4.5±1.7[a]	0.05±0.01[b]	0.29±0.04[a]
FAD + Colcemid	12.6±1.2	66.9±2.1[a]	4.7±1.5[a]	0.05±0.01[b]	0.26±0.05[b]
FAD + Colcemid & EHDP	12.4±1.4	54.6±3.3	2.0±0.4	0.02±0.02	0.16±0.02
FAD + Methyl-ThCA	11.3±1.3	52.1±2.1	1.7±0.3	0.04±0.02	0.12±0.06

MONKEYS	COLLAGEN	"ELASTIN"	CHOLESTEROL	CALCIUM	NON-LIPID PHOSPHORUS
	(in mg/cm length of aorta; average)				
Control (CD=18 months)	1.9	3.7	0.52	0.022	0.024
FAD, no drugs	3.4	6.3	1.57	0.129	0.041
FAD + EHDP	2.0	3.9	0.56	0.019	0.028
FAD + Colcemid	3.0	5.8	1.64	0.210	0.043

[a] Highly significant increases from control values ($p<0.01$)
[b] Significant increases from control values ($p<0.05$)

the aortic accumulations of collagen, elastin, calcium, non-lipid phosphorus and cholesterol occurring in untreated animals on the atherogenic diet. The amino acid, calcium and lipid composition of elastin was normal in rabbits treated with the above drugs.

Figure 8a shows a section through a typical lesion of aorta in a rabbit on FAD for 8 weeks without drug treatment. The markedly raised lesion contained proliferated (lipid-rich) foam cells, marked accumulation of collagen, fragmented and deranged elastica as well as(Fig. 8b) deposition of calcium on the deranged elastica. By contrast, treatment with Colcemid and EHDP combined (Fig.9) and similarly with Methyl-ThCA resulted in almost complete suppression of atherosclerosis, with the small lesions present consisting mainly of a thin layer of intimal foam cells over an otherwise normal aorta and no calcification demonstrable.

In monkeys during the induction period of fibrous atherosclerosis, Colcemid had no effect on the accumulation of the aortic constituents measured (Table III) in contrast to its partial effect in rabbits. However, collagen, elastin, calcium and cholesterol were at normal levels with EHDP treatment.

Figure 10a shows a section through one of the more human-type aortic lesions elicited in monkeys on FAD without drug treatment for 18 months. A fibrous capsule surrounded a core of (lipid-filled) foam cells; the intimo-medial elastica were deranged and fragmented and calcification was present (Fig. 10b) in the intimo-medial area, predominantly over deranged elastica. In agreement with the biochemical findings, EHDP-treated monkeys (30 mg/kg body weight/day) showed only a few small lesions (Fig. 11) consisting of a superficial layer of lipid-filled cells.

When the atherogenic diet was withdrawn and the animals were given the above drugs during the respective periods of feeding the control diet (CD), the following results were obtained (Table IV). In rabbits after the cessation of the atherogenic diet, there was a further marked increase in the aortic content of collagen, the elastin fraction, total cholesterol, calcium and non-lipid phosphorus. Treatment with EHDP as well as with Colcemid alone arrested further progression of all biochemical abnormalities. However, EHDP and Colcemid in combination or Methyl-ThCA alone caused most lesion components to regress completely to normal levels, except

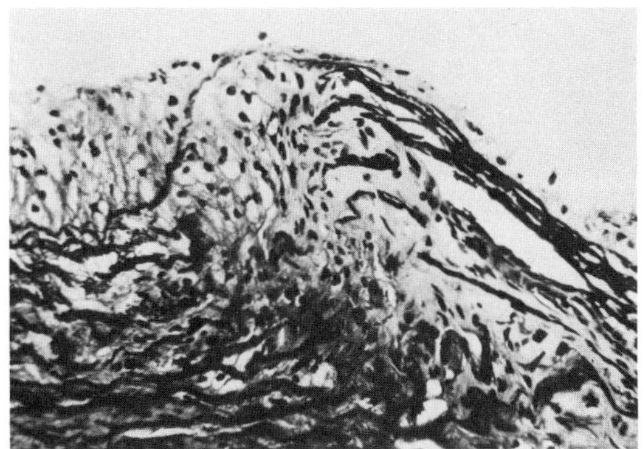

Figure 8a

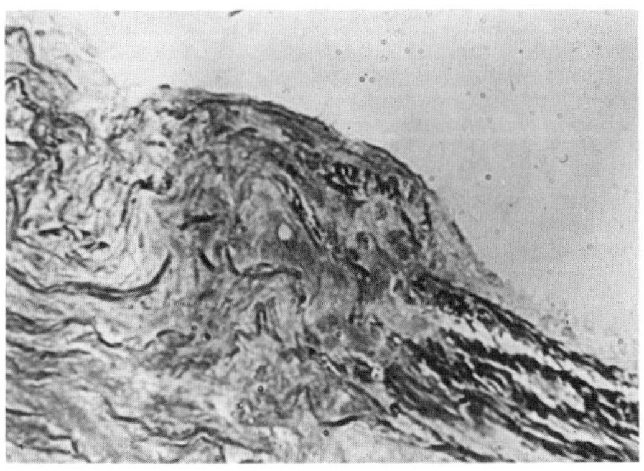

Figure 8b

Figure 8: Sequential sections through a characteristic lesion of thoracic aorta of rabbit on the fibrogenic atherogenic diet (FAD) without drugs for 8 weeks. a. Note proliferated intimal foam cells (top), accumulation of collagen (grey) and deranged and fragmented elastica (black in the intimo-medial area. Verhoeff's Van Gieson, x102. (Reduced 50% for purposes of reproduction.) b. Note calcium depostion (black) on the deranged elastica. Alizarin Red-Light Green, x102. (Reduced 50% for purposes of reproduction.)

for the cholesterol content which regressed only moderately and with the exception of calcium which revealed no regression at all in animals receiving the combined Colcemid-EHDP treatment. But aortic calcium accumulations were biochemically not detectable in animals treated with Methyl-ThCA alone.

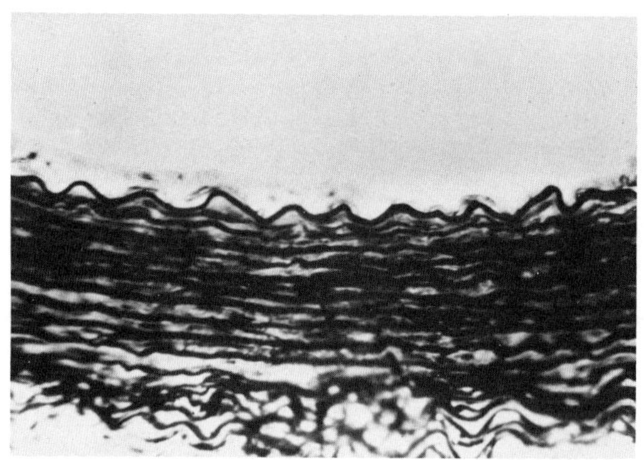

Figure 9: Lesion of thoracic aorta of rabbit on FAD and treated with EHDP & Colcemid. Note absence of collagen accumulation, normal arterial elastica, raising of the intima by a thin layer of (lipid-rich) foam cells. Verhoeff's-Van Gieson, x102. (Reduced 50% for purposes of reproduction.) No calcium deposition was detectable in a sequential section stained with Alizarin-Red.

The biochemical results were in agreement with the histochemical findings. Figure 12a shows an aortic plaque commonly found in untreated rabbits after cessation of the atherogenic diet. Most foam cells had disappeared and the lesion had become more fibrous. There was an increase in collagen deposition and the intimo-medial elastica appeared to be even more fragmented and deranged with an increase in the calcification of the deranged elastica (Fig. 12b). To illustrate the best regression results in rabbits, Figure 13a shows a lesion in a rabbit treated simultaneously with Methyl-ThCA after cessation of FAD. There were a few layers of intimal foam cells over a largely normalized aorta with the calcification of the intimo-medial elastica being reduced to minimal (Fig. 13b). However, in rabbits treated with Colcemid and EHDP combined, calcification of the intimo-medial elastica remained even in areas where all other lesion components had regressed (Fig. 14).

a) 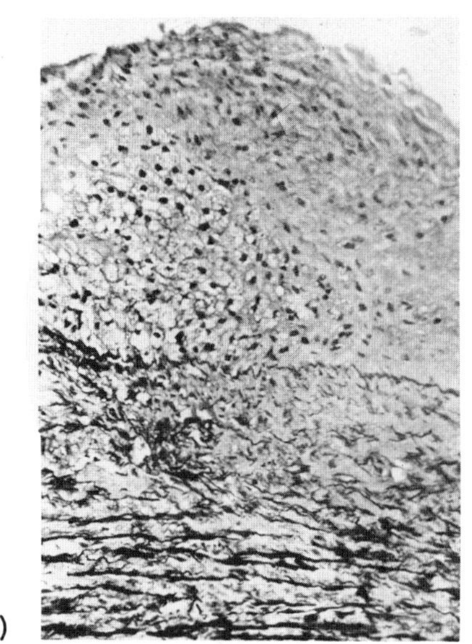

b) 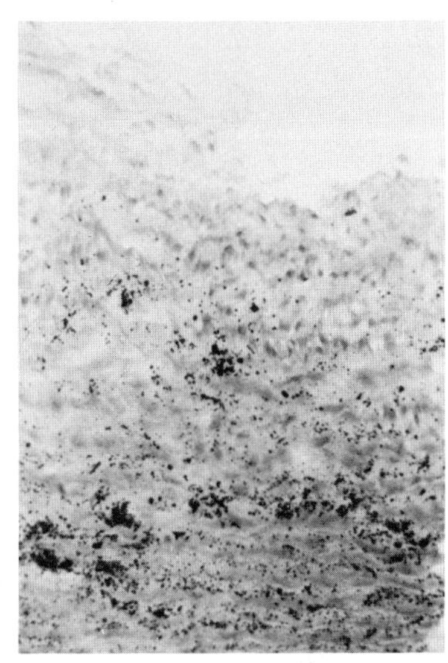

Figure 10: Sequential sections through one of the characteristic fibrous lesions of thoracic aorta in a monkey on FAD without drugs for 18 months. a. Note collagen containing plaque capsule (grey) surrounding a core of foam cells; the intimo-medial elastica (black) is fragmented and deranged. Verhoeff's-Van Gieson, x102. (Reduced 50% for purposes of reproduction.) b. Calcium deposition (black) was present in the intimo-medial area, especially over deranged elastica. Yasue's-Light Green, x102. (Reduced 50% for purposes of reproduction.)

In monkeys only Methyl-ThCA alone and a combination of Colcemid and ThCA were tested for their capacity to promote lesion regression. As compared to normal controls, untreated monkeys hardly showed any decrease in the accumulations of aortic collagen, elastin, cholesterol, calcium and non-lipid phosphorus over a 14 month "regression" period (Table IV). In contrast, both drug regimens resulted over the same regression period in complete removal of all lesion components measured except for cholesterol which still was mildly elevated in the intima-media of whole aorta.

In agreement with the biochemical results, the following histochemical findings were obtained. Like in rabbits (compare Fig. 12a), cessation of the atherogenic diet in untreated monkeys for only 14 months resulted

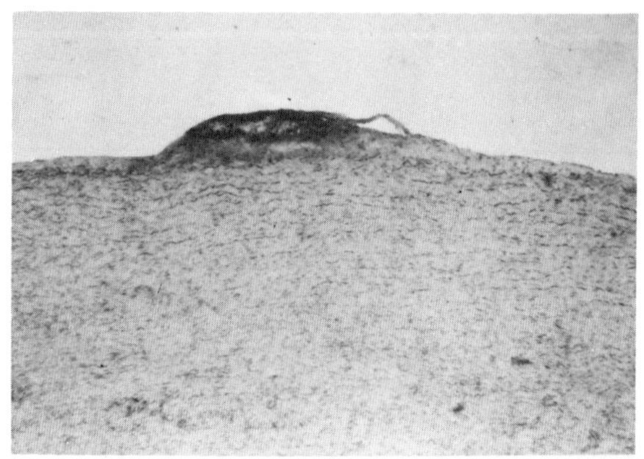

Figure 11: Lesion of thoracic aorta in monkey on FAD and treated with EHDP for 18 months. The lesion consists only of a superficial layer of lipid-filled intimal cells (black). Oil Red O, x40. (Reduced 50% for purposes of reproduction.) No connective tissue changes or calcifications were detectable in sequential sections of this lesion stained with appropriate stains.

in more condensed fibrous plaques (Fig. 15). There was no substantial regression of the lesions except for the disappearance of most foam cells, leaving an essentially fibrous plaque which also revealed marked calcification. In contrast, monkeys treated during the same regression period with either Methyl-ThCA alone or a combination of Colcemid and ThCA revealed only a few small lesions, mainly in the abdominal aorta. These lesions consisted (as shown in the Gomorri-Trichrome stain of abdominal aorta in a monkey treated with the Methyl-ThCA (Fig. 16a) of a near complete normalization of the aortic connective tissue, leaving a few layers of intimal foam cells as a remaining abnormality. Calcification was absent in this lesion (Fig. 16b). Lesions of monkeys treated with the Colcemid-ThCA combination during the regression period had a similar appearance. It is noteworthy that, of all atherosclerotic lesions, only mild accumulations of intimal foam cells - comparable to fatty streaks in man - are regarded as truly reversible, if the conditions of regression prevail long enough (119-121).

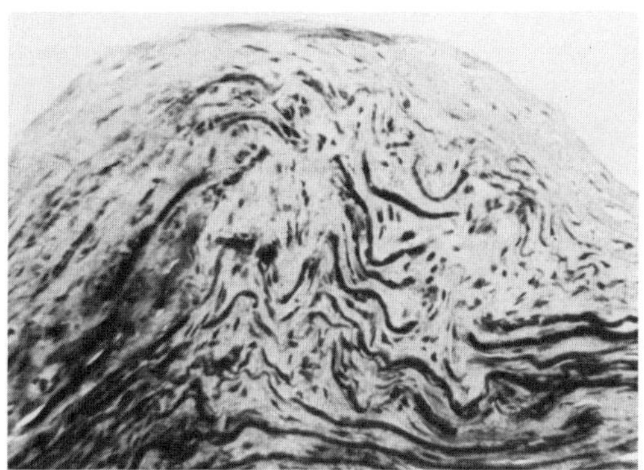

Figure 12a

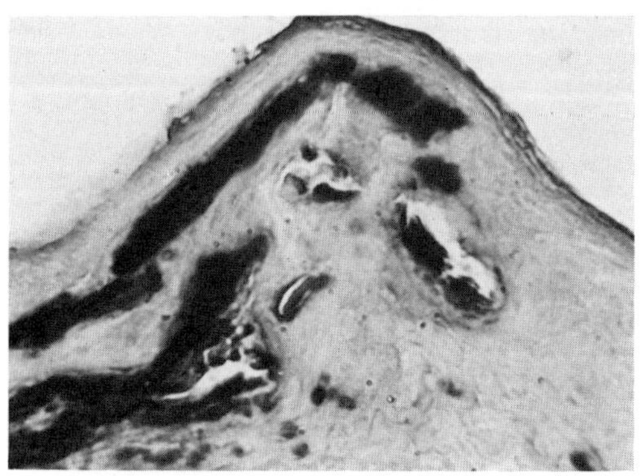

Figure 12b

Figure 12: Sequential sections through a lesion of thoracic aorta of rabbit on FAD for 8 weeks without drugs followed by the control diet (CD) without drugs for 8 more weeks. a. There is a greater accumulation of collagen (grey) and fragmentation and derangement of intimo-medial elastica than in lesions of untreated rabbits produced by FAD alone (compare Figure 8a); most foam cells have disappeared. Verhoeff's-Van Gieson, x102. (Reduced 50% for purposes of reproduction.) b. The calcification (black) of the deranged intimo-medial elastica has increased. Alizarin Red-Light Green, x102. (Reduced 50% for purposes of reproduction.)

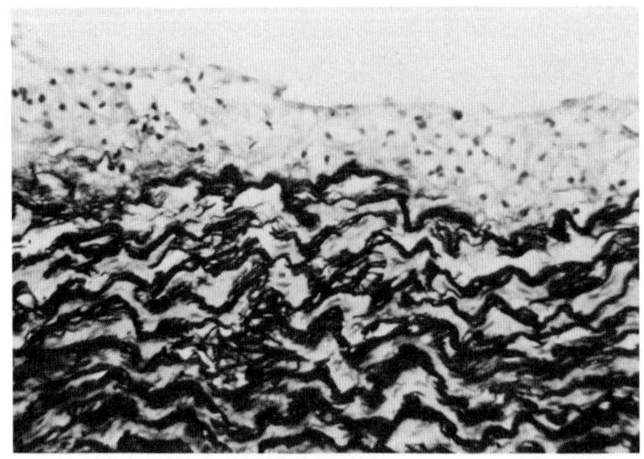

Figure 13a

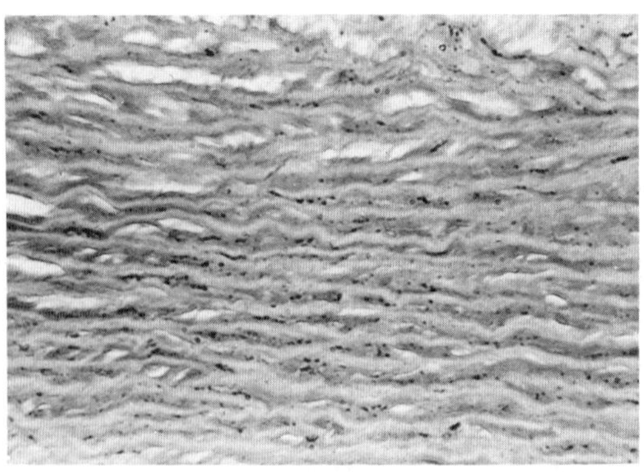

Figure 13b

Figure 13: Sequential sections through a lesion of thoracic aorta of rabbit on FAD without drugs for 8 weeks followed by CD and treated with Methyl-ThCa for 8 more weeks. a. The collagen and elastica are near normal and the lesion consists mainly of a few layers of intimal foam cells. Verhoeff's-Van Gieson, x102. (Reduced 50% for purposes of reproduction.) b. The pre-established calcification was reduced to minimal remaining calcium depositions (black dots), especially on and along the intimo-medial elastic lamellae. Yasue's-Light Green, x128. (Reduced 50% for purposes of reproduction.)

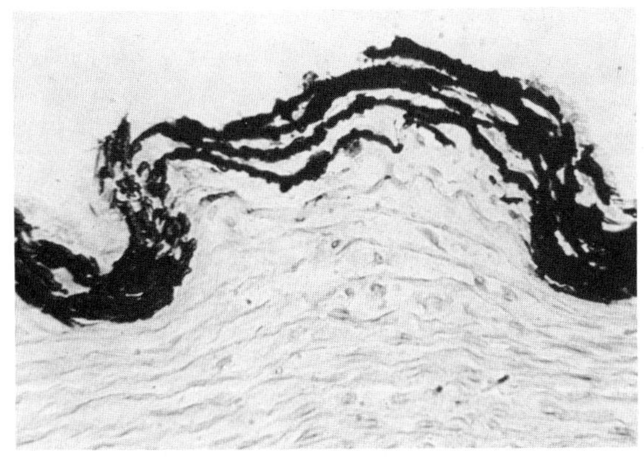

Figure 14: Section through grossly normal appearing thoracic aorta of rabbit on FAD without drugs for 8 weeks followed by CD and treated with Colcemid & EHDP. Note absence of intimal proliferation and absence of collagen accumulation with, however, continued presence of calcification (black) of the intimo-medial elastica. Yasue's Light Green, x102. (Reduced 50% for purposes of reproduction.) Lesion areas of aorta in these animals had a similar appearance as in those animals treated with Methyl-ThCA (see Fig. 13a) except for the persistent calcification of the intimo-medial elastica.

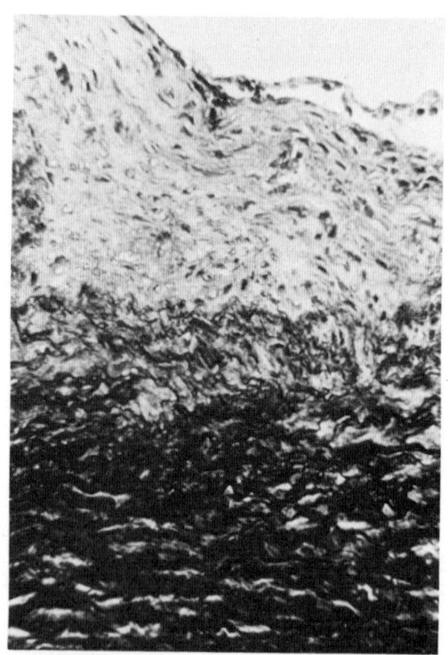

Figure 15: Lesion of thoracic aorta of monkey on FAD without drugs for 18 months followed by 14 more months of CD without drugs. The lesion appeared to be more compact through loss of foam cells; collagen accumulations (grey) and fragmented and deranged intimo-medial elastica are prominent. Verhoeff's-Van Gieson, X102. (Reduced 50% for purposes of reproduction.) Calcium staining of a sequential section from this lesion revealed the continued presence of calcification, especially of lesion elastica.

a) 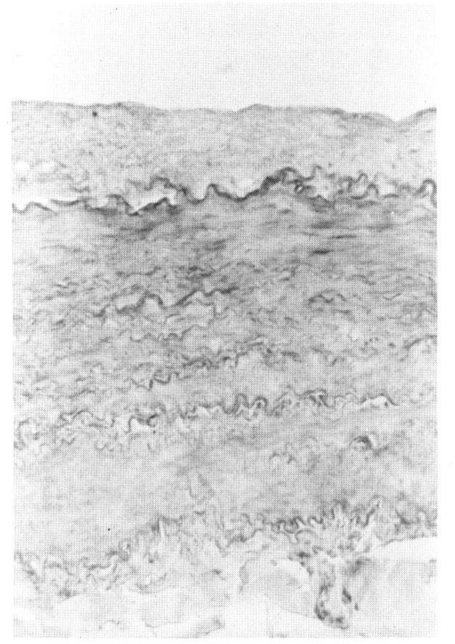

b) 

Figure 16: Sequential sections through a lesion of abdominal aorta of monkey on FAD without drugs for 18 months followed by 14 more months of CD and treated with Methyl-ThCA. a. Collagen and elastica are near normal; the lesion consists mainly of a few layers of intimal foam cells. Gomorri-Trichrome-Aniline Blue, x102. (Reduced 50% for purposes of reproduction.) b. No calcification was detectable in the lesion. Yasue's Light Green, x102. (Reduced 50% for purposes of reproduction.) Lesions of animals treated with the Colcemid-ThCA combination during the regression period has a similar appearance.

Table IV

COMPONENTS OF AORTIC INTIMA-MEDIA FROM ANIMALS ON FAD WITHOUT DRUGS FOLLOWED BY CD WITH AND WITHOUT DRUGS:
RABBITS = FAD 8 WEEKS → CD 8 WEEKS; MONKEYS = FAD 18 MONTHS → CD 14 MONTHS

RABBITS	COLLAGEN	"ELASTIN"	CHOLESTEROL	CALCIUM	NON-LIPID PHOSPHORUS
	(absolute amounts in mg/whole aorta; mean ± SD)				
Control (CD=16 weeks)	12.2±1.3	58.3±1.8	1.7±0.8	0.04±0.01	0.17±0.04
FAD (8 weeks), no drugs	18.7±2.3[a]	82.5±4.3[a]	12.8±2.7[a]	0.12±0.04[a]	0.34±0.05[a]
FAD → CD, no drugs	23.7±3.4[a]	97.2±11.5[a]	9.9±2.0[a]	0.27±0.08[a]	0.73±0.16[a]
FAD → CD + EHDP	16.8±2.1[a]	103.1±12.6[a]	7.5±1.3[a]	0.14±0.05[a]	0.31±0.04[a]
FAD → CD + Colcemid	15.3±4.3[b]	78.4±4.9[a]	5.1±1.5[a]	0.09±0.04[a]	0.23±0.07
FAD → CD + Colcemid & EHDP	12.8±1.6	80.3±5.3[a]	3.6±1.0[a]	0.06±0.02[a]	0.21±0.05
FAD → CD + Methyl-ThCA	12.9±1.3	55.8±5.4	8.2±2.2[a]	0.04±0.02	0.13±0.03

MONKEYS	COLLAGEN	"ELASTIN"	CHOLESTEROL	CALCIUM	NON-LIPID PHOSPHORUS
	(in mg/cm length of aorta; average)				
Control (CD=32 months)	1.8	3.4	0.55	0.020	0.029
FAD (18 months), no drugs	3.4	6.3	1.57	0.129	0.099
FAD → CD, no drugs	2.9	5.4	0.97	0.118	0.085
FAD → CD + methyl-ThCA	1.5	3.4	0.76	0.021	0.029
FAD → Colcemid & ThCA	1.7	3.1	0.60	0.020	0.018

[a]Highly significant increases from control values ($p < 0.01$)

[b]Significant increases from control values ($p < 0.05$)

CONCLUSION

From our experimental studies and those of other investigators cited, the following conclusions can be drawn. While it is important to develop techniques of lowering serum lipids and lipoproteins in order to control vascular disease, one should not overlook alternative methods which may have a direct effect on the vascular wall regardless of serum cholesterol or lipoprotein levels. Of the foremost importance for this purpose appear to be agents which influence the metabolism of vascular connective tissue and calcium. Calcium homeostasis appears to be an important factor in the inhibition of atherogenesis and the reversal of even calcified lesions.

With regard to calcium homeostasis recent studies by Robert *et al.*(122) revealed that lesion formation as well as elastolysis, calcification of arterial elastin and the binding of secondary proteins to elastin are suppressed by daily injections of thyrocalcitonin.

The intimal cyclic AMP-phosphodiesterase system also appears to play a role in atherogenesis and its reversal. The group of the late Dr. Shimamoto from Japan recently showed that atherogenesis could be suppressed and the reversal of pre-established lesions could be promoted by the phosphodiesterase inhibitor EG626 which increases the level of cyclic AMP in the arterial intima (123). The activity of the enzyme phosphodiesterase again is heavily dependent on Ca^{++} (124,125), indicating the importance of calcium homeostasis in the induction and regression of atherosclerotic lesions.

ACKNOWLEDGEMENTS

The work of Dr. Kramsch's laboratory reported in this overview has been supported by U.S. Public Health Grants HL 15512 and HL 13262.

REFERENCES

1. Smith, E.B. and R.H. Smith
In: *Atherosclerosis Reviews*, Vol. 1, R. Paoletti and A.M. Gotto, editors, Raven Press, New York, 1976, p. 119.

2. Lillie, R.D., Pizzolato, P. and Strong, J.P. Virchows Arch. A. Path. Anat. and Histol. 371: 323 (1976)
3. Lansing, A.I., Alex, M. and Rosenthal, T.B. J. Gerontol. 5: 314 (1950)
4. Moon, H.D. and Rinehart, J.F. Circulation 6: 481 (1952)
5. Zugibe, F.T. and Brown, K.D. Circ. Res. 8: 287 (1960)
6. Parker, F. Am. J. Pathol. 36: 19 (1960)
7. Adams, C.W.M. and Tuqan, N.A. J. Pathol. Bacteriol. 82: 131 (1961)
8. Osborn, G.R. The Incubation Period of Coronary Thrombosis. Butterworth and Co., Ltd., London, 1963
9. Friedman, M. Arch. Pathol. 76: 318 (1963)
10. Smith, E.B., Evans, P.H. and Downham, M.D. J. Atheroscler. Res. 7: 171 (1967)
11. Kramsch, D.M. and Hollander, W. Exp. Mol. Pathol. 9: 1 (1968)
12. Smith, E.B. In: Arterial Mesenchyme and Arteriosclerosis, Advances in Experimental Medicine and Biology, Vol. 43, W.D. Wagner and T.B. Clarkson, editors, Plenum Press, New York, 1974, p. 125
13. Trelstad, R.L. Biochem. Biophys. Res. Commun. 57: 717 (1974)
14. Rauterberg, J. and Allam, S.S. Occurrence of type I and type III collagen in normal and atherosclerotic human aortas. Presented at the IVth International Symposium on Atherosclerosis, 1976. Proceedings in press
15. Gay, S. and Balleisen, L. Interaction of collagen types with platelets and transformation of collagen type synthesis in human atherosclerosis. Ibid.
16. Barnes, M.J., Gordon, J.L. and MacIntyre, D.E. Biochem. J. 160: 647 (1976)
17. Nikkari, T. and Heikkinnen, O. Acta Chem. Scand. 22: 3047 (1966)
18. Kramsch, D.M. and Hollander, W. J. Clin. Invest. 52: 236 (1973)
19. Hollander, W., Colombo, M.A., Kramsch, D.M. and Kirkpatrick, B. Adv. Cardiol. 13: 192 (1974)
20. Kramsch, D.M., Hollander, W. and Renaud, S. Circulation 48, IV: 41 (1974)

21. Armstrong, M.L. and Megan, M.B.
Circ. Res. 36: 257 (1975)
22. Wolinsky, H., Goldfischer, S., Daly, M., Kasak, L.E. and Coltoff-Schiller, B.
Circ. Res. 36: 553 (1975)
23. Kramsch, D.M., Franzblau, C. and Hollander, W.
J. Clin. Invest. 50: 1666 (1971)
24. Yu, S.Y.
Lab. Invest. 25: 121 (1971)
25. Keeley, F.W. and Partridge, S.M.
Atherosclerosis 19: 287 (1974)
26. Kramsch, D.M., Franzblau, C. and Hollander, W.
In: Arterial Mesenchyme and Arteriosclerosis, Advances in Experimental Medicine and Biology, Vol. 43, W.D. Wagner and T.B. Clarkson, editors, Plenum Press, New York, 1974, p. 193
27. Ross, R. and Bornstein, P.
J. Cell Biol. 40: 366 (1969)
28. Gotte, L., Menegheli, V. and Castellani, A.
In: Structure and Function of Connective and Skeletal Tissue, S. Fitton-Jackson, R.D. Harkness and G.R. Tristram, editors. Butterworth, London, 1965, p. 93
29. John, R. and Thomas, J.
Biochem. J. 127: 261 (1972)
30. Moczar, M. and Robert, L.
Atherosclerosis 11: 7 (1970)
31. Gertler, A.
Europ. J. Biochem. 20: 541 (1971)
32. Kagan, H.M., Hewitt, N.A., Salcedo, L.L. and Franzblau, C.
Biochim. Biophys. Acta 365: 223 (1974)
33. Robert, A.M., Grosgogeat, Y., Reverdy, V., Robert, B. and Robert, L.
Atherosclerosis 13: 427 (1971)
34. Walton, K.W. and Williamson, N.
Atherosclerosis 8: 599 (1968)
35. Hoff, H.F. and Gaubatz, J.W.
Exp. Molec. Pathol. 26: 214 (1977)
36. Faris, B., Salcedo, L.L., Cook, V., Johnson, L., Foster, J.A. and Franzblau, C.
Biochim. Biophys. Acta 418: 93 (1976)
37. Szigeti, M., Monnier, G., Jacotot, B. and Robert, Conn. Tissue Res. 1: 145 (1972)
38. Robert, L., Robert, B., and Robert, A.M.
Exp. Ann. Biochim. Med. 31: 111 (1972)
39. Wagner, W.D. and Clarkson, T.B.
Proc. Soc. Exp. Biol. Med. 143: 804 (1973)

40. Tokita, K., Kanno, K. and Ikeda, K.
Human aortic elastin with changes during atherogenesis. Presented at the IVth International Symposium on Atherosclerosis, 1976. Proceedings in press
41. Jacotot, B., Beaumont, J.L., Monnier, G., Szigeti, M., Robert, B. and Robert, L.
Nutr. Metabol. 15: 46 (1973)
42. Smith, E.B., Evans, P.H. and Downham, M.D.
J. Atherosclerosis Res. 7: 171 (1967)
43. Jacotot, B., Monnier, G. and Beaumont, J.L.
Clin. Chim. Acta 33: 95 (1971)
44. Stevens, R.L., Colombo, M., Gonzales, J.J., Hollander, W. and Schmid, K.
J. Clin. Invest. 58: 470 (1976)
45. Radhakrishnamurty, B., Ruiz, H.A., Jr., and Berenson, G.S.
J. Biol. Chem. 252: 4831 (1977)
46. Anderson, J.C.
In: International Review of Connective Tissue Research, Vol. 7. D.A. Hall and D.S. Jackson, editors, Academic Press, New York, 1976, p. 251
47. Robert, L. and Robert, B.
Gerontologia 19: 330 (1973)
48. Robert, A.M., Grosgogeat, Y., Reverdy, V., Robert, B. and Robert, L.
Atherosclerosis 13: 427 (1971)
49. Ouzilou, J., Robert, A.M., Robert, L., Bouisson, H. and Pieraggi, M.T.
Paroi Arterielle 1: 105 (1973)
50. Zamoscianyk, H. and Veis, A.
Fed. Proc. 25: 409 (1966)
51. Macarak, E.J., Howard, B.V. and Kefalides, N.A.
Annals N.Y.Acad. Sci. 275: 104 (1976)
52. Ross, R. and Glomset, J.A.
Science 180: 1332 (1973)
53. Layman, D.L., Epstein, E.H., Jr., Dodson, R.F. and Titus, J.L.
Proc. Natl. Acad. Sci. USA 74: 671 (1977)
54. Robert, L. and Robert, B.
In: Connective Tissue, Biochemistry and Pathophysiology. R. Fricke and F. Hartmann, editors. Springer-Verlag, Berlin and New York, 1974, p. 240
55. Whight, T.N. and R. Ross
J. Cell Biol. 59(2): 371a (1973)
56. Ehrlich, H.P. and Bornstein, P.
Nature New Biol. 238: 257 (1972)
57. Grant, M.E. and Prockop, D.J.
New Engl. J. Med. 286: 291 (1972)

58. Fuller, G.C. and Langner, R.O.
Science 168: 987 (1970)
59. Calatroni, A., Donelly, P.V. and DiFerrante, N.
J. Clin. Invest. 48: 332 (1969)
60. Armstrong, M.L.
In: Atherosclerosis Reviews, Vol. 1, R. Paoletti and A.M. Gotto, editors. Raven Press, New York, 1976, p. 137
61. Slack, H.G.B.
Nature 174: 512 (1954)
62. Yu, S.Y. and Yoshida, A.
Lab. Invest., in press
63. Wartman, A., Lampe, T.L., McCann, D.S. and Boyle, A.J.
J. Atheroscler. Res. 7: 331 (1967)
64. Lindner, J.P.
In: Atherosclerosis III, G. Schettler and A. Weizel, editors. Springer-Verlag, Berlin, 1974, p. 218
65. McCullagh, K.G. and Page, I.H.
Ibid, p. 239
66. Mustard, J.F., Packham, M.A., Moore, S. and Kinlough-Rathbone, R.L.
Ibid, p. 253
67. Wahl, L.M., Wahl, S.M., Martin, G.R. and Mergenhagan, S.E.
Fed. Proc. 33: 618 (1974)
68. Schwarz, W. and Guldner, F.H.
Z. Zellforsch. Mikrisk. Anat. 83: 416 (1967)
69. Parakkal, P.F.
J. Cell Biol. 41: 345 (1969)
70. Kramsch, D.M. and Chan, C.T.
Fed. Proc. 35: 598 (1976)
71. Jordan, R.E., Hewitt, N., Lewis, W., Kagan, H.M. and Franzblau, C.
Biochemistry 13: 3497 (1974)
72. Kagan, H.M. and Lerch, R.M.
Biochim. Biophys. Acta 434: 223 (1976)
73. Data to be published.
74. Jacotot, B.
In: Atherosclerosis III, G. Schettler and A.Weizel, editors. Springer-Verlag, Berlin, 1974, p. 207
75. Loewen, W.A.
J. Atheroscler. Res. 9: 35 (1969)
76. Baumstark, J.S.
Arch. Biochem. Biophys. 118: 619 (1967)
77. Franzblau, C.
In: Elastin in Comprehensive Biochemistry, Vol.26C, M. Florkin and E.H. Stotz, editors. Elsevier, Amsterdam, 1971, p. 659

78. Janoff, A. and Scherer, J.
J. Exp. Med. 128: 1137 (1968)
79. Legrand, Y., Caen, J., Boyse, F.M. Raffelson, E.M., Robert, B. and Robert, L.
Biochim. Biophys. Acta 309: 406 (1973)
80. Bjorkerud, S.
Virchows Arch. Abt. A., Pathol. Anat. 347: 197 (1969)
81. Stemerman, M.B. and Ross, R.
J. Exp. Med. 136: 769 (1972)
82. Partridge, S.M. and Keeley, F.W.
In: Arterial Mesenchyme and Arteriosclerosis, Advances in Experimental Medicine and Biology, Vol. 43, W.D. Wagner and T.B. Clarkson, editors, Plenum, New York, 1974, p. 173
83. Ashe, B.M. and Zimmerman, M.
Fed. Proc. 36: 678 (1977)
84. Werb, Z. and Gordon, S.
J. Exp. Med. 142: 361 (1975)
85. Glagov, S.
Presented at the Annual Hugh Lofland Conference on Arterial Wall Metabolism, 1977.
86. Schwartz, C.J.
Ibid
87. Schaffner, T., Elner, V. and Wissler, R.W.
Fed. Proc. 36: 400 (1977)
88. Clark, J.M. and Glagov, S.
Ibid: 393
89. Srinivason, S.R., Lopez, S., Radhakrishnamurty, B. and Berenson, G.S.
Atherosclerosis 12: 321 (1970)
90. Kagan, H.M.
Unpublished data
91. Packham, M.A.
these proceedings
92. Weissman, G. and Weissman, S.
J. Clin. Invest. 39: 1657 (1960)
93. Yu, S.Y. and Blumenthal, H.T.
J. Gerontol. 18: 127 (1963)
94. Urry, D.W., Cunningham, W.D. and Ohnishi, T.
Biochim. Biophys. Acta 292: 853 (1973)
95. Vogel, J.J. and Boylan-Salyers, B.D.
Clin. Orthopaed. 118: 230 (1976)
96. Seligman, M., Eilberg, R.G. and Fishman, L.
Calc. Tiss. Res. 17: 229 (1975)
97. Hornebeck, W. and Partridge, S.M.
Europ. J. Biochem. 51: 73 (1975)
98. Yu, S. and Blumenthal, H.T.
J. Gerontol. 18: 119 (1963)

99. Haust, D. and Geer, J.C.
Amer. J. Pathol. 60: 329 (1970)
100. Bladen, H.A. and Martin, G.R.
Fifth International Congress on Electron Microscopy. Academic Press, New York, p. QQ-5
101. Serafini-Fracassini, A.
J. Atheroscler. Res. 3: 178 (1963)
102. Lian, J.B., Skinner, M., Glinecher, M.J. and Gallop, P.
Biochem. Biophys. Res. Commun. 73: 349 (1976)
103. Walker, W.J.
New Engl. J. Med. 297: 163 (1977)
104. Buchwald, H., Moore, R.B. and Varco, R.L.
In: Lipids, Lipoproteins, and Drugs, Advances in Experimental Medicine and Biology, Vol. 63, Plenum, New York, 1974, p. 221
105. Blankenhorn, D.
In: Proceedings of the International Workshop Conference on Atherosclerosis, London, Ontario, in press
106. Wissler, R.W. and Vesselinovitch, D.
Ann. N.Y. Acad. Sci. 275: 363 (1976)
107. Lee, K.T., Nam, S.C., Kwon, O.H., Kim, S.B. and Goodale, F.
Exp. Molec. Pathol. 2: 1 (1963)
108. Geerdink, R.A., Breel, P.M., Sander, P.C. and Schillhorn-Van Veen, J.H.
Atherosclerosis 18: 173 (1973)
109. Hollander, W., Kramsch, D.M., Paddock, J. and Colombo, M.A.
Circ. Res. 34 (Suppl. I): 131 (1974)
110. Rosenblum, I.Y., Flora, L. and Eisenstein, R.
Atherosclerosis 22: 411 (1975)
111. Wagner, W.D., Clarkson, T.B. and Foster, J.
Atherosclerosis 27: 419 (1977)
112. Fleisch, H., Russel, R.G.G., Bisaz, S., Muehlbauer, R.C. and Williams, D.A.
Europ. J. Clin. Invest. 1: 12 (1970)
113. Minkin, C., Rabadjija, L. and Golhaber, P.
Calc. Tiss. Res. 14: 161 (1974)
114. Wells, H. and Lloyd, W.
Endocrinology 83: 521 (1968)
115. Yin, H.H., Ukena, T.E. and Berlin, R.D.
Science 178: 867 (1972)
116. Harris, E.D., Jr., and Krane, S.M.
Arthritis Rheumatism 14: 669 (1971)
117. Kritchevsky, D., Tepper, S.A., Vesselinovich, D. and Wissler, R.W.
Atherosclerosis 14: 53 (1971)

118. Kramsch, D.M., Hollander, W. and Renaud, S. Circulation 48 (Suppl.4): 40 (1973)
119. McMeans, J.W. J. Med. Res. 31: 41 (1916)
120. McGill, H.C. In: Atherosclerosis III, G. Schettler and A. Weizel, editors. Springer-Verlag, Berlin, 1974, p. 27
121. Stary, H.C. Proceedings of the International Symposium on the State of Prevention and Therapy in Human Arteriosclerosis and in Animal Models, in press
122. Robert, L., Moczar,M., Miskulin, A.M. and Robert, A.M. Ibid
123. Numano, F., Maezawa, H., Shimamoto, T. and Adachi,K. Annals N.Y. Acad. Sci. 275: 311 (1976)
124. Stevens, F.C., Walsh, M., Ho, H.C., Teo, T.S. and Wang, J.H. J. Biochem. 251: 4495 (1976)
125. Walterson, D.M. and Vanaman, T.C. Biochem. Biophys. Res. Comm. 73: 40 (1976)

DRUG SCREENING IN CELL CULTURES

George Rothblat

Department of Physiology/Biochemistry, Medical College of Pennsylvania, Philadelphia, Pennsylvania

Although tissue culture cells have been used for the study of lipid metabolism for a number of years it is within the last five years that the tremendous potential of this experimental system has been fully realized. The data that have been generated from cell culture studies have greatly broadened our basic knowledge of lipid metabolism. It is now an appropriate time to consider the possibilities of cell culture systems as a tool for screening for drugs that affect lipid metabolism.

First, what are the advantages of cell culture? The obvious are cost, volume and speed. A flask of cells costs much less than an animal. In addition, the time frame for studies using cultured cells is almost always much shorter than those using whole animals. A tissue culture experiment seldom runs for more than a few days contrasted to weeks or months for many animal studies. Also, the quantity of the test drug needed for tissue culture screening will be much less than in other experimental systems.

The major disadvantages will be oversensitivity and lack of specificity. The cell in culture is growing in a closed system far removed from the controls and protection from its normal *in vivo* environment. Almost any pertubation of the system could result in either direct or indirect changes in cellular lipid metabolism. Thus, because of the intrinsic sensitivity and lack of specificity, coupled with cost and time factors, cell culture would appear to be primarily useful as a preliminary screening system.

A number of basic decisions must be made when selecting a cell culture-drug screening system. The first decision will relate to the type of lipid to be measured. Simply measuring the synthesis or content of total cellular lipid will result in even greater lack of specificity and therefore probably be of very little use. The second consideration relates to the cell type to be studied. At this point a whole series of interrelated questions can be raised. Does one design a program around aortic smooth muscle cells, or can drugs be effectively screened using fibroblasts or other cell types? Does one use only primary cells or can established cultures, or even transformed cells be used? And finally, from what animal does one obtain the cells. The answers to these questions will obviously reflect the scientific prejudices of the individuals setting up the system. Some considerations that might influence these decisions are: 1. Thus far, no qualitative differences have been observed between smooth muscle cells and fibroblasts in their basic mechanism of lipid metabolism, although quantitative differences have been documented. Specialized cells such as hepatocytes, adipocytes, endothelial cells and endocrine cells may express fundamental differences in lipid metabolism. 2. The growth of cells in culture has been shown to result in shifts of the enzymatic and metabolic patterns of the cells when compared to the original tissues, however, many of these changes appear to occur very rapidly and can be seen even in primary culture. 3. The total reliance on primary cells, particularly human cells, may greatly restrict the availability of cellular material.

The most important decision to be made relates to the particular metabolic parameter to be used when screening drugs. Basically there are three general parameters, synthesis, transport, and accumulation. Since in many instances primary interest will revolve around drugs that affect cholesterol metabolism some of the current concepts of cellular cholesterol metabolism are presented in Figure 1.

The basic system by which cholesterol is metabolized at the cellular level applies to a variety of cell types and is based on the studies of a number of investigators (1-4). In this system cholesterol is incorporated into cells by mechanisms which can be broadly divided into those systems which incorporate the entire lipoprotein molecule (Fig. 1, step 1a) and those in which free cholesterol is incorporated without internalization of the

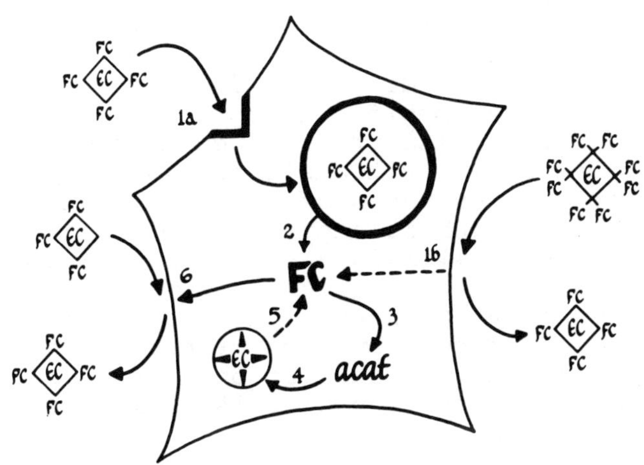

Figure 1: Cellular cholesterol metabolism. Step 1a, lipoprotein internalization by either specific or non-specific receptors.
Step 1b, free cholesterol (FC) uptake by surface transfer.
Step 2, liberation of FC following lysosomal processing.
Step 3, transfer of FC to internal membranes.
Step 4, esterification of FC by Acyl CoA:cholesterol acyltransferase (ACAT) and storage of esterified cholesterol (EC) in lipid inclusion.
Step 5, hydrolysis of EC.
Step 6, efflux of FC by surface transfer mechanisms.

carrier lipoprotein (Fig. 1, step 1b). Lipoprotein uptake can be mediated by specific receptors or can proceed via non-specific endocytosis. The specific receptors are tightly regulated and their number are reduced as internal cholesterol concentration is elevated, thus controlling the amount of cholesterol being incorporated by specific receptor uptake (1). Actually, recent studies suggest that extensive and continued cholesterol uptake and accumulation may only proceed by mechanisms that bypass specific receptors (5). Internalized lipoprotein is incorporated in, and processed by, lysosomes with the ultimate liberation of free cholesterol (Fig. 1, step 2). This liberated free cholesterol becomes available for the regulation of the cellular synthesis of both cholesterol and the specific lipoprotein receptor (1). Free cholesterol is also transported to the microsomal acyl CoA:cholesterol acyltransferase (ACAT) supplying substrate for the synthesis of esterified cholesterol (Fig. 1, step 3) which is stored in cellular lipid inclusions (Fig. 1, step 4) (1,6,7).

An alternative mechanism of free cholesterol transport can proceed by cell surface transfer which does not require lipoprotein internalization (Fig. 1, step 1b). The magnitude and direction of this flux of free cholesterol would be regulated by the composition of the lipoprotein as well as the nature of the lipoprotein/cell surface interaction. Under some experimental conditions the equilibrium favors influx and the incorporated cholesterol can be utilized for the formation of cholesterol ester (Fig. 1, step 1b). Under other conditions the equilibrium is shifted so that surface transfer results in efflux of free cholesterol from the cell (Fig. 1, step 6) resulting in reduced cellular content, often coupled with stimulated synthesis (8,9,10). Finally it appears that esterified cholesterol can only be cleared from fibroblasts or smooth muscle cells by first undergoing hydrolysis (Fig. 1, step 5) (11,12). It has not as yet been established which hydrolytic enzymes are primarily responsible for the hydrolysis of stored cholesteryl ester, but it appears that this hydrolytic process must be coupled with the efflux of the liberated free cholesterol to effectively produce a significant reduction in cellular cholesterol pools.

In the framework of this model one can examine the possible effect of drugs on some of the individual metabolic steps. The first step would be the transport of cholesterol into the cell, either by lipoprotein uptake or by surface transfer (Fig. 1, steps 1a and 1b). A drug might influence transport either by modifying the cell, for example by modifying the receptors on the plasma membrane, or when added to the culture medium the drug could directly influence the lipid or apoprotein composition of the carrier lipoprotein so it no longer functioned as a delivery vehicle for the cholesterol. Alternatively, there is considerable evidence to indicate that specific lipoproteins produced by hypercholesteremic animals stimulate cellular cholesterol uptake and accumulation (6,13,14), thus it should be possible to design drug screening systems in which the test compounds are administered to animals and the serum from these treated animals assayed in a cell culture system to determine if the test drug modified the stimulatory effect of the hyperlipemic lipoproteins. In such a combined animal/tissue culture system, drugs would not be screened directly in cell culture, but the cells might serve as a sensitive indicator for possible drug modifications of serum lipoproteins.

The second step in cellular cholesterol metabolism involves lysosomal processing (Fig. 1, step 2). At this time there is already one compound that has been shown to affect this step, the drug chloroquine. A number of experiments have demonstrated that chloroquine inhibits the hydrolysis of incorporated esterified cholesterol, leading to the accumulation of cholesterol in the lysosome (1,12). Obviously, this is not a desirable effect, however, compounds which stimulated cholesterol ester clearance from the lysosome could be potentially beneficial, particularly since there is evidence indicating that at least some of the accumulated cholesterol present in foam cells is present in lipid laden lysosomes (15,16).

Another potential site of action of a drug would be at the level of ACAT (Fig. 1, step 4). Inhibition of this enzyme should lead to reduced esterified cholesterol synthesis and accumulation. A metabolic step of particular interest is the hydrolysis of stored cholesteryl ester (Fig. 1, step 5). If compounds were available which stimulated hydrolysis it might be possible to both inhibit ongoing cellular cholesteryl ester deposition, and to stimulate the clearance of accumulated cholesteryl ester. The techniques for the screening of drugs affecting either cholesteryl ester synthesis or hydrolysis with tissue culture cells are presently available.

The final site for drug action is free cholesterol efflux (Fig. 1, step 6). If drugs were available which enhanced efflux by either directly serving as an acceptor of free cholesterol or by modifying serum lipoproteins so that they would more efficiently promote efflux, the pool of cellular free cholesterol might be kept sufficiently reduced to prevent esterification and the resultant accumulation of esterified cholesterol. Stimulated efflux would serve to short circuit the pathway leading to cholesteryl ester accumulation by removing the substrate free cholesterol.

I would now like to show three examples of the effect various compounds can have on cholesterol metabolism in cells. The cell type in these experiments was the Fu5AH rat hepatoma cell. This cell line was used because we had previously demonstrated that these cells accumulate large amounts of cholesteryl ester when exposed to hyperlipemic rabbit serum but not when grown in the presence of normal lipemic serum (6,17). These cells appear to have the basic pathway for metabolizing cholesterol that is described in Figure 1. The metabolic parameters which were assayed in these studies were cholesterol ester accumulation and the esterification of incorporated radiolabeled free cholesterol.

The first study used Triton WR 1339 and Tween 80. To obtain hyperlipemic serum by means other than dietary manipulations, a rabbit was injected with Triton WR 1339, a treatment known to induce severe hyperlipemia. When added to the culture medium, this serum failed to produce the cellular response of increased esterification and accumulation of esterified cholesterol previously observed with hyperlipemic serum obtained from cholesterol fed animals (6). However, since Triton treatment results in detectable levels of Triton in the circulation, experiments were conducted to determine if surfactants added *in vitro* to hyperlipemic serum could influence cellular cholesteryl ester accumulation and esterification of free cholesterol. Figure 2 shows the effect on esterification and cholesteryl ester content produced by increasing concentration of two surfactants. Both parameters were markedly reduced by increasing concentration of these compounds. The inhibitory effect was not seen when the surfactants were added to cell cultures for 18 hr and then removed before exposure to hyperlipemic serum. This observation, that pretreatment of cells with surfactant did not inhibit esterified cholesterol accumulation, suggests that the surfactants act by modifying the serum lipoproteins and not by directly affecting cellular metabolism. It is interesting to note that the inhibition of esterified cholesterol

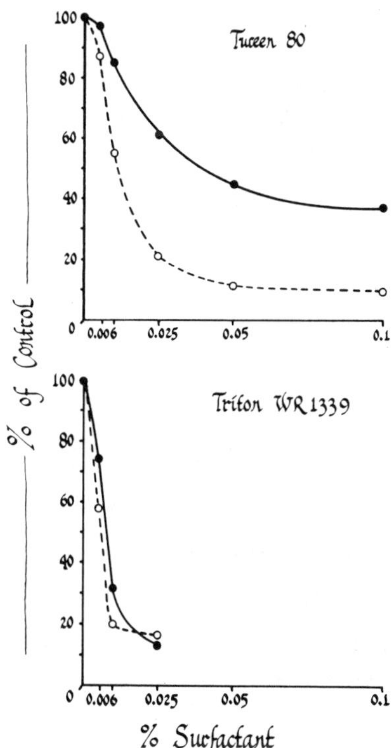

Figure 2: Effect of Tween 80 and Triton WR 1339 on cholesteryl ester accumulation o——o and free cholesterol esterification ●——● in Fu5AH hepatoma cells exposed to 5% hyperlipemic rabbit serum for 24 hr. Cholesterol esterification represents the conversion of incorporated exogenous FC to cellular EC.

accumulation produced by surfactant in this cell system parallels the effect of certain surfactants _in vivo_. A number of studies have shown reduced aortic lipid deposition in cholesterol fed animals injected with selected surfactants (18,19).

Figure 3 shows the effect of increasing lecithin concentrations on cholesteryl ester accumulation in the hepatoma cells. The medium contained a constant level of lipoprotein obtained from hyperlipemic serum. As exogenous lecithin was increased, cholesteryl ester

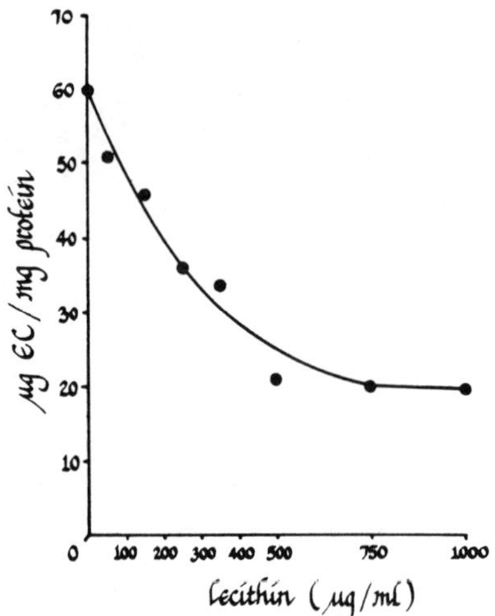

Figure 3: Effect of increasing lecithin concentration on esterified cholesterol accumulation by Fu5AH hepatoma cells exposed for 24 hr to d<1.019 lipoprotein from hyperlipemic rabbit serum. Lipoprotein added to culture medium to supply 100 μg FC/ml.

accumulation decreased. Although the mechanism of action of lecithin in this system is not known, the ability of lecithin to stimulate free cholesterol efflux (10,20) may be responsible for the inhibition of accumulation. Additional studies will be needed to establish if lecithin stimulated efflux of cholesterol results in reduced esterification and accumulation.

The last example uses the drug chlorophenoxyisobutyrate (CPIB). Table 1 shows the free, esterified and total cholesterol content of the cells grown in hyperlipemic serum together with CPIB. The addition of the drug results in a decrease in cholesteryl ester which is paralleled by an increase in free cholesterol. The columns on the right in Table 1 show the uptake and esterification of the exogenous free cholesterol. Although the drug did not markedly reduce free cholesterol uptake, it did significantly inhibit esterification, here expressed as the percent of incorporated free cholesterol which became esterified. Esterification dropped from 39% in controls

Table 1

EFFECT OF CPIB ON CE ACCUMULATION BY Fu5AH CELLS[a,b]

CPIB	Cellular Cholesterol Content (μg/mg Protein)			Exogenous FC[c]	
	FC	CE	TC	μg Incorporated	% Esterified[d]
0	24.0±0.8	36.7±1.2	60.7±1.9	12.6±0.4	39.1±0.1
1mM	29.5±0.7	27.4±1.8	56.9±2.3	11.5±0.2	24.6±0.6
5mM	33.1±2.0	16.3±0.4	49.4±0.4	10.8±0.2	7.9±0.5

[a]Cells incubated 24 hours with 2.5% hyperlipemic rabbit serum labeled with 4-^{14}C-cholesterol, and either 0,1 or 5 mM CPIB.

[b]Mean ± Standard Deviation

[c]Calculated from exogenous FC specific activity

[d]% Esterification=cpm in CE/ (cpm in FC + cpm in CE).

to 8% at the higher dose of CPIB. These results demonstrate that CPIB can reduce cholesteryl ester accumulation in the cells and suggests that it may act by inhibiting ACAT. This observation is consistent with the data of Brecher and Chobanian (21) who demonstrated an inhibitory effect of CPIB on ACAT in aortic homogenates.

These three examples of compounds that modify cellular cholesterol metabolism serve to illustrate that cell culture systems could be useful for drug screening. The recent development of techniques for the growth or maintenance of differentiated cells offer promising new systems. For example, a number of laboratories now maintain hepatocytes in culture which continue to synthesize both lipoproteins and bile acids. In our laboratory we have recently developed systems for the growth of preadipocytes in culture (22). These cells synthesize and release lipoprotein lipase and apparently undergo lipogenesis and lipolysis. Such differentiated cells are good candidates for consideration for the screening of drugs which affect specific aspects of lipid metabolism. Thus in the near future it should be possible to use cultured cells for the screening of drugs that affect not only the basic parameters of lipid metabolism but also specialized functions such as lipoprotein synthesis, bile acid synthesis, lipogenesis and lipolysis.

ACKNOWLEDGEMENT

This research was supported by USPHS research grant HL-20608.

REFERENCES

1. Goldstein, J.L. and M.S. Brown
   Ann. Rev. Biochem. 46: 930 (1977)
2. Koschinsky, T., T.E. Carew and D. Steinberg
   J. Lipid Res. 18: 451 (1977)
3. Miller, N.E., D.B. Weinstein, and D. Steinberg
   J. Lipid Res. 18: 438 (1977)
4. Stein, O., D.B. Weinstein, Y. Stein, and D. Steinberg
   Proc. Nat. Acad. Sci. 73:14 (1976)
5. Goldstein, J.L., R.G.W. Anderson, L.M. Buja, S.K. Basu and M.S. Brown
   J. Clin. Invest.59: 1196 (1977)
6. Rothblat, G.H., L. Arbogast, D. Kritchevsky, and M. Naftulin
   Lipids 11: 97 (1976)

7. Rothblat, G.H., J.M. Rosen, W. Insull, A.O. Yau, and D.M. Small
Exp. Mol. Path. 26: 318 (1977)
8. Sokoloff, L. and G.H. Rothblat
Biochim. Biophys. Acta. 280: 172 (1972)
9. Arbogast, L.Y., G.H. Rothblat, M.H. Leslie, and R.A. Cooper
Proc. Nat. Acad. Sci. 73: 3680 (1976)
10. Stein, O., J. Vanderhoeck and Y. Stein
Biochim. Biophys. Acta. 431: 347 (1976)
11. Rothblat, G.H. and D. Kritchevsky
Biochim. Biophys. Acta. 144: 423 (1967)
12. Stein, O., J. Vanderhoeck and Y. Stein
Atherosclerosis 26: 465 (1977)
13. Bates, S.R. and R.W. Wissler
Biochim. Biophys. Acta. 450: 78 (1976)
14. Pearson, J.D.
Atherosclerosis 24: 233 (1976)
15. Haley, N.J., H. Shio and S. Fowler
Lab. Invest., in press
16. Wolinsky, H.
Ann. N.Y. Acad. Sci. 275: 238 (1976)
17. Rothblat, G.H.
Lipids 9: 526 (1974)
18. Kellner, A., J.W. Correll and A.T. Ladd
J. Exp. Med. 93: 385 (1951)
19. Weigensberg, B.I.
J. Athero. Res. 10: 291 (1969)
20. Burns, C.H. and G.H. Rothblat
Biochim. Biophys. Acta 176: 616 (1969)
21. Brecher, P.I. and A.V. Chobanian
Circ. Res. 35: 692 (1974)
22. Rothblat, G.H. and F.D. DeMartinis
Biochem. Biophys. Res. Comm. 78: 45 (1977)

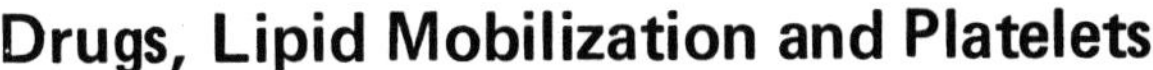

Drugs, Lipid Mobilization and Platelets

MECHANISMS OF LIPOMOBILIZATION

Giuliana Fassina

Institute of Pharmacology, University of Padua
Padua, Italy

The main functions of adipose tissue are (a) synthesis of long-chain fatty acids, (b) storage of exogenous and endogenous fatty acids in triglyceride form, and (c) free fatty acid release to the blood stream where they serve as a caloric substrate (1-4). The last process, hydrolysis of triglycerides and free fatty release, is a key control site for lipid mobilization. It is subject to multiple regulatory factors of nervous and hormonal origin (4-9). Well-known stimulating factors are sympathetic nervous activity, circulating catecholamines, ACTH, glucagon, TSH; depressing agents are insulin and prostaglandin E_1. The breakdown of the control mechanism at the subcellular level leading to an excess of plasma free fatty acids (FFA), is involved (2,7,10-12) not only in hyperlipoproteinemias, ketosis, fatty liver, but also have effects on the coagulating system prone to promote intravascular thrombosis, and effects on the contractility of myocardium and on excitability of the heart in particular conditions, These potential dangers of an excessive lipomobilization from adipose tissue stress the importance of clarifying the subcellular mechanism which regulates the reception and modulation of the multiple stimuli on lipolysis.

A summary of the recent investigations on this regulatory mechanism will follow, with a view to putting forth a more widespread prospective outline for future research.

HORMONE-SENSITIVE TRIGLYCERIDE HYDROLYSIS

The lipolytic process, which is better defined as

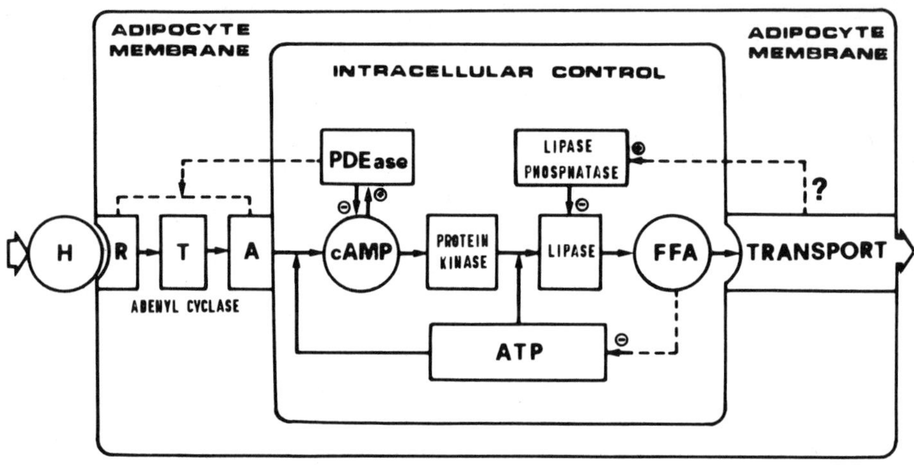

Figure 1: From G. Fassina, Adv. in General and Cellular Pharmacology, Plenum Press, 1977. (4)

hormone-sensitive triglyceride hydrolysis, is subject to a very fine regulation and metabolic equilibrium [recently reviewed by Heindel, Orci and Jeanrenaud (9) and Fassina (4)]. The scheme in Figure 1, even if not very precise, already demonstrates the complexity of the mechanism regulating the process. Such a mechanism may be divided in theory in at least two or maybe three strictly interrelated control systems. The first one, localized at plasma membrane level is the adenylate cyclase system. It acts as interceptor of hormone messages, transmitting them, well-amplified and modulated, into the cell by means of cyclic AMP (3'5'-adenosine monophosphate).

The second control system is that put in motion by cyclic AMP: it involves the activation of a protein kinase which works on the inactive lipase, converting it, by phosphorylation, to the active form. Finally, the activated lipase utilizes triglycerides as substrate. Their hydrolysis gives free fatty acids and glycerol as the final products which are released into the extracellular fluid. This is the final physiological response. Other aspects of the regulatory mechanism are found at the level of phosphodiesterase and of lipase phosphatase. PDEase transforms cyclic AMP to 5'AMP, thereby inactivating it. Lipase phosphatase inactivates the triglyceride lipase.

Further, again at plasma membrane level, a third regulatory system probably intervenes: the one regulating free fatty acid release into the medium or blood stream. In fact, while glycerol release is a simple, passive diffusion process, the exit of free fatty acids is more complex [as reviewed by Heindel, Orci and Jeanrenaud (9)] being possibly a mixture of a diffusion and an energy requiring transport process, as well as one implying the intervention of intracellular and extracellular binding sites. This is of great physiological interest as the increase in intracellular free fatty acid level may be harmful to the adipocyte.

On the whole, this multiple regulation strongly points out that homeostasis of lipomobilization depends not only on the transmission of stimuli into the cells, but also the modulation and the quenching of them, especially when they are too frequent or excessive. This is well in line with the general concept that in any informational system - both biological or not - quenching a signal must be of equal important to its generation. Like the pauses between tones are an important part of music (13).

Technically, as proposed by Galton (14), a cellular process can be compared to an electronic-transfer system which entails a series of amplifying devices together with feedback mechanisms, such as loops. This fine regulation allows multiple routes for biological control: the control elements are not only represented by enzymes, but also by cofactors and substrates. In view of this, if we consider the intracellular pathway leading to lipomobilization similar to that of a microscopic cybernetic system, the first scheme is too simple, as it does not bring out clearly enough other important factors of regulation. Out of these, an important factor is the energy production and consumption, that is, energy balance, on one side; and, on the other side, the role of ion movements, mainly of calcium. Data indicating that hormonal control of lipolysis is related to energy metabolism (15-19) have been reviewed by Heindel, Orci and Jeanrenaud (9) and Fassina (4). Here, attention is focused on the role of ions, mainly of calcium in the lipolytic process. A more complex and up to date scheme of lipolysis regulation is shown later.

THE ROLE OF IONS IN THE HORMONAL CONTROL OF LIPOLYSIS

The correlation of transmembrane ion flux and the

Table 1

THE ROLE OF IONS IN THE HORMONAL CONTROL OF LIPOLYSIS

Changes in transmembrane ion flux and hormones interact to regulate lipolysis
Mosinger, 1970 (20)

Requirement of extracellular Ca^{2+} in ACTH induced lipolysis
Lopez, White and Engel, 1959 (22); Braun and Hechter, 1970 (23); Kuo, 1970 (24)

Requirement of extracellular Ca^{2+} for modulating lipolysis activated by various hormones and db-cAMP
Fassina, 1967 (25); Mosinger and Vaughan, 1967 (26); Efendic, Alm and Löw, 1970 (27); Schimmel, 1973 (28)

Ca^{2+} involved in the antilipolytic action of digitoxin and PGE_1
Fassina and Contessa, 1967 (29)

Lipolytic hormones were all found to stimulate the release of Ca^{2+}
Clausen, 1970 (30)

---

hormonal control of lipolysis has been investigated (20, 21). The results indicate an outstanding role of calcium in the regulation of hormone-induced lipolysis (Tables 1 and 2).

It has been generally postulated that there might be a link between cAMP and calcium, inasmuch as calcium, although not necessary for the formation of the cyclic nucleotide, could be needed for its action (45). In adipose tissue such a concept might hold. But, if this is true, which is the mechanism of Ca^{2+} intervention in the process? Is it a direct one, particularly in hormone stimulus, or only a modulator of it? Or, finally, does the cation interfere in a multiple way, that is, simultaneously or successively, at many steps in the process?

Recent studies on this are: (a) calcium distribution in adipocytes, (b) effect of drugs on $^{45}Ca^{2+}$ movements in relation to subcellular calcium distribution and

Table 2

DRUGS WHICH AFFECT CALCIUM METABOLISM AND INHIBIT HORMONE-INDUCED LIPOLYSIS

Drug	References
Ouabain	Ho, Jeanrenaud and Renold, 1966 (31); Mosinger and Kujalova, 1966 (32); Bleicher, 1966 (33); Vulliemoz, Triner and Nahas, 1968 (34)
Digitoxin, Cassaine (alkaloid showing digitalis-like actions)	Fassina and Contessa, 1967 (29); Dorigo and Fassina, 1969 (35)
Vitamin D_2	Fassina et al., 1969 (36)
Local anaesthetics	Hales, 1970 (37); D'Costa and Angel, 1973 (38); Siddle and Hales, 1974 (39); D'Costa and Angel, 1975 (40)
Sulfonylureas	Brown et al., 1972 (41); Fain, Rosenthal and Ward, 1972 (42); Allen, Largis and Ashmore, 1974 (43); Ebert, Hillebrandt and Schwabe, 1974 (44)

metabolism, (c) effect of Ca^{2+} on enzymes involved in lipomobilization.

SUBCELLULAR DISTRIBUTION OF CALCIUM IN ADIPOCYTES

As in other cells (46) over 90% of the total calcium in adipocytes exists in an unexchangeable pool probably forming part of the glycoprotein complex matrix of fat cell membranes (47). The remaining cell Ca^{2+} fraction is exchangeable with that of the surrounding medium (Figure 2). This amount, however, is not entirely intracellular: half of the exchangeable Ca^{2+} in fat cells appears to be bound near the external surface of cell membrane, in a rapidly exchangeable pool. The intracellular Ca^{2+} (about 0.3 mM) is, as in other cells (48), partially free in the cytoplasm: cytoplasmic Ca^{2+} concentration is in the range of 10^{-6}M. The other part of the

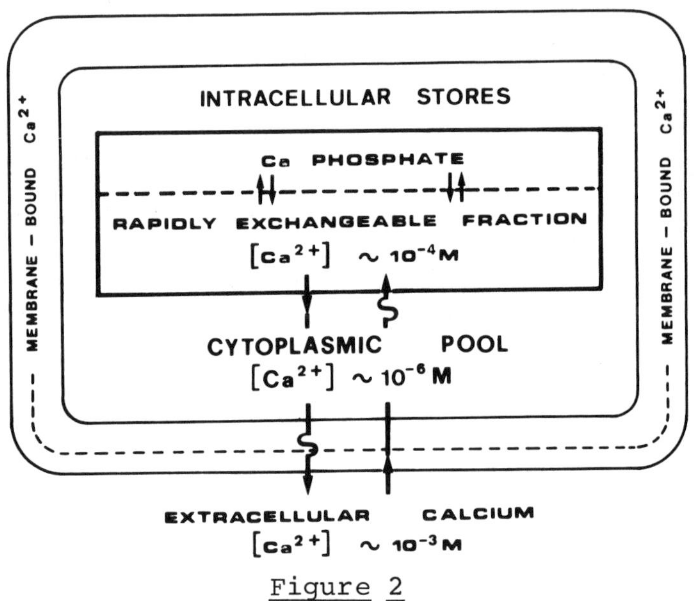

Figure 2

intracellular exchangeable Ca^{2+} is linked to stores capable of accumulating large amounts of it, and of exchanging calcium with that in cytoplasm. One of these sites of calcium storage is the endoplasmic reticulum (47,49). The other one is in mitochondria (50,51). Two pools of calcium are associated with each storage site: an ionized pool (exchangeable) and a stable or complexed one (52, 53).

From a dynamic point of view, it is evident that the cytoplasmic free Ca^{2+} concentration (10^{-6}M) is well below the level of dialyzable Ca^{2+} in the extracellular fluid (10^{-3}M), so that a calcium gradient exists from outside to inside the cells (Figure 2). The low cytoplasmic Ca^{2+} concentration can be maintained and adjusted by transmembrane Ca^{2+} flux, and, in parallel or alternatively, by redistribution of calcium between intracellular stores and the cytoplasm (47). This intracellular system of regulation is linked to a carrier-mediated energy dependent transport across membranes (50). With regard to this, it is interesting to point out that fat cell membranes (47,54), like mitochondria, contain a highly active Ca^{2+}-sensitive adenosine triphosphatase.

Table 3

EFFECT OF LIPOLYTIC AND ANTILIPOLYTIC DRUGS ON CALCIUM MOVEMENTS

DRUGS	EFFECTS
Epinephrine	Increased efflux from adipocytes (energy-dependent)
	Release from mitochondria
Insulin	Reduced efflux in response to epinephrine
	Increased uptake by microsomes
	Partial conversion of stable to exchangeable pool in mitochondria

Data from references 47,52,53,57-59.

EPINEPHRINE

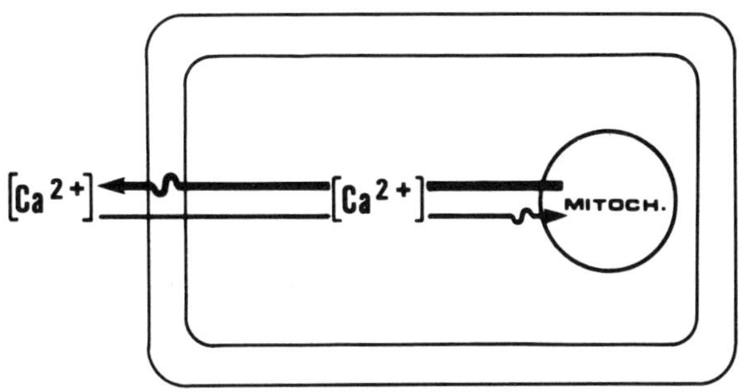

Figure 3: Data from: Severson et al., 1976; Kissebah et al., 1975; Gaion and Krishna, 1976,1977.

EFFECT OF DRUGS STIMULATING OR INHIBITING LIPOLYSIS ON CALCIUM DISTRIBUTION IN FAT CELLS

This complex network of calcium exchanges, which entails expenditure of energy, could be an important shunt in the hormonal control system on lipolysis. Several drugs stimulating or inhibiting lipolysis have been shown to modulate calcium transport in fat cells in correlation with their effect on lipolysis. Lipolytic hormones appear to greatly increase the turnover of calcium in adipose tissue: they were all found to stimulate the release of $^{45}Ca^{2+}$ from epididymal fat pads (30) as well as its uptake (55,56). More recent studies on adipocytes, fat cell ghosts and subcellular fractions, evaluated in detail the kinetics of the Ca^{2+} flux under hormonal and drug influence. Epinephrine was shown (47,57, 58,59) to induce a very rapid efflux of $^{45}Ca^{2+}$ from the cell to the extracellular medium (Table 3 and Figure 3). This could derive from a diminished calcium incorporation into mitochondria (53), resulting in a higher cytoplasmic Ca^{2+} level. An analogous increased efflux of calcium from mitochondria was induced in other tissues also by cyclic AMP (60).

The inhibitors of lipolysis, such as insulin and procaine-HCl, reduced the Ca^{2+} efflux in response to epinephrine (47) and acted in favor of an increase in calcium intracellular concentration. Insulin was also shown to induce a redistribution between intracellular calcium pool (52) by increasing the exchangeable fraction in mitochondria and the ability of microsomes to bind and accumulate calcium (Table 3 and Figure 4). Thus, epinephrine increases calcium efflux from adipocytes, while insulin modifies its intracellular movements. These effects could modify the activity of enzymes involved in lipomobilization.

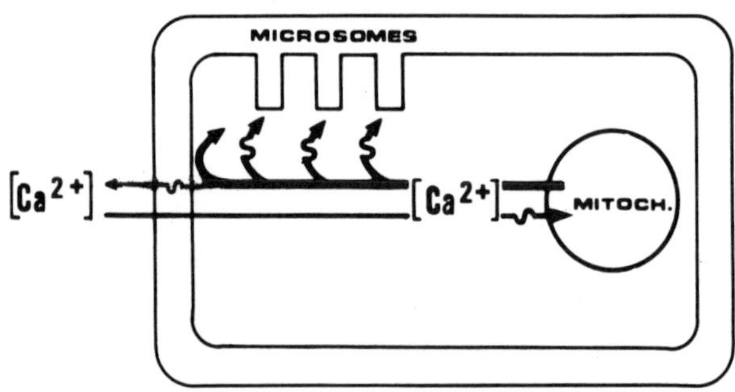

Figure 4: Data from: McDonald, Bruns and Jarett, 1976.

Table 4

EFFECT OF CA^{2+} ON ENZYME ACTIVITIES IN ADIPOCYTES

Protein kinase	↓	Kissebah et al., 1974 (63), 1975 (64)
Lipase phosphatase	↑	Kissebah et al., 1974 (63), 1975 (64)
Guanylate cyclase	↑	Gaion and Krishna, 1977 (58,59)

EFFECT OF CALCIUM ON ENZYMES INVOLVED IN LIPOMOBILIZATION

Several cell functions seem to be sensitive to changes in calcium concentration (61). This ion is essential for many enzymatic activities. Also, the properties of cell membranes are influenced by calcium present in them. Calcium movements induced by drugs could then modify not only the activity of soluble enzymes, but also the membrane functions, such as their fluidity, permeability to substrates, and activities of membrane-bound enzymes.

In the adipocyte, Ca^{2+} affects several enzyme activities (62). Above all, we must remember that the activity of protein kinase and of lipase phosphatase is modulated by calcium ions to favor inhibition of lipolysis (63,64). It is probable, even if not yet demonstrated, that - as in other tissues (65) - Ca^{2+} may also negatively affect the adenylate cyclase activity. Another interesting effect of calcium is on the guanylate cyclase system, responsible for variations in cyclic GMP levels (Table 4). Synthetic cyclic GMP was able to stimulate lipolysis, even to a lesser extent than cyclic AMP (66,67). Gaion and Krishna (57-59) have demonstrated an increase of cyclic GMP which is parallel to the release of Ca^{2+} by epinephrine in adipocytes. These two events are very rapid (within a period of less than one minute) and precede the variations both in cAMP and in lipolysis. Therefore these authors (59) suggest an interesting participation of cyclic GMP and Ca^{2+} to the hormone-stimulated lipolysis, probably as modulators of transmission.

FINAL COORDINATION

Thus, these preliminary data are indicative that calcium movements and cyclic nucleotides are probably connected to the transmission and modulation of hormone messages in adipose tissue too, as suggested for other tissues and functions (45,48).

The data briefly summarized here, seem to suggest a certain correlation of drug effect on Ca^{2+} movements (Table 3) with those on enzymatic activities involved in lipolysis (Table 4) and affected by Ca^{2+}. Thus, they could be tentatively coordinated in the following scheme (Figure 5), showing a regulatory system more complex than that previously described. This is only indicative, but could suggest new lines of research. The pattern of the hormone-sensitive lipolytic process is outlined in detail, together with the structures involved in calcium

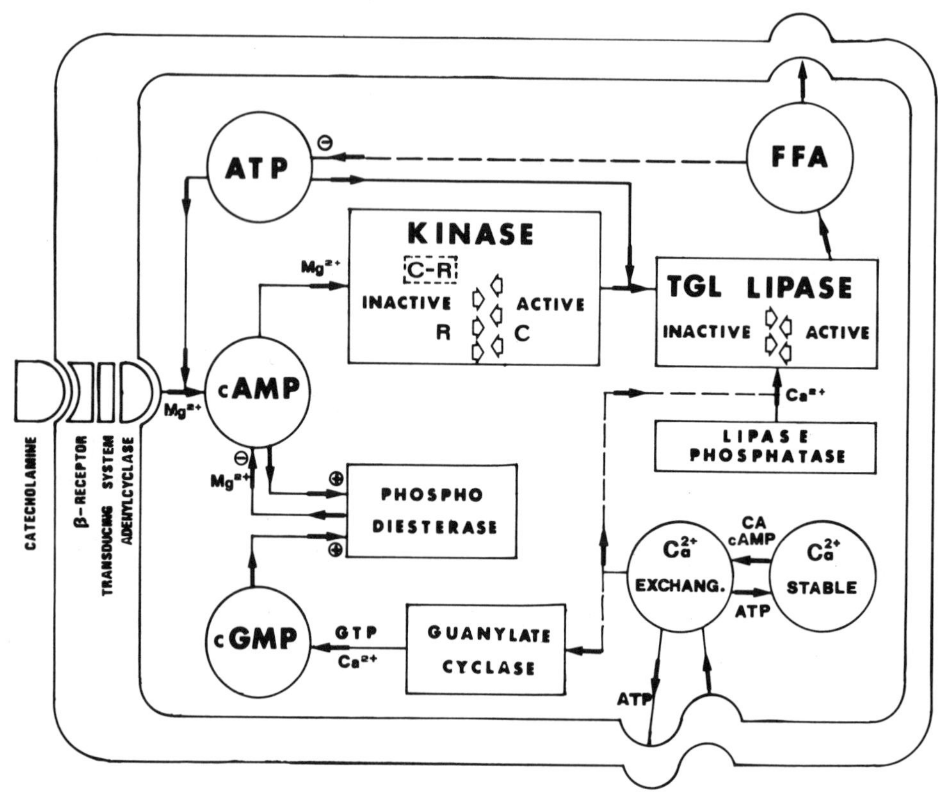

Figure 5

movement. These structures, able to deposit calcium and supporting its movements in and out of the adipocytes, are arranged in only two pools: the stable one, which includes mitochondria microsomes and plasma membrane; the exchangeable one, present in each of the aforementioned organelles and easily exchangeable with the cytoplasmic one. An increase of intracellular calcium could inhibit lipolysis acting on lipase phosphatase, which inactivates lipase. This could be the main mechanism of the antilipolytic effect of insulin (63). In fact, insulin facilitates an increase in intracellular calcium concentration (47); lipase phosphatase is stimulated by insulin and this activity is well-correlated with the inhibition of lipolysis (47,68).

An increase of intracellular calcium concentration could also promote the guanylate cyclase activity, with a consequent rise in cyclic GMP (69,70). The increased cGMP could in turn modify the levels of cyclic AMP through phosphodiesterase. In fact, cGMP was shown to stimulate PDEase activity (71,72). To be more precise (73) low concentrations of cGMP activated the soluble cAMP phosphodiesterase, while high concentrations of GMP inhibited it. Particulate cAMP phosphodiesterase activity was inhibited, but only by high concentrations of cGMP (73).

As previously mentioned (Table 3), epinephrine and insulin have complex effects on calcium movements, acting at more than one level. Moreover, such effects probably happen successively. Thereby they could induce sequential variations on the aforementioned enzyme activities, thus offering a proper modulation of lipolytic stimuli not only at the first stage, but also at the last stages of the process.

REFERENCES

1. Renold, A.E. and Cahill, G.F., Jr., editors, Adipose Tissue, Handbook of Physiology, Sect. 5, Am. Physiol. Soc. 1965
2. Jeanrenaud, B. and Hepp, P., editors, Adipose Tissue. Regulation and Metabolic Functions, Suppl. 2, Thieme Verlag and Academic Press, 1970
3. Björntorp, P. and J. Östman. In: Advances in Metabolic Disorders, R. Levine and and R. Luft, editors, volume 5, Academic Press, New York, 1971, pp. 277-327

4. Fassina, G.
In: Advances in General and Cellular Pharmacology, T. Narahashi and C.P. Bianchi, editors, Plenum Press, New York, 1977, pp. 155-185
5. Jeanrenaud, B.
In: Rev. of Physiol. Biochem. and Exp. Pharmacology, volume 60, Springer Verlag, Berlin, 1968, pp.57-410
6. Butcher, R.W.
In: Adipose Tissue. Regulation and Metabolic Functions, B. Jeanrenaud and D. Hepp, editors, Thieme Verlag and Academic Press, 1970, pp. 5-10
7. Steinberg, D.
In: Pharmacological Control of Lipid Metabolism, W.L. Holmes, R. Paoletti and D. Kritchevsky, editors, Volume 26, Advances Exp. Med. Biol., Plenum Press, New York, 1972, pp. 77-88
8. Fain, J.N.
Pharmacol. Rev. 25: 67, 1973
9. Heindel, J.J., L. Orci and B. Jeanrenaud
In: Pharmacology of Lipid Transport and Atherosclerotic Processes, E.J. Masoro, editor, IEPT, Sect. 24, volume 1, Pergamon Press, New York, 1975, pp. 175-373
10. Vague, J. and R.M. Denton
Physiopathology of Adipose Tissue, Excerpta Medica Foundation, Amsterdam, 1969
11. Havel, R.J.
In: Pharmacological Control of Lipid Metabolism, W.L. Holmes, R. Paoletti and D. Kritchevsky, editors, Volume 26, Advances Exp. Med. Biol., Plenum Press, New York, 1972, pp. 57-70
12. Mayes, P.A.
In: Pharmacology of Lipid Transport and Atherosclerotic Processes, E.J. Masoro, editor, IEPT, Sect. 24, vol.1, Pergamon Press, New York, 1975, pp. 125-174
13. Kakiuchi, S., R. Yamazaki, Y. Teshima, K. Uenishi, and E. Miyamoto
In: Advances in Cyclic Nucleotide Research, G.I. Drummond, P. Greengard and G.A. Robison, editors, vol. 5, Raven Press, New York, 1975, pp. 163-178
14. Galton, D.J.
S. Afr. Med. J. 49: 469 (1975)
15. Fassina, G., P. Dorigo and I. Maragno
In: Adipose Tissue, Regulation amd Metabolic Functions B. Jeanrenaud and D. Hepp, editors, Thieme Verlag and Academic Press, 1970, pp. 88-92
16. Angel, A., K.S. Desai and M.L. Halperin
J. Lipid Res. 12: 203 (1971)
17. Heindel, J.J., S.W. Cushman and B. Jeanrenaud
Am. J. Physiol. 266: 16 (1974)

18. Fassina, G., P. Dorigo and R.M. Gaion
In: Lipids, Lipoproteins and Drugs, D. Kritchevsky R. Paoletti and W.L. Holmes, editors, Vol. 63, Adv. Exp. Med. Biol., Plenum Press, New York, 1975, pp. 105-122
19. Giudicelli, Y., R. Pecquery, D. Provin, B. Agli, and R. Nordmann
Bioch. Biophys. Acta 486: 385 (1977)
20. Mosinger, B.
In: Adipose Tissue, Regulation and Metabolic Functions, B. Jeanrenaud and D. Hepp, editors, Thieme Verlag and Academic Press, 1970, pp. 71-75
21. Hales, C.N. and M.C. Perry
In: Adipose Tissue, Regulation and Metabolic Functions, B. Jeanrenaud and D. Hepp, editors, Thieme Verlag and Academic Press, 1970, pp. 63-65
22. Lopez, E., J.E. White and F.L. Engel.
J. Biol. Chem. 234: 2254 (1959)
23. Braun, T. and O. Hechter
In: Adipose Tissue, Regulation and Metabolic Functions, B. Jeanrenaud and D. Hepp, editors, Thieme Verlag and Academic Press, 1970, pp. 11-19
24. Kuo, J.F.
Biochim. Biophys. Acta 208: 509 (1970)
25. Fassina, G.
Life Sci. 6: 2191 (1967)
26. Mosinger, B. and M. Vaughan
Biochim. Biophys. Acta 144: 566 (1967)
27. Efendic, S., B. Alm and H. Löw
Horm. Metab. Res. 2: 287 (1970)
28. Schimmel, R.J.
Biochim. Biophys. Acta 326: 272 (1973)
29. Fassina, G. and A.R. Contessa
Biochem. Pharmacol. 16: 1447 (1967)
30. Clausen, T.
In: Adipose Tissue, Regulation and Metabolic Functions, B. Jeanrenaud and D. Hepp, editors, Thieme Verlag and Academic Press, 1970, pp. 66-70
31. Ho, R.J., B. Jeanrenaud and A.E. Renold
Experientia 22: 86 (1966)
32. Mosinger, B. and V. Kujalova
Biochim. Biophys. Acta 116: 174 (1966)
33. Bleicher, S.J.
J. Clin. Invest. 45: 988 (1966)
34. Vulliemoz, Y., L. Triner and G.G. Nahas
Life Sci. 7: 1063 (1968)
35. Dorigo, P. and G. Fassina
Life Sci. 8: 1143 (1969)

36. Fassina, G., I. Maragno, P. Dorigo, and A.R. Contessa
Europ. J. Pharmacol. 5: 286 (1969)
37. Hales, C.N.
Diabetologia 6: 47 (1970)
38. D'Costa, M.A. and A. Angel
Clin. Res. 21: 1057 (1973)
39. Siddle, K. and C.N. Hales
Biochem. J. 142: 345 (1974)
40. D'Costa, M.A. and A. Angel
Can. J. Physiol. Pharmacol. 53: 603 (1975)
41. Brown, J.D., A.A. Steele, D.B. Stone and F.A. Steele
Endocrinology 90: 47 (1972)
42. Fain, J.N., J.W. Rosenthal and W.F. Ward
Endocrinology 90: 52 (1972)
43. Allen, D.O., E.E. Largis and J. Ashmore
Diabetes 23: 51 (1974)
44. Ebert, R., O. Hillebrandt and U. Schwabe
Naunyn-Schmiedeberg's Arch. Pharmacol. 286: 181 (1974)
45. Rasmussen, H.
Science 170: 404 (1970)
46. Borle, A.B.
J. Gen. Physiol. 53: 43 (1969)
47. Kissebah, A.H., P. Clarke, N. Vydelingum, H. Hope-Gill, B. Tulloch, and T.R. Fraser
J. Clin. Invest. 5: 339 (1975)
48. Rasmussen, H., P. Jensen, W.L. Lake, N. Friedman and D. Goodman
In: Advances in Cyclic Nucleotide Research, G.I. Drummond, P. Greengard and G.A. Robison, editors, volume 5, Raven Press, New York, 1975, pp. 375-394
49. Hales, C.N., J.B. Luzio, J.A. Chandler and L. Herman
J. Cell Sci. 15: 1 (1974)
50. Martin, R., R. Clausen and J. Gliemann
Biochem. J. 152: 121 (1975)
51. Severson, D.L., R.M. Denton, H.T. Pask and P.J. Randle
Biochem. J. 140: 225 (1974)
52. McDonald, J.M., D.E. Bruns, and L. Jarett
Biochem. Biophys. Res. Commun. 71: 114 (1976)
53. Severson, D.L., R.M. Denton, B.J. Bridges and P.J. Randle
Biochem. J. 154: 209 (1976)
54. Dorigo, P.
Biochem. Pharmacol. 21: 1329 (1971)

55. Akgun, S. and D. Rudman
Endocrinology 84: 926 (1969)
56. Alm, B., S. Efendic and H. Löw
Horm. Metab. Res. 2: 142 (1970)
57. Gaion, R.M. and G. Krishna
Pharmacologist 18: 591 (1976)
58. Gaion, R.M. and G. Krishna
In: Abstracts, Sixth International Symposium on Drugs Affecting Lipid Metabolism, Philadelphia, these proceedings
59. Gaion, R.M. and G. Krishna
Pharmac. Exptl. Therap., in press
60. Borle, A.B.
J. Membrane Biol. 16: 221 (1974)
61. Lakshminarayanaiah, N. and C.P. Bianchi
In: Advances in General and Cellular Pharmacology, T. Narahashi and C.P. Bianchi, editors, Vol. 2, Plenum, New York, 1977, p. 1-70
62. Rizack, M.A.
J. Biol. Chem. 239: 392 (1964)
63. Kissebah, A.H., N. Vydelingum, B.R. Tulloch, H. Hope-Gill, and T.R. Fraser
Horm. Metab. Res. 6: 247 (1974)
64. Tulloch, B.R., A. Kissebah, N. Vydelingum, P. Clarke, H. Hope-Gill, and T.R. Fraser
In: Advances in Cyclic Nucleotide Research, G.I. Drummond, P. Greengard, and G.A. Robison, editors, vol. 5, Raven Press, New York, 1975, p. 807 (abst.)
65. Steer, M.L., D. Atlas, and A. Levitzki
N.Engl. J. Med. 290: 409 (1975)
66. Braun, T., O. Hechter, and H.P. Bar
Proc. Soc. Exptl. Biol. 132: 233 (1969)
67. Murad, F., V. Manganiello and M. Vaughan
J. Biol. Chem. 245: 3352 (1970)
68. Khoo, J., D. Steinberg, B. Thompson and S.E. Mayer
J. Biol. Chem. 248: 3823 (1973)
69. Illiano, G., G.P. Tell, M.I. Siegel and P. Cuatrecasas
Proc. Nat.Acad.Sci. USA 70: 2443 (1973)
70. Vydelingum, N., A.H. Kissebah, V. Wynn and A. Simpson
Diabetologia 11: 382 (1975)
71. Beavo, J.A., J.G. Hardman and E.W. Sutherland
J. Biol. Chem. 246: 3841 (1971)
72. Klotz, U. and K. Stock
Naunyn-Schmiedeberg's Arch. Pharmacol. 274:54 (1972)
73. Sakai, T., W.J. Thompson, V. Lavis and R.H. Williams
Arch. Biochem. Biophys. 162: 331 (1974)

NICOTINIC ACID AND INHIBITION OF FAT MOBILIZING LIPOLYSIS. PRESENT STATUS OF EFFECTS ON LIPID METABOLISM

Lars A. Carlson

King Gustaf V Research Institute and the Department of Internal Medicine, Karolinska Hospital, Stockholm, Sweden

In the beginning of the 1960's inhibition of fat mobilizing lipolysis (FML) was introduced as a tool in experimental medicine and as a new principle in the treatment of certain metabolic disorders (1,2). There were two major reasons for this at that time. First, we had found that nicotinic acid has a very powerful pharmacological fat mobilizing lipolysis inhibitory (FMLI) property thereby reducing the levels of circulating plasma free fatty acids (FFA) (3,4). Secondly, models for the metabolic consequences of excessive FFA mobilization were just being developed (Figure 1). These models predicted that excessive FFA mobilization might cause certain unwanted metabolic effects such as hyperlipidemia and ketosis. Therefore it became of clinical interest to consider the use of inhibitors of FFA mobilization in acute as well as chronic situations. Today these models are in principle still believed to be valid. The major causes and effects of excessive FFA mobilization are summarized in Tables 1 and 2. Some areas where the use of compounds with FMLI property might be of benefit are summarized in Table 3.

FMLI - FAT MOBILIZING LIPOLYSIS INHIBITORS

Some FMLI are listed in Table 4. From the pharmacological point of view the carboxylic acids seem to

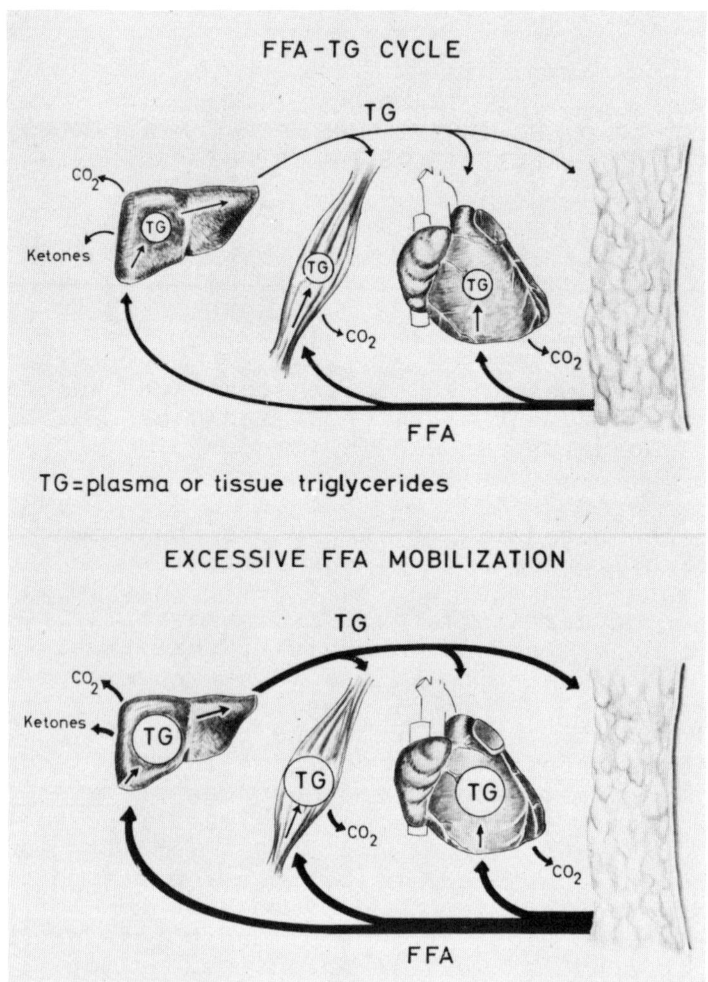

<u>Figure 1</u>: Models for the <u>normal</u> (top) and <u>excessive</u> (bottom) mobilization of FFA as they were developed in the 1960's (1). Note in particular the increased secretion of triglycerides and ketone bodies from the liver in response to excessive FFA mobilization.

Table 1

EXCESSIVE MOBILIZATION OF FFA

Common Causes
Catecholamines "Insulin deficiency" Other hormonal/nutritional imbalance
Effects
Raised plasma FFA levels Increased tissue extraction
Associated Effects in AT
Decreased LLA[1] Decreased FIAT[2]

[1] LLA = Lipase Activity

[2] FIAT = Fatty acid Incorporation into Adipose Tissue

have been the most promising as yet, but an ideal compound has so far not been developed and tested clinically. We assessed several nicotinic acid derivatives synthesized by Stjernström and coworkers at Astra Pharmaceutical Company (5,6). One of the most promising as FMLI was 5-fluoronicotnic acid. About 100-200 mg was as effective in lowering FFA as 1000 mg of nicotinic acid and caused very little, if any, flush. However, when we tried 5-fluoronicotinic acidin patients with hyperlipidemia we distressingly enough did not obtain the expected lowering of lipoprotein levels (7). On the other hand 5-fluoronicotinic acid has been used successfully as a FMLI in patients with acute myocardial infarction as described below.

It is of great interest that phenoxy-acids are FMLI considering their usefulness as plasma triglyceride lowering compounds (8,9,10). It has been shown that this inhibition is associated with a reduction of the level of cyclic AMP in adipose tissue (8,9).

Table 4

EXAMPLES OF INHIBITORS OF FAT MOBILIZING LIPOLYSIS

Insulin
Prostaglandin E_1
Nucleo-tides-sides
Adenosine derivatives
Adrenergic Blockers
Cyclic Carboxylic Acids
Nicotinic acid
Salicylic acid
Pyrazoles
Thiazoles
Phenoxy acids
Clofibrate
Gemfibrozil

FMLI NICOTINIC ACID DERIVATIVES AND MYOCARDIAL INFARCTION

Raised FFA levels may be of prognostic importance during acute myocardial infarction both with regard to the occurrence of ventricular arrhythmias and to the size of the infarct. The "Oliver hypothesis" suggests that high plasma concentrations of FFA may induce ventricular arrhythmias in the ischaemic heart (11,12). By using the potent nicotinic acid derivative discussed above, 5-fluoronicotinic acid, in acute myocardial infarction, Oliver and coworkers were able to demonstrate a reduction in arrhythmias as a result of the reduction of the high FFA levels (13). These studies lend strong support to the "Oliver hypothesis" and indicate an important area for FMLI. The fact that high FFA levels may stimulate O_2 consumption of the heart (14) and that nicotinic acid reduces catecholamine stimulated calorigenesis (15) led Kjekshus and Mjøs (16) to study the effect of FMLI on experimental myocardial infarction. They found that nicotinyl alcohol, which is rapidly oxidized to nicotinic acid and therefore a powerful FMLI, simultaneously with lowering of FFA reduced the size of infarcts in dogs

Table 2

PATHOPHYSIOLOGY OF EXCESSIVE MOBILIZATION OF FFA

Elevated FFA Levels

Inhibition of glucose extraction (Randle)
Induction of arrhythmias (IHD)
Thrombogenicity

Increased Tissue Extraction of FFA

Intracellular TG accumulation
→ fatty degeneration

Increased ketone formation
→ ketosis

Increased secretion of VLDL
→ hyperlipidemia

Stimulation of O_2 consumption
→ hypermetabolism

Table 3

CLINICAL FIELDS WHERE INHIBITION
OF FFA MOBILIZATION MAY BE OF BENEFIT

Hyperlipidemia

Diabetes
(hyperglycemia, ketosis)

Myocardial infarction
(size, arrhythmias)

Trauma and "stress"

FAMILIAL HYPERCHOLESTEROLEMIA

Type IIA Hyperlipoproteinemia

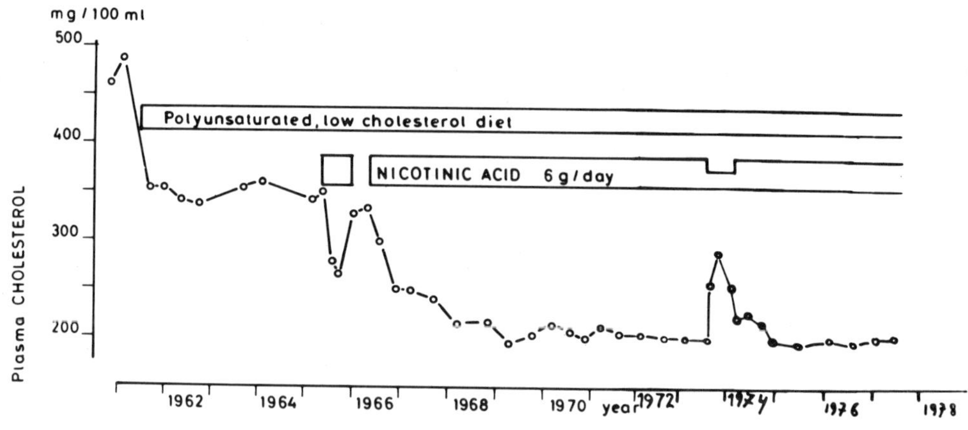

Case AT (♂ born 1911) Myocardial infarction 1961

<u>Figure</u> <u>2</u>: Effect of long term treatment with nicotinic acid, 6 g/day, on plasma cholesterol in a patient with familial hypercholesterolemia initially presenting with tendinous xanthomata, which completely disappeared after two years of nicotinic acid therapy (21). Note the sensitivity to dose change in 1973.

<u>Table</u> <u>5</u>

NICOTINIC ACID EFFECTS ON PLASMA LIPOPROTEINS

Chylomicrons	↓
VLDL	↓
LP-β	↓
LDL	↓
HDL	(↑)

where the left anterior descending coronary artery had been occluded. These findings have been confirmed with other FMLI (17). The use of FMLI early in acute myocardial infarction has indeed obtained further promotion from these studies.

NICOTINIC ACID AND HYPERLIPIDEMIA: EFFECTS ON LIPOPROTEIN CLASSES

The plasma cholesterol lowering effect of nicotinic acid was first reported by Altschul *et al* in 1955 (18). Once tolerated this drug has in high doses, 3-15 g per day, excellent effects in types IIA, IIB, III, IV and V hyperlipoproteinemia (19,20). As an example of the usefulness of nicotinic acid in long term treatment of hyperlipidemia the response in a patient with familial hypercholesterolemia (type IIA) is shown in Figure 2. Studies in fasting patients with hyperlipoproteinemia (19,20,21,22) as well as during alimentary lipemia (23, 24) have shown that nicotinic acid has the effects on the different plasma lipoprotein classes listed in Table 5. However, two remarks should be given. When the level of low density lipoproteins (LDL) in plasma is low and that of very low density (VLDL) high, the LDL levels may rise in response to treatment with nicotinic as well as other drugs (22,25). The clinical implications of this were discussed elsewhere (26). The high density lipoprotein (HDL) may increase during treatment of hyperlipidemia with nicotinic acid, particularly if the pretreatment levels are low as in type V and type IV hyperlipoproteinemia (22,26).

NICOTINIC ACID AND HYPERLIPIDEMIA: MODES OF ACTION

Originally Altschul and coworkers studied the effect of nicotinic acid on plasma cholesterol because they believed that "increase of intravital oxidation decreases blood cholesterol" and nicotinic acid and its amide "raise the level of DPN, a constituent of the respiratory enzyme system, and they may thus influence the cholesterol metabolism by intensified oxidation" (19). They found that the acid but not the amide had a potent cholesterol lowering effect (19). Earlier studies on the mode of action of nicotinic acid in particular its effect on cholesterol synthesis and catabolism were reviewed in Altschul's book of 1964 (19). A more recent handbook on the metabolic effects of nicotinic acid appeared in 1971 (27).

EFFECT OF NICOTINIC ACID ON FRACTIONAL TURNOVER AND CONCENTRATION OF LDL IN TYPE IIA

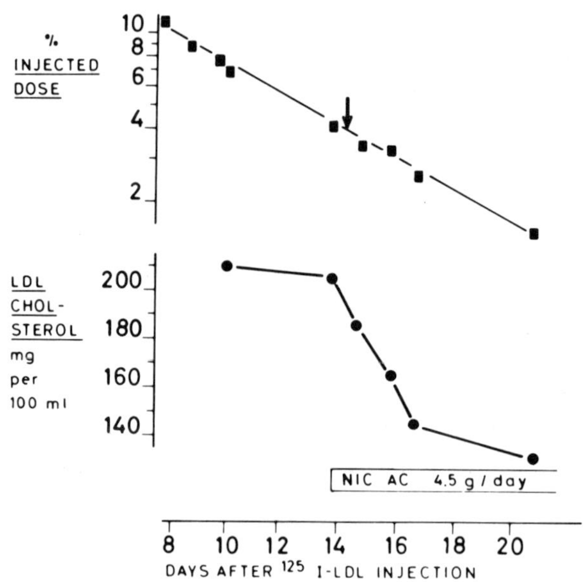

Figure 3: Effect of nicotinic acid on the concentration of LDL cholesterol and the fractional turnover of ^{125}I-labelled LDL (expressed as % of injected dose present in plasma). Autologous ^{125}I-LDL (d=1.030-1.050) was injected at day 0, a mono-exponential disappearance of ^{125}I-LDL was observed to start at day 6. Nicotinic acid was started at day 14 and within 2 days the LDL concentration was reduced by 30% without concomitant apparent change in the fractional catabolism of LDL. The reduction in LDL by 1/3 is therefore best explained by 1/3 reduction in its synthesis possibly caused by a decrease of the hepatic production of VLDL-apoB by 1/3.

Here I will only briefly summarize some of the effects of nicotinic acid in adipose tissue which may influence the synthesis or catabolism of chylomicra, VLDL and LDL.

As depicted in Figure 1 an excessive FML may raise the synthesis of VLDL by increasing the production of

Table 6

NICOTINIC ACID. POSSIBLE MECHANISMS IN ADIPOSE TISSUE FOR LOWERING PLASMA CONCENTRATIONS OF CHYLOMICRA, VLDL AND LDL

Mechanism	Primary effect	Effects on VLDL Concentration	Effects on LDL
Inhibition of lipolysis	Synthesis of VLDL ↓↓	VLDL concentration ↓	ApoB → LDL ↓ LDL concentration ↓
Increase of LLA[1]	Catabolism of VLDL and chylomicra ↑↑	VLDL and chylomicron concentration ↓	ApoB → LDL± LDL concentration±
Increase of FIAT[2]	Catabolism of VLDL and chylomicra ↑↑	VLDL and chylomicron concentration ↓	ApoB → LDL± LDL concentration±

[1]LLA = Lipoprotein Lipase Activity

[2]FIAT = Fatty acid Incorporation into Adipose Tissue.

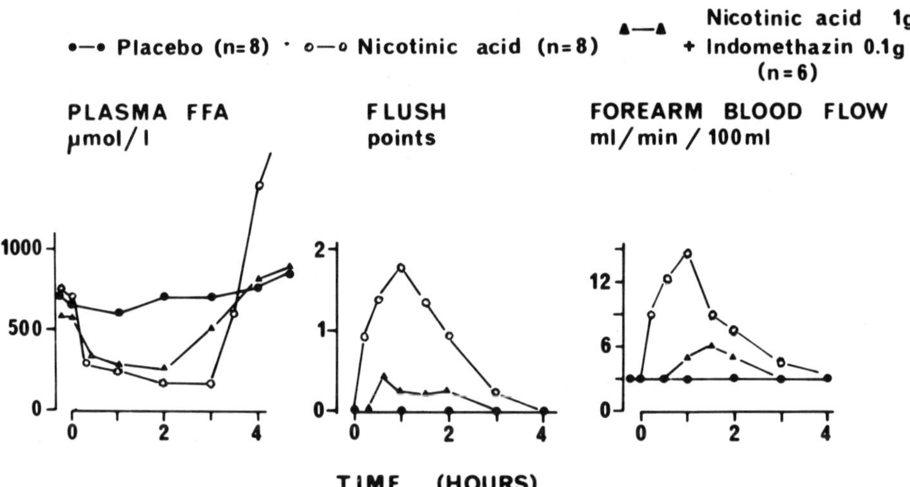

Figure 4: Effects of placebo, nicotinic acid (1 g) and nicotinic acid (1 g) + indomethazine (0.1 g) given at three different occasions in a double blind study as a single dose at 0 hours on concentration of FFA, fascial flush and forearm blood flow (venous occlusion pletysmography). Note the reduction in flush and forearm blood flow caused by indomethazine. Mean values are given.

one of its main components, the triglycerides. Conversely, a reduction of both excessive and normal FML may reduce the triglyceride synthesis in the liver and thereby diminish the hepatic production of VLDL. This may be one possible mechanism for a FMLI like nicotinic acid to reduce the concentration of VLDL in blood. Furthermore because of the precursor product relation between VLDL and LDL:

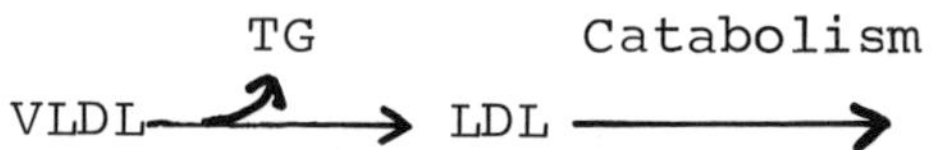

it is easy to see how a diminished production of VLDL also would cause a reduction in the production of LDL. By such a mechanism the level of the LDL lipoprotein class would also fall in response to FMLI. In fact studies with iodine labelled LDL before and during nicotinic acid treatment (Figure 3) indicate that the nicotinic acid induced reduction of LDL levels is not caused by an increased catabolism of LDL but due to a reduced synthesis which most likely was due to a reduced synthesis of its immediate precursor VLDL as discussed above. However, there is evidence that the 24 hour FFA flux is not reduced during treatment with nicotinic acid, particularly because of nocturnal "overshoot" in FFA levels (23,28). These studies were, however, done under metabolic ward conditions and it may be that nicotinic acid is more effective in free living persons to cause a reduction of the 24 hour FFA turnover.

For various reasons it seems likely that nicotinic acid must exert other mechanisms than FMLI in order to have all the effects listed in Table 5. For instance the pronounced effect on chylomicrons could hardly be explained by a reduction of chylomicron formation, particularly not caused by reduced FFA turnover. It seems much more likely that nicotinic acid also increases the catabolism of triglyceride rich lipoproteins. The important reactions in this catabolism are

$$\text{plasma TG} \xrightarrow{\text{LLA}} \text{FA} \xrightarrow{\text{FIAT}} \text{tissue TG}$$

lipoprotein lipase activity (LLA) splits off the fatty acids from the triglycerides and the next step is the fatty acid incorporation in adipose tissue (FIAT) and other tissues. Both LLA in adipose tissue (29,30,31) and FIAT (32,33) are raised by nicotinic acid. Both these effects may cause a stimulation of the catabolism of chylomicra as well as of VLDL. This would be expected to lower the circulating level of these lipoproteins but not to effect the concentration of LDL. It is of interest in this connection that clofibrate has identical but weaker effects as nicotinic acid in adipose tissue: FML ↓, LLA ↑ and FIAT ↑ .

The complexity of the effects of nicotinic acid in adipose tissue and the influence of these effects on serum lipoproteins is summarized in Table 6.

NICOTINIC ACID AND FLUSH

One of the often unpleasant side effects of nicotinic acid is the flush. The well-known tachyphylaxis for this effect suggested to us that it might be due to release of some substance synthesized *in vivo* and not due to a direct effect of nicotinic acid. The nicotinic acid flush appeared very similar to the flush we had observed after prostaglandin E_1 (PGE_1) (34). We therefore in a randomized double-blind study evaluated the effect of an inhibitor of PGE_1 synthesis, indomethazine, on the flush.

Figure 4 shows that both the flush and the increase in forearm blood flow caused by nicotinic acid were considerably reduced by indomethazine while the FFA lowering was almost unaffected. Later studies have also revealed that nicotinic acid causes a release of PGE_1 from the forearm.

ACKNOWLEDGEMENT

This work was supported by grants from the Swedish Medical Research Council (19X-204).

REFERENCES

1. Carlson, L.A., Boberg, J. and Högstedt, B. In: Handbook of Physiology. Adipose Tissue, A.E. Renold and C.F. Cahill, editors, 1965, pp. 625-644.
2. Carlson, L.A. Diabetologia 5: 361-365 (1969)
3. Carlson, L.A. and Örö, L. Acta Med. Scand. 172: 641-645 (1962)
4. Carlson, L.A. Acta Med. Scand. 173: 719-722 (1963)
5. Carlson, L.A., Hedbom, Ch., Helgstrand, E., Sjöberg, B. and Stjernström, N.E. In: Drugs Affecting Lipid Metabolism, W.L. Holmes, L.A. Carlson, and R. Paoletti, editors, Plenum, New York, 1969, pp. 85-92.
6. Carlson, L.A., Hedbom, Ch., Helgstrand, E., Misiorny, A., Sjoberg, B., Stjernström, N.E. and Westin, G. Acta Pharm. Suecia 9: 221-228 (1972)
7. Carlson, L.A., unpublished observations
8. Carlson, L.A., Walldius, G. and Butcher, R.W. Atherosclerosis 16: 349-357 (1972)
9. D'Costa, M.A. and Angel, A. J. Clin. Invest. 55: 138-148 (1975)
10. Carlson, L.A. Proc. Roy. Soc. Med. 69: 101-103 (1976)
11. Kurien, V.A. and Oliver, M.F. Lancet 2: 122 (1966)

12. Oliver, M.F., Kurien, V.A. and Greenwood, T.W. Lancet 1: 710 (1968)
13. Rowe, M.J., Neilson, J.M.M. and Oliver, M.F. Lancet 1: 295 (1975)
14. Challoner, D.R. and Steinberg, D. Am. J. Physiol. 210: 280 (1966)
15. Havel, R.J., Carlson, L.A., Ekelund, L.-G. and Holmgren, A. Metabolism 13: 1402-1412 (1964)
16. Kjekshus, J.K. and Mjøs, O.D. J. Clin. Invest. 52: 1770 (1973)
17. Mjøs, O.D., Miller, N.E., Riemersma, R.A. and Oliver, M.F. Circulation 53: 494-500 (1976)
18. Altschul, R., Hoffer, A. and Stephen, J.D. Arch. Biochem. 54: 558 (1955)
19. Niacin in Vascular Disorders and Hyperlipemia, R. Altschul, editor, Charles C. Thomas, Springfield, 1964.
20. Carlson, L.A. and Orö, L. Atherosclerosis 18: 1-9 (1973)
21. Carlson, L.A. In: Drugs Affecting Lipid Metabolism, W.L. Holmes, L.A. Carlson, and R. Paoletti, editors, Plenum, New York, 1969, pp. 327-338
22. Carlson, L.A., Froberg, S. and Orö, L. Atherosclerosis 16: 359-368 (1972)
23. Froberg, S.O., Boberg, J., Carlson, L.A. and Ericsson, M. In: Metabolic Effects of Nicotinic Acid and its Derivatives, K.F. Gey and L.A. Carlson, editors, Hans Huber Publisher, Bern, 1971, pp. 167-181
24. Barboriak, J.J. and Meade, R.C. Atherosclerosis 13: 199 (1971)
25. Carlson, L.A., Olsson, A.G., Orö, L., Rössner, S. and Walldius, G. In: Atherosclerosis III, G.Schettler and A. Weizel, editors, Springer-Verlag, Berlin, 1974, pp. 768-781
26. Carlson, L.A., Olsson, A.G. and Ballantyne, D. Atherosclerosis 26: 603-609 (1977)
27. Metabolic Effects of Nicotinic Acid and its Derivatives, K.F. Gey and L.A. Carlson, Hans Huber Publisher, Bern, 1971
28. Schlierf, G. and Hess, G. Artery 3: 174-179 (1977)
29. Nikkilä, E.A. In: Metabolic Effects of Nicotinic Acid and Its Derivatives, K.F. Gey and L.A. Carlson, editors, Hans Huber Publisher, Bern, 1971, p. 487.

30. Otway, S., Robinson, D.C., Rogers, M.P. and Wing, D.R.
In: Metabolic Effects of Nicotinic Acid and Its Derivatives, K.F. Gey and L.A. Carlson, editors, Hans Huber Publisher, Bern, 1971, p. 497
31. Shafrir, E. and Biale, Y.
In: Metabolic Effects of Nicotinic Acid and Its Derivatives, K.F. Gey and L.A. Carlson, editors, Hans Huber Publisher, Bern, 1971, p. 515
32. Carlson, L.A., Eriksson, I. and Walldius, G.
Acta Med. Scand. 194: 363-369 (1973)
33. Walldius, G.
Acta Medica Scandinavica, Supplement 591(1976)
34. Carlson, L.A., Ekelund, L.-G and Orö, L.
Acta Med. Scand. 183: 423-430 (1968)

DRUG EFFECTS ON PLATELET AGGREGATION AND PROSTAGLANDIN FORMATION

J.B. Smith, C.M. Ingerman and M.J. Silver

Cardeza Foundation and Department of Pharmacology, Thomas Jefferson University, Philadelphia, Pennsylvania, U.S.A.

INTRODUCTION

In this paper, we intend to present our current understanding of the mechanisms of induction and inhibition of platelet aggregation and prostaglandin formation. We will try to show how this new understanding may help us rationally design effective antithrombotic therapies. We will not review the many drugs that inhibit platelet aggregation. For this, the reader is referred elsewhere (1).

To begin with, we must recognize that although platelets do play a major part in arterial thrombosis, other factors including the vessel wall and the plasma coagulation system are involved. Information obtained from *in vitro* studies of the mechanisms of platelet aggregation relate almost exclusively to platelets, since tests are usually done on samples prepared from anticoagulated blood. The relative contributions of the clotting system or of the vessel wall to thrombosis can only be surmised from such studies for example, by adding thrombin or constituents of the vessel wall. With these points in mind, we shall deal first with our present understanding of the mechanisms of induction and inhibition of platelet aggregation and prostaglandin formation as studied *in vitro*, and then consider the much more complicated mechanisms that may operate *in vivo*.

PROSTAGLANDINS INDUCE PLATELET AGGREGATION

Until very recently, ADP has occupied the center stage as a platelet aggregating agent. Within a second or two of its addition to citrated platelet-rich plasma, ADP causes the normally disc-shaped platelets to extend pseudopods and to adhere to each other or aggregate. This can be conveniently measured since the amount of light transmitted through platelet-rich plasma increases rapidly as the platelets clump together (2). Most other nucleotides including UDP, GDP, CDP and IDP have little activity as inducers of aggregation (3) although analogues of ADP including 2-chloro-ADP (4) and 2-azido-ADP (5,6), which are more potent aggregating agents, have been synthesized.

In 1974, it was found that two naturally-occuring prostaglandin endoperoxides, PGG_2 and PGH_2, cause platelet aggregation (7). None of the other naturally-occurring prostaglandins which have been isolated have been found to induce aggregation, although recently several analogues of PGH_2, including an azo analogue (8) and two methano-epoxy analogues (9,10), have been synthesized which do so (Figure 1).

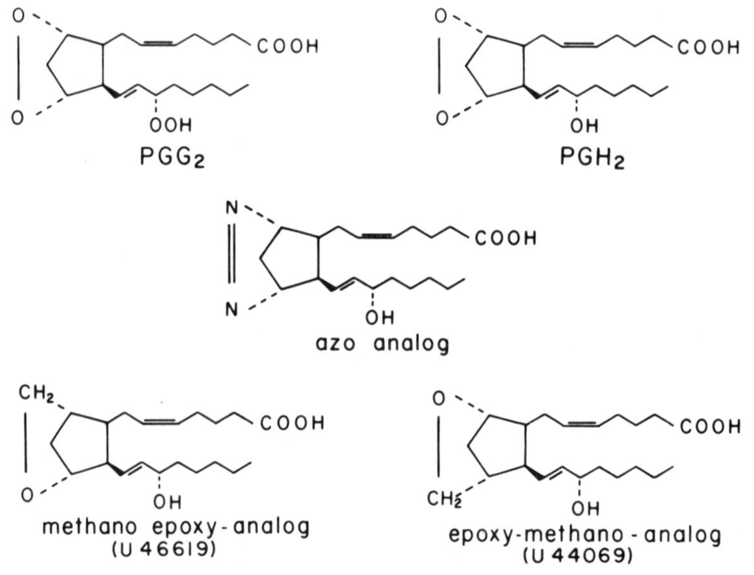

Figure 1: Structure of prostaglandins that aggregate platelets. For further details see text.

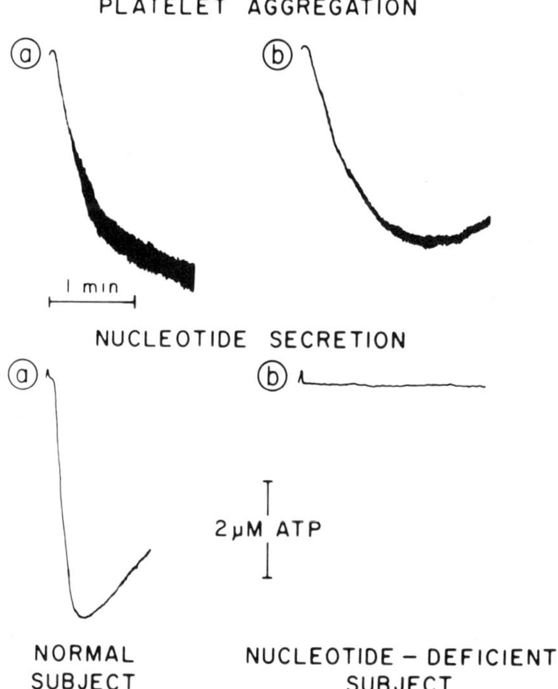

Figure 2: Aggregation and nucleotide secretion induced in human citrated platelet-rich plasma by PGG_2. Traces marked a) show the responses obtained when 5 μM PGG_2 was incubated with normal citrated platelet-rich plasma. Traces marked b) were obtained while studying a patient with platelet nucleotide deficiency.

Aggregation of platelets by PGG_2 is accompanied by the release of ADP from granules within the platelets, and it was suggested that aggregation by PGG_2 is mediated by this released ADP (11). However, by using a new machine, the lumiaggregometer, we have been able to show that PGG_2 can cause aggregation without nucleotide release (12). This machine simultaneously measures platelet aggregation by monitoring changes in light transmission and nucleotide secretion by determining the light flashes produced by the reaction of ATP with luciferin-luciferase. Figure 2a illustrates that, in normal subjects, 5 μM PGG_2 induces both platelet aggregation

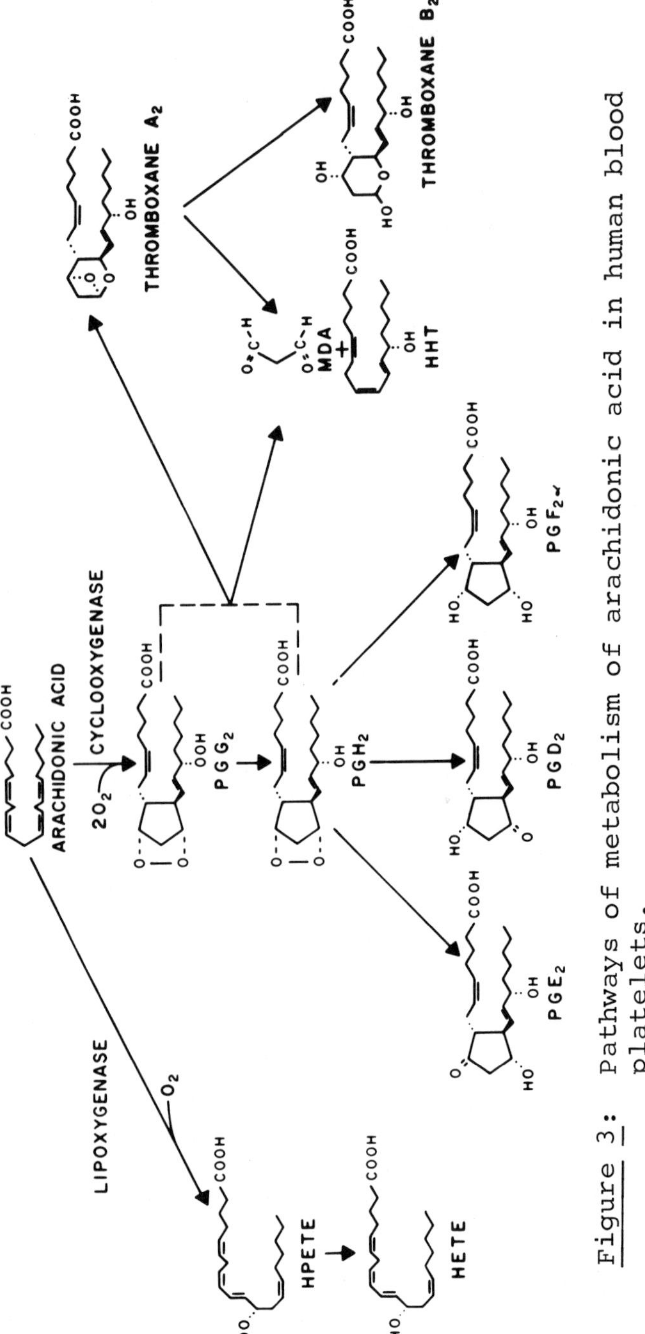

Figure 3: Pathways of metabolism of arachidonic acid in human blood platelets.

and nucleotide secretion. However, in platelet-rich plasma obtained from a patient whose platelets lack stored nucleotides, PGG_2 induces aggregation without nucleotide release (Figure 2b). Even in normal subjects, doses of PGG_2 below 2 μM can cause reversible platelet aggregation without nucleotide release.

Aggregation of platelets by PGG_2 is in many ways similar to that produced by the proteolytic enzyme, thrombin. As little as 0.1 U/ml (about 10^{-9}M) thrombin induces aggregation in citrated platelet-rich plasma (13) and thrombin also causes the release of ADP from platelets (14). However, the aggregation of platelets by thrombin can occur in the presence of ATP, an ADP-antagonist (15) and thrombin aggregates non-mammalian thrombocytes which are not aggregated by ADP (16).

Although both PGG_2 and thrombin can aggregate platelets without releasing ADP, of course normally they will release ADP. Furthermore, both of these agents act synergistically with the ADP they release (17,18,19).

THROMBOXANE A_2 INDUCES AGGREGATION

In 1973, it was demonstrated that arachidonic acid can induce platelet aggregation (20,21) and it seemed probably that this was due to its conversion by the platelets into the prostaglandin endoperoxides PGG_2 and PGH_2. The finding, during arachidonate-induced aggregation, of endoperoxide-like material which was reducible with stannous chloride to $PGF_{2\alpha}$ also supported this view (22). Furthermore, it was shown that arachidonate can aggregate platelets depleted of releasable ADP (23). More specific insight into the role of the endoperoxides in platelet aggregation was obtained through work of Hamberg, Samuelsson and co-workers. When incubated with human platelets, arachidonic acid was shown to be transformed via the main pathways summarized in Figure 3 (24). In one pathway, arachidonic acid was converted by a lipoxygenase first into a C_{20}-hydroperoxy fatty acid (HPETE) and then into a C_{20}-hydroxy fatty acid (HETE). In a second pathway, arachidonic acid was transformed by a cyclooxygenase into PGG_2 which subsequently was almost exclusively converted into a hemiacetal derivative, now named thromboxane B_2, a C_{17}-hydroxy fatty acid (HHT) and malondialdehyde. The significance of the metabolic transformation of PGG_2 into thromboxane B_2 became apparent through the discovery of a biologically-active intermediate in this conversion (25). This intermediate had a half-life of 32 sec in saline and could be trapped as a derivative by the addition of nucleophilic reagents. Additional experiments indicated that the intermediate had a bicyclic oxane-oxetane ring system and it was given the name thromboxane A_2 because of its origin and structure.

Thromboxane A_2 has not yet been isolated but indirect evidence indicates that its biological effects are similar to but more potent than those of PGG_2.

The incubation of washed human platelets with thrombin is accompanied by the synthesis of large amounts of the end products of both pathways of arachidonic acid metabolism (26). This is because the arachidonic acid substrate is released from platelet phospholipids in response to thrombin (27). We have recently been able to show that the phospholipase activity which releases this arachidonic acid is remarkably specific. Neither oleic or linoleic acids, which are present together with arachidonic acid in the 2 position of platelet phospholipids, are released from platelets by thrombin (28).

In contrast to thrombin, the nucleotide ADP is a very poor inducer of platelet prostaglandin formation (29). Incubation of PGG_2 with platelets is accompanied by the formation of small amounts of thromboxane B_2 which results from both added PGG_2 and PGG_2 formed endogenously (unpublished observations).

OTHER PROSTAGLANDINS INHIBIT PLATELET AGGREGATION

Although PGG_2 is a potent inducer of platelet aggregation, some other prostaglandins may inhibit aggregation at concentrations one hundred fold less (Figure 4). Of the many naturally-occurring prostaglandins tested by Kloeze (30) for their ability to inhibit ADP-induced aggregation, PGE_1 was found to be an outstanding inhibitor. However, PGE_1 is rapidly metabolized *in vivo* (31) and this severely limits its use as an antithrombotic agent. The second compound in Figure 3 (ONO-747) was developed on the premise that the introduction of an ethyl group at the 17-carbon atom would reduce the rate of formation of the inactive 15-keto-PGE_1 by the 15-hydroxy prostaglandin dehydrogenase present in large amounts in the lungs. This compound is about ten times more active than PGE_1 *in vitro* and retains its anti-

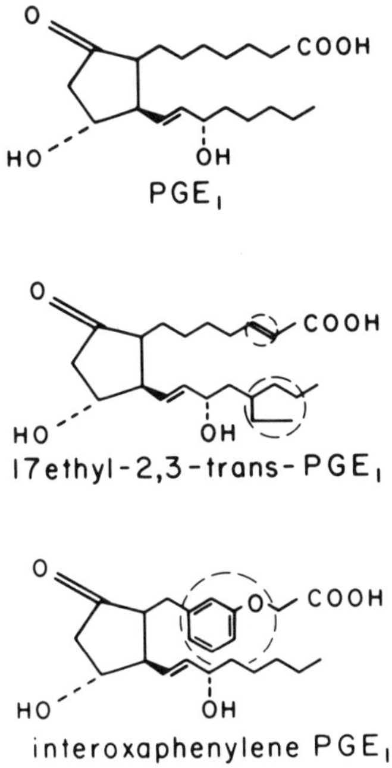

Figure 4: Structures of prostaglandins that inhibit platelet aggregation. For further details see text.

platelet effect (examined *ex vivo*) for about 10 min. after intravenous infusion (32). The third compound was designed primarily to reduce β-oxidative breakdown of the carboxyl side chain, another major route of inactivation of prostaglandins, it was also felt that the bulky m-phenylene group might reduce the rate of formation of the 15-keto-prostaglandin by steric hindrance. This compound is about ten times more active than PGE_1 *in vitro* and retains its effect for about 15 min after intravenous injection (33).

Another naturally-occurring prostaglandin, PGD_2, is about twice as potent as PGE_1 as an inhibitor of platelet aggregation *in vitro* (34,35). There is strong evidence that both of these prostaglandins inhibit aggregation by elevating platelet cyclic AMP (34,36). Prostaglandins are more potent by far than any other known agent in increasing platelet cyclic AMP and inhibiting platelet aggregation.

INHIBITORS OF CYCLOOXYGENASE ACTIVITY ALSO INHIBIT PLATELET AGGREGATION

The other major group of drugs which is being studied extensively as inhibitors of platelet aggregation are the cyclooxygenase inhibitors such as aspirin and indomethacin. These compounds inhibit the conversion of arachidonic acid into PGG_2 and consequently block arachidonate-induced aggregation in vitro (20) and arachidonate-induced death in vivo (37). These compounds have little effect on aggregation induced by either ADP (38) or by PGG_2 itself (7), presumably because both ADP and PGG_2 are weak stimulators of the phospholipase activity that releases arachidonic acid for endogenous platelet prostaglandin formation. Paradoxically, these compounds only have weak effects on the aggregation (38) or the release of ADP induced by thrombin, although this latter process does involve arachidonic acid release and endogenous prostaglandin formation (39). It seems that, just as thrombin and PGG_2 can induce platelet aggregation that is not mediated by ADP, thrombin can also induce aggregation and release that is independent of PGG_2.

THE VESSEL WALL CAN INDUCE OR INHIBIT AGGREGATION

It has been realized for some time that constituents of the vessel wall, which become available as a result of vessel injury, may initiate platelet aggregation. It was observed first that platelets adhere to newly-exposed collagen in vivo (40) and then demonstrated that collagen induces platelet aggregation in vitro (41). Aggregation by collagen is associated with the release of ADP from the platelets and for some time it was assumed that this released ADP was solely responsible for the aggregation. However, more recently, it was found that aspirin inhibits the release of ADP and aggregation induced by collagen (42) and that collagen induces platelet prostaglandin formation (29). This and other evidence has led to the hypothesis that the formation of PGG_2 is mainly responsible for the release of ADP by collagen, and aggregation results when PGG_2 and ADP act synergistically.

In the last year it has become clear that we have been neglecting the fact that constituents continuously released from the vessel wall may act to inhibit platelet aggregation. Credit for elucidation of this activity goes to Moncada, Vane and co-workers (43,44,45). Prostacyclin (PGI_2) is probably being continuously released

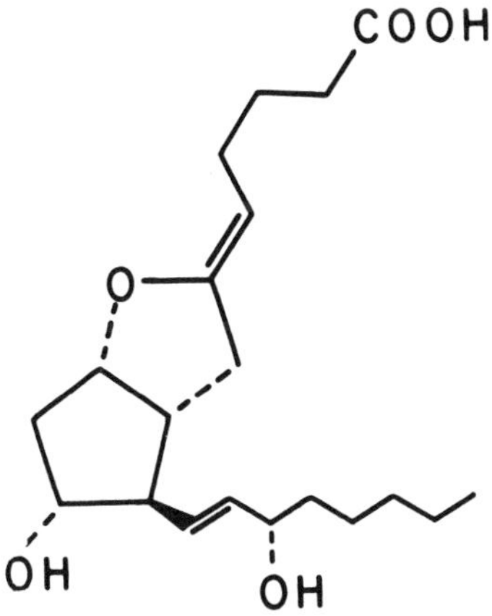

Figure 5: Structure of prostacyclin.

from endothelial cells and it causes the elevation of platelet cyclic AMP (46,47,48,49). Prostacyclin is the most potent inhibitor of aggregation presently known (Figure 5).

DRUG EFFECTS *IN VIVO*

Before discussing the possible value of any drug as an antithrombotic agent, we must consider some of the events that may be involved in thrombosis. The endothelium, which normally may release a powerful inhibitor of aggregation, becomes damaged. Collagen fibres become exposed; the platelets adhere to them and generate PGG_2. The PGG_2 induces the release of platelet ADP and causes platelet aggregation. PGG_2 is also transformed into thromboxane A_2 by platelets, or perhaps into prostacyclin by endothelial cells. Thrombin formation is initiated. The thrombin releases platelet ADP, causes platelet aggregation, induces more PGG_2 formation and begins to clot fibrinogen. Clearly, it is going to be difficult to find a single drug which counteracts this biological cascade.

Will it be of value to administer a synthetic prostaglandin to prevent thrombosis when the endothelium may be releasing prostacyclin continuously? One thought on this is that the platelets produce a hydroperoxy fatty acid HPETE during aggregation and hydroperoxy fatty acids inhibit prostacyclin formation (45). If the formation of prostacyclin is therefore "shut off" during thrombosis, obviously it will be of value to use the synthetic prostaglandin.

Will cyclooxygenase inhibitors such as aspirin prevent thrombosis? Although these drugs inhibit platelet aggregation that involves the formation of PGG_2 they are only weak inhibitors of aggregation and release induced by thrombin or of the aggregation induced by ADP. Furthermore, they may reduce the production of prostacyclin by the endothelial cells and thereby increase the extent to which thrombin can induce aggregation. Incidentally, this might explain why aspirin has little effect on bleeding except in patients who have defective mechanisms of thrombin generation (50). If arterial thrombosis is largely dependent on the production of PGG_2 and thromboxane A_2, and independent of thrombin generation, aspirin should prevent thrombosis.

What new approaches can we pursue in the light of our knowledge of prostacyclin and thromboxane formation? Well, of course, the speculations are rampant. Are lipid hydroperoxides harmful because they inhibit prostacyclin formation? Will we prevent thrombosis if we selectively inhibit thromboxane formation? Will it be of value to consume 8,11,14-eicosatrienoic acid which is neither the precursor of thromboxane A_2 nor prostacyclin, but is the precursor of PGE_1? Can we synthesize stable analogues of prostacyclin or antagonists of thromboxane?

Somewhere, amongst the answers to these questions, lies a potential therapeutic approach to the thrombosis problem. This burgeoning field has opened up because of the knowledge of platelet aggregation and prostaglandin formation acquired in the last seven years.

REFERENCES

1. Mustard, J.F. and Packham, M.A. Drugs 9: 19 (1975)
2. Mustard, J.F. and Packham, M.A. Pharmacol. Rev. 22: 97 (1970)
3. Chambers, D.A., Salzman, E.W. and Neri, L.L. In Platelets in Hemostasis. Exp. Biol. Med. 3: 62 (1968)

4. Maguire, M.H. and Michael, F.
Nature 217: 571 (1968)
5. Cusack, N.J. and Born, G.V.R.
Thrombos. Haemostas 38: 241 (1977)
6. Macfarlane, D.E. and Mills, D.C.B.
Thrombos. Haemostas 38: 241 (1977)
7. Hamberg, M., Svensson, J., Wakabayashi, T. and Samuelsson, B.
Proc. Natl. Acad. Sci.U.S.A. 71: 345 (1974a)
8. Corey, E.J., Nicolaou, K.C., Machida, Y., Malmsten, C.L. and Samuelsson, B.
Proc. Natl. Acad. Sci. U.S.A. 72: 3355 (1975)
9. Bundy, G.L.
Tetrahedron Lett. 24: 1957 (1975)
10. Malmsten, C.
Life Sciences 18: 169 (1976)
11. Malmsten, C., Hamberg, M., Svensson, J. and Samuelsson, B.
Proc. Natl. Acad. Sci. U.S.A. 72: 1446 (1975)
12. Charo, I.F., Feinman, R.D., Detwiler, T.C., Smith, J.B., Ingerman, C.M. and Silver, M.J.
Nature, in press
13. Thomas, D.P.
Nature 215: 298 (1967)
14. Haslam, R.J.
Nature 202: 765 (1964)
15. Macfarlane, D.E. and Mills, D.C.B.
Blood 46: 309 (1975)
16. Belamarich, F.A., Shepro, D. and Kien, M.
Nature 220: 509 (1968)
17. Niewiarowski, S. and Thomas, D.P.
Nature 212: 1544 (1966)
18. Packham, M.A., Guccione, M.A., Chang, P.L. and Mustard, J.F.
Amer. J. Physiol. 225: 38 (1973)
19. Smith, J.B., Ingerman, C. and Silver, M.J.
Adv. Prostagl. Thromb. Res. 2: 747 (1976)
20. Silver, M.J., Smith, J.B., Ingerman, C. and Kocsis, J.J.
Prostaglandins 4: 863 (1973)
21. Vargaftig, B.B. and Zirinis, P.
Nature 244: 114 (1973)
22. Smith, J.B., Ingerman, C., Kocsis, J.J., and Silver, M.J.
J. Clin. Invest. 53: 1468 (1974)
23. Kinlough-Rathbone, R.L., Reimers, H.J., Mustard, J.F. and Packham, M.A.
Science 192: 1011 (1976)

24. Hamberg, M. and Samuelsson, B.
Proc. Natl. Acad. Sci. U.S.A. 71: 3400 (1974)

25. Hamberg, M., Svensson, J. and Samuelsson, B.
Proc. Natl. Acad. Sci. U.S.A. 72: 2994 (1975)

26. Hamberg, M., Svensson, J. and Samuelsson, B.
Proc. Natl. Acad. Sci. U.S.A. 71: 3824 (1974b)

27. Bills, T.K., Smith, J.B. and Silver, M.J.
Biochim. Biophys. Acta 424: 303 (1976)

28. Bills, T. K., Smith, J.B. and Silver, M.J.
J. Clin. Invest. 60: 1, (1977)

29. Smith, J.B., Ingerman, C., Kocsis, J.J. and Silver, M.J.
J. Clin. Invest. 52: 965 (1973)

30. Kloeze, J.
Biochim. Biophys. Acta 187: 285 (1969)

31. Hamberg, M. and Samuelsson, B.
J. Biol. Chem. 246: 6713 (1971)

32. Ojima, M. and Fujita, K.
Adv. Prostagl. Throm. Res. 2: 781 (1976)

33. Nelson, N.A., Jackson, R.W., Au, A.T., Wynalda, D.J. and Nishizawa, E.E.
Prostaglandins 10: 795 (1975)

34. Smith, J.B. and Macfarlane, D.E.
In The Prostaglandins, P.W. Ramwell, editor, Volume 2, Plenum Press, New York, 1974, p. 293

35. Nishizawa, E.E., Miller, W.L., Gorman, R.R. and Bundy, G.L.
Prostaglandins 9: 109 (1975)

36. Mills, D.C.B. and Macfarlane, D.E.
Thromb. Res. 5: 401 (1974)

37. Silver, M.J., Hoch, W., Kocsis, J.J., Ingerman, C. and Smith, J.B.
Science 183: 1085 (1974)

38. O'Brien, J.R.
Lancet 1: 894 (1968)

39. Smith, J.B. and Willis, A.L.
Nature New Biology 231: 235 (1971)

40. Kjaerheim, A. and Hovig, T.
Thromb. Diath. Haemorrh. 7: 1 (1962)

41. Hovig, T.
Thromb. Diath. Haemorrh. 9: 264 (1963)

42. Weiss, H.J., Aledort, L.M. and Kochwa, S.
J. Clin. Invest. 47: 2169 (1968)

43. Moncada, S., Gryglewski, R., Bunting, S. and Vane, J.R.
Nature 263: 663 (1976)

44. Moncada, S., Higgs, E.A. and Vane, J.R.
Lancet 1: 18 (1977)

45. Gryglewski, R., Bunting, S., Moncada, S., Flower, R.J. and Vane, J.R.
Prostaglandins 12: 685 (1976)
46. Johnson, R.A., Morton, D.R., Kinner, J.H., Gorman, R.R., McGuire, J.C. and Sun, F.F.
Prostaglandins 12: 915 (1976)
47. Gorman, R.R., Bunting, S. and Miller, O.V.
Prostaglandins 13: 377 (1977)
48. Tateson, J.E., Moncada, S. and Vane, J.R.
Prostaglandins 13: 389 (1977)
49. Weksler, B.B., Marcus, A.J. and Jaffe, E.A.
Proc. Natl. Acad. Sci. U.S.A., in press
50. Smith, J.B., Silver, M.J., Ingerman, C.M. and Kocsis, J.J.
Thromb. Res. 5: 291 (1974)

DRUG EFFECTS ON PLATELET ADHERENCE TO COLLAGEN AND DAMAGED VESSEL WALLS

M.A. Packham, J.-P. Cazenave, R.L. Kinlough-Rathbone and J.F. Mustard

Department of Biochemistry, University of Toronto, Toronto, Ontario; and Department of Pathology, McMaster University, Hamilton, Ontario, Canada

ABSTRACT

The interaction of platelets with damaged vessel walls leads to the formation of platelet-fibrin thrombi and may also contribute to the development of atherosclerotic lesions because platelets adherent to exposed collagen release a mitogen that stimulates smooth muscle cell proliferation. The first step in thrombus formation, platelet adherence to an injured vessel wall, can be studied quantitatively by the use of platelets labeled with ^{51}chromium. In these investigations, rabbit aortas were damaged by passage of a balloon catheter and segments of the aortas were everted on probes that were rotated in platelet suspensions. Collagen-coated glass cylinders were also used. Adherence was measured in a medium containing approximately physiologic concentrations of calcium, magnesium, protein and red blood cells. Conditions of testing influence the effect of non-steroidal anti-inflammatory drugs, sulfinpyrazone, and dipyridamole on platelet adherence. Aspirin and sulfinpyrazone were not inhibitory when tested in a medium with a 40% hematocrit; this indicates that products formed by platelets from arachidonate probably do not play a major part in the adherence of the first layer of platelets to the surface, although they may be involved in thrombus formation. Indomethacin, dipyridamole, prostaglandin E_1, methylprednisolone and penicillin G and related antibiotics did inhibit platelet adherence although the concentrations required were higher than would likely be achieved *in vivo* upon administration to human patients. None of the non-steroidal anti-inflammatory drugs inhibited the release of granule contents from adherent platelets. Pretreatment of the damaged vessel wall with aspirin increased platelet adherence, presumably because it prevented the formation of PGI_2 by the vessel wall. Platelet adherence to undamaged or damaged vessel walls was enhanced by prior exposure of the wall to thrombin. Platelet reactions with aggregating agents and platelet survival can be modified by changes in dietary lipids but there is very little evidence concerning the effects of lipids on platelet adherence. If some forms of dietary fat damage the endothelium, platelet interaction with the damaged area and release of the mitogen for smooth muscle cells would contribute to the development of atherosclerotic lesions.

RESPONSE OF PLATELETS TO VESSEL WALL INJURY

The interaction of platelets with blood vessel walls, particularly with damaged vessel walls, has attracted more and more attention since it has become apparent that platelets play a role in the development of atherosclerosis associated with vessel wall injury (1-5). Although the mechanisms through which platelets or platelet aggregates cause endothelial injury are not established, there is no question concerning the fact that platelets release or form materials which affect the vessel wall. These materials include vasoactive compounds - ADP, serotonin, histamine, epinephrine - from platelet granules (6); the enzymes collagenase (7) and elastase (8); factors that increase endothelial permeability (9-12); prostaglandins and thromboxanes (13-15) and, as demonstrated by the work of Ross and his colleagues (5,16), a factor that is mitogenic for smooth muscle cells. This mitogenic factor released by platelets when they react at an injury site on a vessel wall undoubtedly plays a role in the development of atherosclerotic lesions. Moore and his colleagues (17) have demonstrated that platelets are involved in the development of atherosclerotic lesions in response to repeated vessel injury. In their experiments, thrombocytopenic rabbits were compared with normal rabbits; both groups were fed standard rabbit chow without lipid supplement. In response to a cannula inserted through the femoral artery into the aorta and left *in situ* for several months, the normal rabbits developed extensive atherosclerotic lesions whereas the thrombocytopenic rabbits had fewer and much smaller lesions. It seems likely that in the normal rabbits, platelets interacted repeatedly with the mechanically damaged wall, releasing the mitogenic factor at the injury site and thus promoting the development of the lesions. It has also been shown that thrombocytopenia prevents the intimal thickening that occurs after balloon injury of the rabbit aorta (18).

The interaction of platelets with the subendothelium at an injury site on a vessel wall not only results in the release or loss of materials from the platelets but also leads to platelet aggregation. Platelets adhere to the microfibrils in the subendothelium, to the basement membrane, and to collagen and it has been demonstrated that platelets which adhere to collagen release the contents of their storage granules (19). These contents include the platelet aggregating agents ADP and serotonin (6). Digestion of the subendothelial surface of the rabbit aorta with collagenase greatly reduces the adhesion of platelets to the surface and prevents the formation of platelet aggregates (19). In addition, when platelets interact with collagen, the arachidonate pathway is activated; this results in the formation of prostaglandin endoperoxides (PGG_2 and PGH_2) and thromboxane A_2 These unstable compounds are also capable of causing platelet aggregation (20-23).

The released ADP and the products formed from arachidonate cause disc-shaped platelets flowing past the injury site to change shape and adhere to the platelets already adherent to collagen and to each other, forming a mass of aggregated platelets. The coagulation pathway is also activated in a number of ways. Exposed collagen activates factor XII (24) and, according to some investigators (25) factor XI is activated on the surface of platelets aggregated by collagen although contradictory results have been reported (26). In addition, platelet factor 3 becomes available on the surface of the aggregated platelets (27) and accelerates two steps of the coagulation pathway (28). Factor XII has also been reported to be activated on the surface of platelets aggregated by ADP (29) and tissue thrombo-plastin from the injured cells of the vessel wall activates the extrinsic coagulation pathway (30).

Activation of the coagulation pathways leads to the formation of thrombin around the platelet aggregate. Thrombin has several effects. It causes the release of platelet storage granule contents (6) and, by activating the phospholipase A_2, promotes the formation of the prostaglandin endoperoxides and thromboxane A_2 (21,31); in addition, thrombin induces platelet aggregation through another, independent mechanism (32,33). Thus thrombin acts in a number of ways to cause further platelet aggregation and release of granule contents, including the mitogenic factor, at the injury site. Thrombin also causes fibrinogen to polymerize to fibrin and platelets adhere to the polymerizing fibrin (34) which stabilizes the platelet mass. Platelets do not adhere to fully polymerized fibrin and thus the fibrin mesh around the aggregated platelets may limit the size of the thrombus. Red cells are trapped in the thrombus and polymorphonuclear leukocytes are attracted by the chemotactic factors that form when platelets aggregate (35,36).

Platelets do not normally interact with undamaged vessel walls so the first consideration must be the factors that may damage the wall and expose the subendothelium. These include bacteria and endotoxin, viruses, antigen-antibody complexes, some hormones, thrombin, platelet aggregates, homocystine, carbon monoxide (which is a constituent of the smoke from tobacco) and hypercholesterolemia (hyperlipidemia)(28,37-43). Hemodynamic effects may also be responsible for injury (44). At the present time we do not know which drugs may be useful to lessen vessel wall injury but modification of plasma lipids by diet or drugs may reduce the risk of endothelial injury caused by some lipids.

In addition to modifying the effects of some of the factors responsible for vessel wall injury, it may be possible to interfere with some of the subsequent events. Theoretically, it might be feasible to inhibit the initial adherence of platelets to the subendothelium, to inhibit aggregation, to inhibit the release of granule contents, or to inhibit the activation of the arachidonate pathway. Inhibition of the activity of thrombin would also have a major effect on thrombus formation and on the release of materials from platelets. Agents which block any of these steps would be expected to diminish the extent of thrombus formation at an injury site and prevent the release of platelet granule contents, including the mitogenic factor for smooth muscle cells.

METHODS FOR MEASURING PLATELET ADHERENCE

It is useful to have techniques for quantifying platelet adherence to damaged vessel walls because of the potential benefit of developing methods to inhibit this first step in the interaction of platelets with the subendothelium. Quantitative methods for measuring platelet adherence have permitted investigations of the factors and conditions that influence adherence and of the effects of drugs on platelet adherence. The two principal methods that have been developed are the morphometric technique of Baumgartner and his colleagues (19) and the radio-isotopic method of Cazenave and his coworkers (45). These techniques have been applied to studies of platelet adherence to the subendothelium of rabbit aortas damaged with a balloon-catheter (19,45) and to surfaces coated with collagen, one of the main subendothelial constituents to which platelets adhere and the principal one that induces the platelet release reaction (45-47). In Baumgartner's method, the surface is examined microscopically for platelets in contact with the surface, platelets spread out on the surface, and platelet thrombi on the surface; in most experiments plasma or whole blood containing an anticoagulant has been used in a perfusion type of system.

In the method developed by Cazenave and coworkers (45), the platelets are labeled with ^{51}chromium, washed and resuspended in Tyrode's solution or Eagle's minimal essential medium. These solutions contain approximately physiologic concentrations of calcium and magnesium. The enzyme apyrase is included in the media to destroy any released ADP and hence inhibit platelet aggregation, both on the surface and in the platelet suspension. Albumin and red blood cells are also included in the media. Collagen-coated glass cylinders, or everted segments of rabbit aorta are mounted on probes that are rotated in the suspensions of washed platelets at 37° for 10 min. at 200 rpm. The probes are rinsed in an EDTA solution before determination of the amount of radioactive chromium (indicative of adherent platelets) associated with them; this treatment ensures that if even a few small aggregates are present on the surfaces, they are removed. In contrast to the studies of Baumgartner and his colleagues (19,46), our investigations have been directed only at an investigation of the adherence of individual platelets to the surfaces, rather than the formation of thrombi on the surfaces. Although most experiments have been done with rabbit platelets, similar results have been obtained with human platelets and collagen-coated surfaces.

One of the advantages of using ^{51}Cr-labeled platelets for adherence studies is that a much larger surface area can be examined than is possible with morphometric techniques. The method is also much less time-consuming than the morphometric technique. Measurement of the radioactivity associated with the surface gives a precise estimate of platelet adherence because ^{51}Cr is not lost when platelets adhere or release their granule contents (47). We have not observed any appreciable loss of label that would be evident if platelet lysis occurred to any significant extent. In addition, any ^{51}Cr lost from the platelets is not taken up by collagen, or the endothelium or subendothelium. Thus we believe that ^{51}Cr-labeling is a simple and accurate method for the measurement of platelet adherence. In contrast, labeled serotonin is not suitable for platelet adherence studies because it is released when the platelets interact with collagen and is readily taken up by the vessel wall. Studies of platelet adherence by other investigators have also been done with ^{51}Cr-labeled platelets (48-50).

EXPERIMENTAL CONDITIONS THAT AFFECT PLATELET ADHERENCE

The effect of divalent cations, particularly calcium and magnesium, on platelet adherence is illustrated in Table 1. The chelating agents citrate, EGTA and EDTA strongly inhibited adherence to the collagen-coated surface and to the everted surface of the damaged rabbit aorta. Although Baumgartner and his colleagues (19,51) have also reported that platelet adherence to the subendothelium is abolished when 0.1% EDTA is used as an anticoagulant in blood, several studies of platelet adherence have been reported in which this chelating agent has been used (52-54). In our experiments (45) (Table 1) 13 mM citrate inhibited adherence to almost the same extent as EDTA, but Baumgartner and his co-workers (19) have reported that a concentration of more than 25 mM citrate is required to inhibit adherence in their system. Because of the evident role of divalent cations in platelet adherence, studies in which chelating agents have been used to prevent coagulation of whole blood or platelet-rich plasma may not be relevant to the *in vivo* situation. We have found that the presence of chelating agents sometimes modifies the apparent effects of drugs on platelet adherence (55).

The protein concentration in the medium also affects platelet adherence. Increasing the albumin concentration

Table 1

EFFECTS OF CHELATING AGENTS ON ADHERENCE OF ^{51}Cr-LABELED RABBIT PLATELETS

Chelating agent		Adherence (% of control)*	
		Collagen-coated surface	Damaged aorta
Citrate	13 mM	25 ± 1.0	8.3 ± 0.9
EGTA	4 mM	24 ± 0.6	2.8 ± 1.1
EDTA	4 mM	22 ± 0.9	4.5 ± 0.7

^{51}Cr-labeled platelets were suspended in Tyrode solution containing 4% albumin, 40% red blood cells, and apyrase.

*Mean ± S.E. of 8 segments (collagen) or 10 segments (aorta) (see references 45,47, and 55 for a detailed description of the method used). Adherence was determined from the amount of ^{51}chromium that became associated with the surface when it was rotated in the platelet suspension. The number of platelets that adhered in the control samples (no chelating agent added) was assigned a value of 100% and adherence values for the other samples were expressed as percentages of these control values.

from 0.35% to 4% diminished the number of adherent platelets and reduced the variance of the results.

Baumgartner and Muggli (19) have discussed the role of protein in the medium on the result of platelet adherence studies, pointing out that the presence of protein "profoundly influences the adhesion reaction," in comparison to adhesion in a suspending medium devoid of protein. Red blood cells increase the number of adherent platelets in the Couette flow system (45) and similar observations concerning the effect of red blood cells have been made in other types of flow systems (19,56-58) and by other investigators (59) with the rotating probe device. The role of red cells appears to be to increase the diffusion of platelets to the surface by physical effects on the platelets.

DRUG EFFECTS ON PLATELET ADHERENCE

The experimental conditions used to study platelet adherence affect the results obtained with non-steroidal anti-inflammatory drugs and other drugs that inhibit platelet functions. Thus, differences in methodology may account for the contradictory reports in the literature concerning the effects of drugs on platelet adherence (52-55,60-62). The effect of the hematocrit of the suspending medium is shown in Table 2. In this medium, containing 0.35% albumin, aspirin inhibited adherence to the damaged vessel wall when the hematocrit of the suspending medium was 20% but not when it was 40%. In contrast, the inhibitory effect of sulfinpyrazone at this concentration was demonstrable, although greatly reduced, when the red blood cell concentration was raised to 40%. The inhibitory effect of dipyridamole was less affected by the increase in hematocrit. In experiments with collagen-coated surfaces in a medium containing 4% albumin and a 40% hematocrit, aspirin and sulfinpyrazone had no apparent effect on adherence although indomethacin was partially inhibitory, even at a concentration of 1μM (Table 3). Similar results have been obtained with everted damaged rabbit aortas. Since all of these non-steroidal anti-inflammatory drugs, and sulfinpyrazone, inhibit the arachidonate pathway in platelets (63-66) and thus prevent the formation of the prostaglandin endoperoxides (PGG_2 and PGH_2) and of thromboxane A_2, it can be concluded that products formed by platelets when the arachidonate pathway is activated do not play a major part in platelet adherence. Indomethacin may act through

Table 2

EFFECT OF HEMATOCRIT ON INHIBITION OF RABBIT PLATELET ADHERENCE TO DAMAGED AORTA BY DRUGS

Drug	Hematocrit (%)	Adherence (% of control) (mean ± S.E.)	P
ASA, 100 μM	20	53 ± 6	< 0.05
ASA, 100 μM	40	100 ± 5	N.S.
Sulfinpyrazone, 100 μM	20	42 ± 6	< 0.05
Sulfinpyrazone, 100 μM	40	82 ± 3	< 0.05
Dipyridamole, 100 μM	20	44 ± 8	< 0.05
Dipyridamole, 100 μM	40	68 ± 3	< 0.05

^{51}Cr-labeled platelets were suspended in Eagle's medium containing 0.35% albumin, 5 mM HEPES buffer and apyrase. Drugs were incubated for 10 min. with the platelet suspension before addition of red blood cells. Platelet count 700,000 per mm^3.

See footnote of Table 1 for method of calculating adherence. Two types of control samples were used: one with 20% hematocrit and one with 40% hematocrit. Adherence was calculated as a percentage of the value of the appropriate control sample.

Table 3

EFFECT OF NON-STEROIDAL ANTI-INFLAMMATORY DRUGS ON RABBIT PLATELET ADHERENCE TO A COLLAGEN-COATED SURFACE

Drug		Adherence* (% of control)	P
None		100	
Indomethacin	100 μM	69	<0.001
Indomethacin	1 μM	69	<0.001
ASA	250 μM	95	N.S.
Sulfinpyrazone	250 μM	97	N.S.

^{51}Cr-labeled platelets were suspended in Tyrode solution containing 4% albumin, 5 mM HEPES buffer and apyrase. Drugs were incubated for 10 min. with the platelet suspension before addition of red blood cells to give a hematocrit of 40%. Platelet count 300,000 per mm^3.

* See footnote of Table 1 for method of calculating adherence.

another, unknown mechanism in exerting its inhibitory effect. In agreement with these observations, Baumgartner and Muggli (60) reported that aspirin did not alter platelet adherence to the subendothelium either *in vitro* with citrated blood to which aspirin had been added or *in vivo* in experiments in which rabbits were given aspirin orally. Davies et al. (61) also did not observe inhibition by aspirin in an *in vitro* system with damaged rabbit aortas perfused with suspensions of washed platelets and red blood cells. However, using conditions that are much less physiologic, inhibition of platelet adherence by aspirin, sulfinpyrazone or other non-steroidal anti-inflammatory drugs can be demonstrated (52-55,62). The relevance of these observations to adherence *in vivo* is questionable.

Table 4

INHIBITION OF THE ADHERENCE OF ^{51}Cr-LABELED RABBIT PLATELETS TO A COLLAGEN-COATED SURFACE

Drug		Adherence* (% of control)
None (control)		100
Dipyridamole	100 μM	72
RA 433	100 μM	46
Prostaglandin E_1	1 μM	41
Methylprednisolone	10 mM	16
Methylprednisolone	1 mM	79
Penicillin G	13.6 mM	38
Cephalothin	13.6 mM	32

The suspending medium was Tyrode solution containing 4% albumin, 40% red blood cells and apyrase. See footnote of Table 1 for method of calculating adherence. $P<0.001$ in all experiments.

It should be emphasized, however, that aspirin and the other drugs in this group of cyclo-oxygenase inhibitors do produce some inhibition of thrombus formation at injury sites on vessel walls (60,67,68).

Other drugs that have been found to inhibit platelet adherence *in vitro* are listed in Table 4. In many cases, the inhibitory concentrations are much higher than can be safely achieved upon administration to human subjects. Dipyridamole and its analog RA 433 inhibit the phosphodiesterase of platelets that normally catalyses the hydrolysis of cyclic AMP (68,69). As a consequence, the level of cyclic AMP in the platelets rises and it seems possible that this may be responsible for part of the inhibition of adherence. Evidence for this is the strong inhibitory effect of prostaglandin E_1 (PGE_1) on platelet adherence, even at very low concentrations (45). PGE_1 is known to raise platelet cyclic AMP levels by stimulating adenylate cyclase on the platelet membrane (68,70, 71). Prostaglandin E_1 inhibits not only platelet adherence but also the platelet release reaction, platelet aggregation and the initial shape change of platelets that follows the addition of aggregating agents (68,72). It may be that its ability to prevent the platelets from changing shape is responsible for the inhibition of adherence. However, PGE_1 has too short a half-life in the circulation for any practical purposes (73,74).

Methylprednisolone also inhibits platelet adherence but the concentrations required are higher than those that would be achieved upon administration of this drug to human patients. Other experiments have shown that methylprednisolone in these concentrations inhibits platelet shape change in response to most aggregating agents and this may account for its inhibitory effect on adherence (75). In other cell systems, corticosteroids have been shown to inhibit the initiation of the arachidonate pathway (76) and they may also have this effect in platelets. Penicillin G and related antibiotics strongly inhibit platelet adherence to a collagen-coated surface and to the damaged aorta (77). These antibiotics inhibit most platelet reactions and are thought to coat the surface of platelets and thus prevent platelets from interacting with aggregating and release-inducing agents (68,77-79). Their inhibition of platelet adherence to collagen and damaged vessel walls and their inhibition of platelet aggregation may be responsible for the abnormal bleeding observed in patients given extremely high doses of these antibiotics (79-81).

EFFECTS OF DRUGS ON RELEASE OF GRANULE CONTENTS FROM ADHERENT PLATELETS

All of the drugs we have examined for possible effects on platelet adherence are known to inhibit collagen-induced platelet aggregation, studied by light transmission changes in an aggregometer, and to inhibit the release of platelet granule contents in this system (33, 68,72,75,77,82-84). However, when collagen is added to platelet-rich plasma or a suspension of platelets in an aggregometer cuvette, very few of the platelets interact directly with collagen. The light transmission changes and the release of granule contents represent the reactions of the non-adherent platelets. These reactions are

Table 5

RELEASE OF ^{14}C-SEROTONIN FROM RABBIT PLATELETS ADHERENT TO A COLLAGEN-COATED SURFACE

Inhibition	Adherence* (% of control)	Release of ^{14}C-serotonin from adherent platelets (% of total in unreacted platelets)
None (control	100	35
ASA, 100 μM	102	49
Indomethacin, 100 μM	78	56
Sulfinpyrazone, 1 mM	62	73
EDTA, 10 mM	34	0

*Platelets were doubly labeled with ^{51}chromium and ^{14}C-serotonin. The suspending medium was Tyrode solution containing 4% albumin, 40% red blood cells and apyrase. The platelet count was 300,000 per mm^3. Adherence was determined as described in the footnote of Table 1.

caused by the ADP released from the adherent platelets and the thromboxane A_2 formed by them (32,33). Experiments were done with doubly labeled platelets (^{51}chromium and ^{14}C-serotonin) to determine whether or not the non-steroidal anti-inflammatory drugs could prevent the release of granule contents from platelets that adhered to collagen in the rotating probe system (Table 5). ^{51}Chromium is not readily lost from platelets; ^{14}C-serotonin is taken up into platelet amine storage granules and is released when platelets interact with collagen or thrombin. Other constituents of platelet granules (including ADP and the factor that is mitogenic for smooth muscle cells) are released in parallel with serotonin (85,86), so release of ^{14}C-serotonin represents the release of these other platelet constituents also.

Platelet adherence was measured by determining the amount of ^{51}chromium that became associated with the collagen-coated surface when it was rotated in the platelet suspension (45). The extent of release from adherent platelets was measured by comparing the ratio of ^{51}chromium to ^{14}C-serotonin in the platelets before the reaction with the ratio in the adherent platelets after the reaction. Experiments were done with and without drugs that inhibit the cyclo-oxygenase of the arachidonate pathway; the concentrations used were strongly inhibitory in the aggregometer system (32,33,87). Although indomethacin and the high concentration of sulfinpyrazone used inhibited adherence, none of the drugs inhibited the release of ^{14}C-serotonin from the adherent platelets (Table 5). The extent of release was actually enhanced by aspirin, indomethacin and sulfinpyrazone.

The finding that these drugs do not inhibit the release of serotonin from the adherent platelets indicates that they probably do not inhibit release of the mitogen when platelets adhere to collagen in a damaged vessel wall. Therefore these drugs should not be expected to have a significant effect on the smooth muscle cell proliferation that occurs in association with the development of atherosclerotic lesions in response to injury or removal of the endothelium. Indeed, Baumgartner and Studer (88) and Clowes and Karnovsky (89) have reported that aspirin does not inhibit the smooth muscle cell proliferation that occurs after removal of the endothelium in experimental animals.

In contrast, chelation of divalent cations with EDTA prevented release of ^{14}C-serotonin from the adherent rabbit platelets (Table 5).

EFFECT OF ASPIRIN ON THE VESSEL WALL

When a vessel wall is injured platelets adhere and release materials that affect the vessel wall but, in addition, the vessel wall can form materials that affect platelet reactions. Of most interest at the moment is prostaglandin I_2 (also termed PGX or prostacyclin). Several groups have shown that the vessel wall can form PGI_2 from the prostaglandin endoperoxides PGG_2 and PGH_2 (13,90,91). PGI_2 is a potent inhibitor of platelet aggregation and the release reaction and, like PGE_1, it raises platelet cyclic AMP levels (92,93). The precursors of PGI_2, the prostaglandin endoperoxides, arise through the arachidonate pathway, occurring either in the platelets or in the injured vessel wall or in both. The conversion of arachidonate to PGG_2 is catalysed by the cyclo-oxygenase enzyme and hence drugs such as aspirin that inhibit this enzyme would be expected to block the formation of PGI_2. The effect of PGI_2 on platelet adherence has not been studied but by analogy with PGE_1, it would be expected to inhibit adherence.

The effect of aspirin pretreatment of platelet or of the damaged vessel wall was investigated with the rotating probe system. Unreacted aspirin was removed by suspending the platelets in a fresh medium or rinsing the aorta segment before platelet adherence was measured. Pretreatment of the platelets with aspirin did not affect the number of platelets that adhered to the damaged surface of the aorta but pretreatment of the damaged wall with aspirin increased platelet adherence significantly in comparison with control values (94). This observation is in keeping with the concept that aspirin would block PGI_2 formation by the vessel wall so that any inhibitory effect of PGI_2 on platelet adherence could not occur. Thus in this type of study it is possible to show that aspirin can actually promote platelet adherence to the damaged wall. Baumgartner and his colleagues (95) have also observed enhanced adherence of single platelets to the subendothelium in the presence of aspirin. A number of years ago, Ts'ao (96) observed that in rabbit vessels subjected to a standardized injury, platelet adherence to damaged endothelial cells was more frequent when the animals had been treated with aspirin. It should be emphasized, however, that the rotating probe technique (45) measures the adherence of individual platelets to the damaged wall and does not estimate thrombus formation, which does appear to be inhibited by aspirin (67,95).

Further experiments (94) have shown that if the wall is not damaged, aspirin pretreatment does not affect platelet adherence. Of course, adherence to an undamaged endothelial surface is very low and there is no stimulus to activate the arachidonate pathway either in the platelets or in the wall. Thus it seems unlikely that the intact vessel wall continuously forms PGI_2 and one should look elsewhere for an explanation for the non-thrombogenic property of the endothelium. Previously it was attributed to the surface coat on the endothelial cells (97).

EFFECT OF THROMBIN ON THE VESSEL WALL

Since platelets have been observed to adhere to glass surfaces that have been exposed to thrombin (98), it seemed possible that a vessel wall exposed to thrombin might also become attractive to platelets. Exposure of undamaged endothelium to thrombin, followed by rinsing and rotation in a platelet suspension led to much increased platelet adherence to the thrombin-treated surface (94,99). It is not known whether thrombin affects the endothelial cells so that they lose their nonthrombogenic surface, or whether it adheres to them and presents an adherent surface to the circulating platelets. Possibly both effects occur. Heparin prevented the effect of thrombin on platelet adherence to the undamaged aorta. Aubrey and his colleagues (100) have shown that thrombin promotes platelet adherence to endothelial cells in culture.

Platelet adherence to injured aortic surfaces was also promoted by pretreatment of the aorta with thrombin, and adherence was inhibited by heparin. Thus inhibition of thrombin formation or of its activity would be expected to have inhibitory effects not only on the coagulation pathway but on any aspects of platelet adherence in which thrombin is involved and possibly also on the thrombin-induced release of granule contents, including the mitogenic factor. In accord with the concept that thrombin may promote platelet adherence and release of granule contents, Clowes and Karnovsky (101) found that heparin blocked the smooth muscle cell proliferation associated with vessel wall injury in rats.

ROLE OF LIPIDS IN PLATELET ADHERENCE TO THE VESSEL WALL

The effects of lipids in the interaction of platelets with vessel walls are not well understood. There are three lines of evidence about the effect of lipids on platelet function: (a) changes in the response to platelets to agents that cause aggregation and release; (b) effects on platelet adherence to collagen and the subendothelial structures; (c) effects on platelet survival. Table 6 summarizes the reported effects of dietary fats on platelet aggregation, tested *in vitro*. When animals or humans are fed diets rich in polyunsaturated fatty acids such as linoleic acid, the sensitivity of the platelets to aggregating agents such as ADP is decreased, as shown by Hornstra and his colleagues (102). The exact

Table 6

EFFECTS OF DIETARY LIPIDS IN THE SENSITIVITY OF PLATELETS TO AGGREGATION

Dietary lipid	Effect on platelet aggregation	Reference
Low fat	decreased	110
Linoleic	decreased	102,111,112
Dihomo-γ-linolenic	decreased	103,104
γ-linolenic	decreased	103
Cholesterol	increased	113,114
Stearic or butter	increased*	108
Arachidonic	increased	107

*Aggregation in response to thrombin was increased, but aggregation in response to ADP or collagen was decreased in these experiments with rats.

mechanism responsible for this effect is not known. Furthermore, it has been demonstrated by some investigators (103,104) (but not by others, 105) that feeding dihomo-γ-linolenic acid decreases platelet responsiveness. This fatty acid is thought to exert its effect by serving as a precursor of prostaglandin E_1 which is known to inhibit most platelet reactions. Recently it has been shown that this fatty acid has a significant inhibitory effect on platelet adhesion to collagen (106). In contrast, when human subjects were fed diets enriched in arachidonic acid, the second phase of platelet aggregation in response to ADP was enhanced (107), possibly because enrichment of the platelet membrane phospholipids with arachidonate led to increased production of thromboxane A_2 when the platelet phospholipase A_2 was stimulated by the close platelet-to-platelet contact induced by ADP. When platelets were harvested from rats given diets rich in butter or stearic acid, the platelets were much more sensitive to thrombin-induced platelet aggregation than platelets from rats given diets that were rich in corn oil (108). In these experiments, butter fat or saturated fatty acids were found to make the rats more susceptible to endotoxin-induced thrombosis.

Since platelet survival appears to reflect vessel wall injury, the effects of dietary fat on platelet survival are of interest. In the early 1960's, Mustard and Murphy (109) found that when human subjects were given diets rich in butter fat and egg-yolk, platelet survival was shorter than it was when the same subjects were given a low fat diet or a diet rich in vegetable fat. Recently, Ross and Harker (43) reported that when hypercholesterolemic diets were given to monkeys, endothelial damage occurred and platelet survival was shortened. Thus it is possible that dietary fat may have at least two effects: (a) modification of platelet function and (b) modification of the interaction of platelets with the vessel wall, thereby producing effects on platelet survival. If some forms of dietary fat do damage the endothelium, this would lead to increased stimulus to the development of atherosclerosis through the release of the mitogenic factor from platelets.

REFERENCES

1. Mustard, J.F. and Packham, M.A.
Thromb. Diath. Haemorrh. 33: 444 (1975)
2. Mustard, J.F., Moore, S., Packham, M.A. and Kinlough-Rathbone, R.L.
In: Proceedings of the First International Atherosclerosis Conference," Prog. Biochem. Pharmacol., Karger, Basel (in press).
3. Ross, R., Glomset, J. and Harker, L.A.
Am. J. Pathol. 86: 675 (1977)
4. Davignon, J.
In: Hypertension: Physiopathology and Treatment
J. Genest, E. Koiw and O. Kuchel, editors, McGraw-Hill, 1977, in press.
5. Ross, R. and Glomset, J.A.
New Engl. J. Med. 7:369 (1976)
6. Holmsen, H.
In: Biochemistry and Pharmacology of Platelets, Ciba Foundation Symposium 35, Elsevier, New York, 1975, p. 175
7. Chesney, C.M., Harper, E. and Colman, R.W.
J. Clin. Invest. 53: 1647 (1974)

8. Legrand, Y., Pignaud, G. and Caen, J.P. Haemostasis 6: 180 (1977)
9. Packham, M.A., Nishizawa, E.E. and Mustard, J.F. Biochem. Pharmacol. (Suppl.): 171 (1968)
10. Nachman, R.L., Weksler, B. and Ferris, B. J. Clin. Invest. 51: 549 (1972)
11. Moncada, S., Ferreira, S.H. and Vane, J.R. Nature 246: 217 (1973)
12. Kuehl, F.A., Jr., Humes, J.L., Egan, R.W., Ham, E.A., Beveridge, G.C. and van Arman, C.G. Nature 265: 170 (1977)
13. Bunting, S., Gryglewski, R., Moncada, S. and Vane, J.R. Prostaglandins 12:897 (1976)
14. Svensson, J. and Hamberg, M. Prostaglandins 12: 943 (1976)
15. Needleman, P., Kulkarni, P.S. and Raz, A. Science 195: 409 (1977)
16. Ross, R., Glomset, J., Kariya, B. and Harker, L. Proc. Natl. Acad. Sci. USA 71: 1207 (1974)
17. Moore, S., Friedman, R.J., Singal, D.P. Gauldie, J., Blajchman, M.A. and Roberts, R.S. Thrombos. Haemostasis 35: 70 (1976)
18. Friedman, R.J., Stemerman, M.B., Wenz, B., Moore, S., Gauldie, J., Gent, M., Tiell, M.L. and Spaet, T.H. J. Clin. Invest., in press
19. Baumgartner, H.R., Muggli, R., Tschopp, T.B. and Turitto, V.T. Thrombos. Haemostasis 35: 124 (1976)
20. Smith, J.B., Ingerman, C., Kocsis, J.J. and Silver, M.J. J. Clin. Invest. 53: 1468 (1974)
21. Willis, A.L., Vane, F.M., Kuhn, D.C., Scott, C.G. and Petrin, M. Prostaglandins 8: 453 (1974)
22. Hamberg, M. and Samuelsson, B. Proc. Natl. Acad. Sci. USA 71: 3400 (1974)
23. Hamberg, M., Svensson, J. and Samuelsson, B. Proc. Natl. Acad. Sci. USA 72: 2994 (1975)
24. Niewiarowski, S., Stuart, R.K. and Thomas, D.P. Proc. Soc. Exp. Biol. Med. 123: 196 (1966)
25. Walsh, P.N. Br. J. Haematol. 22: 237 (1972)
26. Schiffman, S., Rimon, A. and Rapaport, S.I. Br. J. Haematol. 35: 429 (1977)
27. Joist, J.H., Dolezel, G., Lloyd, J.V., Kinlough-Rathbone, R.L. and Mustard, J.F. J. Lab. Clin. Med. 84: 474 (1974)

28. Mustard, J.F. and Packham, M.A.
In: Inflammation, Immunity and Hypersensitivity, H.Z. Movat, editor, Harper and Row, New York, 1971, p. 528
29. Walsh, P.N.
Blood 43: 597 (1974)
30. Nemerson, Y. and Pitlick, F.A.
In: Progress in Hemostasis and Thrombosis, T.H. Spaet, editor, Vol. 1, Grune and Stratton, New York, 1972, p. 1
31. Bills, T.K. Smith, J.B. and Silver, M.J.
J. Clin. Invest. 60: 1 (1977)
32. Packham, M.A., Kinlough-Rathbone, R.L., Reimers, H.-J., Scott, S. and Mustard, J.F.
In: Prostaglandins in Hematology, M.J. Silver, J.B. Smith, J.J. Kocsis, editors, Spectrum Publications, New York, 1977, p. 247
33. Kinlough-Rathbone, R.L., Packham, M.A., Reimers, H.J., Cazenave, J.-P. and Mustard, J.F.
J. Lab. Clin. Med., in press
34. Niewiarowski, S., Regoeczi, E., Stewart, G.J., Senyi, A. and Mustard, J.F.
J. Clin. Invest. 51: 685 (1972)
35. Weksler, B.B. and Coupal, C.E.
J. Exp. Med. 137: 1419 (1973)
36. Turner, S.R., Tainer, J.A. and Lynn, W.S.
Nature 257: 680 (1975)
37. Dalldorf, F.G., Pate, D.H. and Langdell, R.D.
Arch. Pathol. 85: 149 (1968)
38. Burch, G.E.
Am. Heart J. 87: 407 (1974)
39. Hardin, N.J., Minick, C.R. and Murphy, G.E.
Am. J. Pathol. 73: 301 (1973)
40. Lough, J. and Moore, S.
Lab. Invest. 33: 130 (1975)
41. Harker, L.A., Ross, R., Slichter, S.J. and Scott, C.R.
J. Clin. Invest. 58: 731 (1976)
42. Thomsen, H.K.
Atherosclerosis 20: 233 (1974)
43. Ross, R. and Harker, L.
Science 193: 1094 (1976)
44. Fry, D.L.
Circ. Res. 22: 165 (1968)
45. Cazenave, J.-P., Packham, M.A., Davies, J.A., Kinlough-Rathbone, R.L. and Mustard, J.F.
In: The Significance of Platelet Function Tests in the Evaluation of Hemostatic and Thrombotic Tendencies, Workshop on Platelets, H.J. Day, M.B. Zucker, H. Holmsen, editors, Philadelphia, 1976, in press

46. Muggli, R. and Baumgartner, H.R.
Thromb. Diath. Haemorrh. 34: 333 (1975)
47. Cazenave, J.-P., Packham, M.A. and Mustard, J.F.
J. Lab. Clin. Med. 82: 978 (1973)
48. Dosne, A.-M., Drouet, L. and Dassin, E.
Microvasc. Res. 11: 111 (1976)
49. Schlossman, D.
Acta Radiol. Diag. 14: 97 (1973)
50. Lagergren, H., Olsson, P. and Swedenborg, J.
Surgery 75: 643 (1974)
51. Baumgartner, H.R., Stemerman, M.B. and Spaet, T.H.
Experentia 27: 283 (1971)
52. Brass, L.F., Faile, D. and Bensusan, H.B.
J. Lab. Clin. Med. 87: 525 (1976)
53. Cowan, D.H., Robertson, A.L., Jr., Giroski, P. and Shook, P.
Abstracts, 6th International Symposium on Drugs Affecting Lipid Metabolism, these proceedings
54. Lyman, B., Rosenberg, L. and Karpatkin, S.
J. Clin. Invest. 50: 1854 (1971)
55. Cazenave, J.-P., Packham, M.A., Guccione, M.A. and Mustard, J.F.
J. Lab. Clin. Med. 86: 551 (1975)
56. Goldsmith, H.L.
In: Progress in Hemostasis and Thrombosis, T.H. Spaet, editor, Vol. 1, Grune and Stratton, New York, 1972, p. 97
57. Turitto, V.T. and Baumgartner, H.R.
Microvasc. Res. 9: 335 (1975)
58. Leonard, E.F., Grabowski, E.F. and Turitto, V.T.
Ann. N.Y. Acad. Sci. 201: 329 (1972)
59. Brash, J.L., Brophy, J.M. and Feuerstein, I.A.
J. Biomed. Mat. Res. 10: 429 (1976)
60. Baumgartner, H.R. and Muggli, R.
Thromb. Diath. Haemorrh. Suppl. 60: 345 (1974)
61. Davies, J.A., Essien, E., Kinlough-Rathbone, R.L., Cazenave, J.-P. and Mustard, J.F.
Blood 46: 1003 (1975)
62. Cazenave, J.-P., Packham, M.A., Guccione, M.A. and Mustard, J.F.
J. Lab. Clin. Med. 83: 797 (1974)
63. Willis, A.L.
Science 183: 325 (1974)
64. Roth, G.J. and Majerus, P.W.
In: Prostaglandins in Hematology, M.J. Silver, J.B. Smith and J.J. Kocsis, editors, Spectrum Publications, New York, 1977, p. 345
65. Malmsten, C., Hamberg, M., Svensson, J. and Samuelsson, B.
Proc. Natl. Acad. Sci. USA 72: 1446 (1975)

66. Ali, M. and McDonald, J.W.D.
J. Lab. Clin. Med. 89: 868 (1977)
67. Danese, C.A., Voleti, C.D. and Weiss, H.J.
Thromb. Diath. Haem. 25: 288 (1971)
68. Mustard, J.F. and Packham, M.A.
In: Current Drug Reviews: Cardiology, Vol. 3, Australasia, Adis Press, in press
69. Mills, D.C.B. and Smith, J.B.
Biochem. J. 121: 185 (1971)
70. Wolfe, S.M. and Shulman, N.R.
Biochem. Biophys. Res.Commun. 35: 265 (1969)
71. Haslam, R.J.
In: Biochemistry and Pharmacology of Platelets, Ciba Foundation Symposium 35, Elsevier, New York, 1975, p. 121
72. Kinlough-Rathbone, R.L., Packham, M.A. and Mustard, J.F.
Brit. J. Haematol. 19: 559 (1970)
73. Ferreira, S.H. and Vane, J.R.
Nature 216: 868 (1967)
74. Mannucci, P.M. and Pareti, F.I.
J. Lab. Clin. Med. 84: 828 (1974)
75. Cazenave, J.-P., Davies, J.A., Senyi, A.F., Blajchman, M.A., Hirsh, J. and Mustard, J.F.
Blood 48: 1009 (1976)
76. Hong, S.-C.L. and Levine, L.
Proc. Natl. Acad. Sci. USA 73: 1730 (1976)
77. Cazenave, J.-P., Guccione, M.A., Packham, M.A. and Mustard, J.F.
Br. J. Haematol. 35: 131 (1977)
78. Cazenave, J.-P., Packham, M.A., Guccione, M.A. and Mustard, J.F.
Proc. Soc. Exptl. Biol. Med. 142: 159 (1973)
79. McClure, P.D., Casserly, J.G., Monsier, C. and Crozier, D.
Lancet 2: 1307 (1970)
80. Brown, C.H.,III, Natelson, E.A., Bradshaw, M.W., Alfrey, C.P., Jr. and Williams, T.W., Jr.
Antimicrobial Agents and Chemotherapy 7: 652 (1975)
81. Brown, C.H., III, Bradshaw, M.W., Natelson, E.A., Alfrey, C.P., Jr., and Williams, T.W., Jr.
Blood 47: 949 (1976)
82. Packham, M.A., Warrior, E.S., Glynn, M.F., Senyi, A.F. and Mustard, J.F.
J. Exp. Med. 126: 171 (1967)
83. Zucker, M.B. and Peterson, J.
J.Lab. Clin. Med. 76: 66 (1970)
84. Evans, G., Packham, M.A., Nishizawa, E.E., Mustard, J.F. and Murphy, E.A.
J. Exp. Med. 128: 877 (1968)

85. Zucker, M.B.
Thromb. Diath. Haemorrh. 28: 393 (1972)
86. Ihnatowycz, I.O., Cazenave, J.-P., Moore, S. and Mustard, J.F.
Thrombos. Haemostas. 38: 229 (1977)
87. Kinlough-Rathbone, R.L., Reimers, H.J., Mustard,J.F. and Packham, M.A.
Science 192: 1011 (1976)
88. Baumgartner, H.R. and Studer, A.
Workshop on Thrombosis and Atherosclerosis, Tokyo, 1976, personal communication
89. Clowes, A.W. and Karnovsky, M.J.
Lab. Invest. 36: 452 (1977)
90. Ho, P.P.K., Herrmann, R.G., Towner, R.D. and Walters, C.P.
Biochem. Biophys. Res. Comm. 74: 514 (1977)
91. Moncada, S., Herman, A.G., Higgs, E.A. and Vane, J.R.
Thromb. Res. 11: 323 (1977)
92. Gorman, R.R., Bunting, S. and Miller, O.V.
Prostaglandins 13: 377 (1977)
93. Tateson, J.E., Moncada, S. and Vane, J.R.
Prostaglandins 13: 389 (1977)
94. Cazenave, J.-P., Kinlough-Rathbone, R.L., Packham, M.A. and Mustard, J.F., unpublished observations
95. Baumgartner, H.R., Tschopp, T.B. and Weiss,H.J.
Thrombos, Haemostas. 37: 17 (1977)
96. Ts'ao, C.
Am. J. Pathol. 59: 327 (1970)
97. Mason, R.G., Sharp, D., Chuang, H.Y.K. and Mohammad, S.F.
Archiv. Pathol. Lab. Med. 101: 61 (1977)
98. Jenkins, C.S.P. and Packham, M.A., unpublished observations
99. Essien, E.M., Cazenave, J.-P., Moore, S. and Mustard, J.F., submitted for publication
100. Aubrey, B.J., Owen, W.G., Fry, G.L., Cheng, F.H. and Hoak, J.C.
Blood 46: 1046 (1975)
101. Clowes, A.W. and Karnovsky, M.J.
Nature 265: 625 (1977)
102. Hornstra, G.
Haemostasis 2: 21 (1973-74)
103. Sim, A.K. and McCraw, A.P.
Thrombos. Res. 10: 385 (1977)
104. Willis, A.L., Comai, K., Kuhn, D.C. and Paulsrud, J.
Prostaglandins 8: 509 (1974)
105. Oelz, O., Seyberth, H.W., Knapp, H.R. and Oates, J.A.
In: Advances in Prostaglandin and Thromboxane Research, B. Samuelsson, R. Paoletti, editors, Vol. 2 Raven,New York, 1976, p. 787

106. Kernoff, P.B.A., Davies, J.A., McNicol, G.P., Willis, A.L. and Stone, K.J.
Thrombos. Haemostas. 38: 194 (1977)

107. Seyberth, H.W., Oelz, O., Kennedy, T., Sweetman, B.J., Danon, A., Frohlich, J.C., Heimberg, M. and Oates, J.A.
Clin. Pharmacol. Therap. 18: 521 (1975)

108. Renaud, S., Kinlough, R.L. and Mustard, J.F.
Lab. Invest. 22: 339 (1970)

109. Mustard, J.F. and Murphy, E.A.
Br. Med. J. 1: 1651 (1962)

110. Iacono, J.M., Binder, R.A., Marshall, M.W., Schoene, N.W., Jencks, J.A. and Mackin, J.F.
Haemostasis 3: 306 (1974)

111. Fleischman, A.I., Justice, D., Bierenbaum, M.L., Stier, A. and Sullivan, A.
J. Nutrition 105: 1286 (1975)

112. Hornstra, G., Lewis, B., Chait, A., Turpeinen, O., Karvonen, M.J. and Vergroesen, A.J.
Lancet 1: 1155 (1973)

113. Wu, K.K., Armstrong, M.L., Hoak, J.C. and Megan, M.B.
Thrombos. Res. 7: 917 (1975)

114. Oversohl, K., Bassenge, E. and Schmid-Schonbein, H.
Thrombos. Res. 7: 481 (1975)

SELECTED ANIMAL MODELS FOR SYSTEMATIC ANTI-ATHEROSCLEROTIC DRUG DEVELOPMENT

Charles E. Day, Paul E. Schurr, and
William A. Phillips

Atherosclerosis Research, The Upjohn Company
Kalamazoo, Michigan, U.S.A.

INTRODUCTION

Even though intensive research into the control of atherosclerosis has been carried out for at least the last quarter century, no one has discovered a way unequivocally to either halt the progression or enhance the regression of this disease. This failure may in part be attributable to an inappropriate application of existing animal models and a lack of suitable models simulating human atherogenic conditions.

In this report we will evaluate several animal models that we feel may be applied to the discovery and development of effective agents to control atherosclerosis. Although we have found this system of models useful in our own drug development program, we recognize that there are myriad possibilities for other and possibly better model systems to find new anti-atherosclerotic drugs and are not recommending the use of one system above another. However, we do advocate that for whatever system is employed it be based on the best rationale available at the time.

Several assumptions will be made for which evidence to support them will not be reviewed, since such evidence has been treated exhaustively in numerous other sources. The foremost assumption is that serum low density lipoproteins (LDL) and very low density lipoproteins (VLDL) are atherogenic. An equally important theorem is that serum high density lipoproteins (HDL) are antiatherogenic. Another assumption is that, in general, _in vivo_ models are far superior to _in vitro_ systems because of considerations such as absorption, distribution, metabolism, and excretion of drugs in whole animals. In addition, it is assumed, without presenting the data to support that assumption, that arterial cholesterol content is a valid indicator of the degree of atherosclerosis in an artery in certain animal models.

Other assumptions include species variability with respect to lipoprotein metabolism and atherosclerosis development. Because of this marked variability it is extremely difficult to extrapolate activity in one species to another unrelated species. An inherent assumption in our approach is that initially random high volume screening remains the best way to discover new compounds with antiatherosclerotic activity. We are not suggesting that these assumptions are either correct or necessarily good ones. We wish simply to inform the reader of the biases under which we currently operate. Inevitably these underlying biases will change as new and better data are generated on which to build a more reasonable approach.

Several terms will be used that require a brief definition. Hypobetalipoproteinemic will be used to describe any agent that reduces atherogenic serum lipoproteins, either LDL or VLDL or both, as measured by some suitable assay such as apolipoprotein B concentration or turbidimetry after heparin precipitation. Agents that increase serum HDL levels are designated as hyperalphalipoproteinemic, and hypocholesterolaric is used to describe drugs that decrease cholesterol deposition in arteries as determined by direct assay of arterial cholesterol content. Antiatherosclerotic is reserved solely for compounds that have the demonstrated ability to significantly reduce or prevent grossly visible atherosclerosis _in vivo_. These agents may be important in prophylactic as well as therapeutic treatment of atherosclerosis.

The animal models that we have the most experience with and will evaluate in this report are the rat, Japanese quail, and cynomolgus monkey.

NORMAL RAT

The rat and mouse have been used extensively for many years in both industrial and academic atherosclerosis research. Their main use has been to evaluate the effect of test compounds on total serum cholesterol or triglycerides. In one respect this has been unfortunate since most (80%) of the serum cholesterol in these rodents is carried in the HDL. In reality researchers have been using rats and mice to search for compounds that reduce the antiatherogenic HDL. This is not a desirable use for these animals.

A more rational purpose for the normal rat in atherosclerosis research would be to look for agents that increase HDL concentration. Therefore, instead of a reduction one should look for an increase in serum total cholesterol. However, an increase in total cholesterol is still not indicative of a specific increase in HDL. Some direct assay for HDL must be used to ascertain a specific increase in this moiety. By reexamining old screening data generated years ago in normal rats and then retesting active hypercholesterolemic agents for their effect on HDL, we have discovered numerous agents that significantly and specifically elevate serum HDL cholesterol levels. In this regard the normal rat can be quite useful for detecting agents with potential antiatherosclerotic activity.

Caution should be exercised in the development of hyperalphalipoproteinemic drugs since the mechanism by which HDL is increased may be crucial for an eventual effect on atherosclerosis. Our working hypothesis is that HDL exerts its antiatherogenicity by mobilizing cholesterol from peripheral tissue stores back to the liver where its cholesterol load can be excreted in the bile or degraded to bile acids and excreted. Should a hyperalphalipoproteinemic agent act by blocking hepatic uptake of HDL for example, then, presumably, that agent would have no effect, or possibly even an undesirable effect, on atherogenesis. We, therefore, strongly recommend that all confirmed hyperalphalipoproteinemic agents discovered in animal models such as the rat be routinely tested in another animal model for their effect on the inhibition of experimental atherosclerosis.

Presently, there is little evidence to suggest that the normal rat will not be a good model for the initial discovery of hyperalphalipoproteinemic agents. It will take some time though to demonstrate whether such activity in rats correlates positively with activity in other species including man.

HYPERCHOLESTEROLEMIC RATS

One of the primary needs in atherosclerosis research is a small and readily available animal model with serum lipoprotein metabolism and profile simulating that of man. To our knowledge such a model does not presently exist, and the hypercholesterolemic rat certainly is not that model. Because of this lack of a suitable model we resorted to the cholesterol-cholic acid induced hypercholesterolemic rat to screen for agents with hypobetalipoproteinemic activity. Most of the serum cholesterol in this model is transported in a cholesterol ester rich but triglyceride poor lipoprotein particle that floats at density 1.006 g/ml (1). Therefore, the hypercholesterolemic rat is not a good model for pharmacologic studies aimed at modifying LDL levels. Although we have no experience with guinea pig models, the guinea pig fed for short periods of time on a cholesterol diet may be a better model for LDL studies (2,3).

Several thousand compounds have been screened by our group in the hypercholesterolemic rat model as described earlier (4), and numerous active compounds have been discovered. An example of one such agent is adamantyloxyphenylpiperidine (5,6). However, the same caution should be exercised with hypobetalipoproteinemic agents as suggested for hyperalphalipoproteinemic drugs. Their effect on atherosclerosis will be mediated through the mechanism of action of their effect on LDL. Therefore, we again recommend that all hypobetalipoproteinemic agents be routinely checked for antiatherosclerotic activity. It is our experience that only a small percentage of both hyperalpha- and hypobetalipoproteinemic agents detected in the rat assays inhibit the development of atherosclerosis as measured in the SEA Japanese quail.

JAPANESE QUAIL

Japanese quail are a small inexpensive animal that develops atherosclerosis when fed a cholesterol containing diet. Since less than half the Japanese quail on a cholesterol diet develop grossly visible lesions, a strain of quail susceptible to experimental atherosclersis (SEA) were produced by selective breeding (7-9). SEA quail presently are used by us for the routine assay of hundreds of compounds per year for antiatherosclerotic and hypocholesterolaric activity (10). All compounds detected as active in the hyperalpha- and hypobetalipoproteinemic screens are routinely assayed for anti-atherosclerotic activity in SEA quail. Adamantyloxyaniline is an example of one agent that possesses both hypobetaliproteinemic activity in the rat and antiatherosclerotic plus hypocholesterolaric activity in SEA quail (11). We are investigating several classes of compounds that possess both lipoprotein modifying activity in rats and antiatherosclerotic activity in quail.

CYNOMOLGUS MONKEYS

A wealth of data is available on the comparative pathology of atherosclerosis in numerous nonhuman primates. The general concensus from these studies is that the lesions seen in nonhuman primates more closely resemble human atherosclerosis than do those of more phylogenetically unrelated species such as rabbits or chickens. Because of both the pathologic and phylogenetic similarity to man, it is reasonable to prefer data from nonhuman primates to that from other animal models such as rats or quail. However, there is relatively little data on lipoproteins and their metabolism in nonhuman primates, and in the absence of much solid evidence one is forced to assume a working hypothesis that lipoprotein metabolism is closer to that of man as well.

Of the nonhuman primates the cynomolgus monkey (Macaca fascicularis) is a particularly good model for coronary artery disease (12,13). In addition, this species is currently available at a reasonable price and is relatively easy to maintain in captivity. Also, early lipoprotein data (13,14) indicated that more than half of the serum cholesterol was transported in the LDL making it feasible to assay for both hypobeta- and hyperalphalipoproteinemic activity in this species. For these reasons we have established a small colony of cynomolgus monkeys for the secondary screening of lipoprotein modifying and antiatherosclerotic agents. Although our experience with these animals is limited, they look quite promising as a useful tool in antiatherosclerosis drug development.

SUMMARY

We have developed an integrated system for anti-atherosclerosis drug development utilizing rats, SEA quail, and cynomolgus monkeys as animal models. In general, the way the system is presently functioning is that thousands of compounds per year are randomly screened for hypobeta- or hyperalphalipoproteinemic activity in rats, and hundreds of compounds per year are screened in SEA quail for antiatherosclerotic and hypocholesterolaric activity. A few selected compounds that have activity in both rats and quail are then tested for lipoprotein modifying activity in cynomolgus monkeys. Nontoxic compounds having very good lipoprotein modifying activity in the monkey will then be recommended for clinical trials in man. We do not anticipate that this battery of testing will guarantee activity in man, but are hoping that it will at least increase the probability for finding a truly effective antiatherosclerotic drug to control the human disease.

REFERENCES

1. Day, C.E., B. Barker, and W.W. Stafford. Comp. Biochem. Physiol. 49B: 501-505 (1974).

2. Mills, G.L., M.J. Chapman, and F.McTaggart. Biochim. Biophys. Acta 260: 401-412 (1972)

3. Chapman, M.J. G.L. Mills, and J.H. Ledford. Biochem. J. 149: 423-436 (1975)

4. Schurr, P.E., J.R. Schultz, and C.E. Day. In: Atherosclerosis Drug Discovery. Edited by C.E. Day, Plenum Press, New York (1976), pp. 215-229.

5. Day, C.E., P.E. Schurr, W.E. Heyd, and D. Lednicer. In: Atherosclerosis Drug Discovery. Edited by C.E. Day, Plenum Press, New York (1976), pp. 231-249.

6. Schurr, P.E. and C.E. Day. Lipids 12: 22-28 (1977)

7. Day, C.E. and W.W. Stafford. In: Lipids, Lipoproteins and Drugs: Proceedings Fifth International Symposium on Drugs Affecting Lipid Metabolism. Edited by D.Kritchevsky,

R. Paoletti, and W.L. Holmes, Plenum Press, New York (1975), pp. 339-347.

8. Chapman, K.P., W.W. Stafford, and C.E. Day. In: Atherosclerosis Drug Discovery. Edited by C.E. Day, Plenum Press, New York (1976), pp. 347-356.

9. Day, C.E. Lab. Animal Sci. 6: 28-30 (1977)

10. Day, C.E., W.W. Stafford, and P.E. Schurr. Lab Animal Sci., in press

11. Day, C.E., W.W. Stafford, and P.E. Schurr. Protides of the Biological Fluids, in press

12. Kramsch, D.M. and W. Hollander. Exp. Molec. Path. 9: 1-22 (1968)

13. Malinow, M.R. P. McLaughlin, L. Papworth, H.K. Naito, L. Lewis, and W.P. McNulty. In: Atherosclerosis Drug Discovery. Edited by C.E. Day, Plenum Press, New York (1976), pp. 3-31.

14. Srinivasan, S.R. J.R. McBride, Jr., B. Radhakrishnamurthy, and G.S. Berenson. Comp. Biochem. Physiol. 47B: 711-716 (1974)

Cholesterol Metabolism in Man

THE EDINBURGH-STOCKHOLM STUDY OF CORONARY HEART DISEASE RISK FACTORS: A SUMMARY

R.L. Logan[1], R.A. Riemersma[1], M.F. Oliver[1], A.G. Olsson[2], S. Rossner[2], G. Walldius[2], L. Kaijser[2], L.A. Carlson[2], L. Lockerbie[3], and W. Lutz[3]

[1]Department of Cardiology, Royal Infirmary, Edinburgh; [2] King Gustav V Research Institute, Karolinska Hospital, Stockholm; [3] Medical Computing and Statistics Group, University of Edinburgh

INTRODUCTION

The mortality from coronary heart disease (CHD) (ICD 410) in men aged 40 years is 3 times higher in Edinburgh than in Stockholm. This assessment is based on two community surveys of CHD incidence (1,2) and WHO mortality data (3). A pilot survey of CHD risk factors (4) suggested that there are significantly higher serum triglycerides, blood pressure, insulin production and cigarette smoking in Edinburgh compared with Stockholm but that serum cholesterol and weight are similar.

PROCEDURES

A more detailed study of CHD risk factors has now been undertaken on two random samples of 40 year old men in each city (Edinburgh 107 men; Stockholm 82 men). All clinical measurements were conducted under controlled and identical conditions and at the same time of year. Sera for serum lipoprotein analysis were flown stored on ice from Edinburgh to Stockholm each week and were analyzed on a blind basis at the same time as those from

Stockholm men. Free fatty acid (FFA) and gas-liquid chromatographic analysis of plasma cholesterol esters and triglyceride fatty acids were conducted in Edinburgh on frozen specimens. GLC analysis of adipose tissue fatty acids was done in Stockholm. Sera for analysis of glucose, FFA, free glycerol (FG), insulin, and glucagon were flown from Stockholm to Edinburgh each week and again the analyses were conducted blind. Blood for liver function tests and serum proteins was also flown from Stockholm for analysis in Edinburgh.

RESULTS

Physical Characteristics

Edinburgh men were significantly shorter than Stockholm men ($p < 0.001$) but there was no signficant difference in the weight. There was no signficant difference in fat cell diameter but triceps skin-fold thickness was greater in Edinburgh men ($p < 0.01$).

There were more men in Edinburgh (28%) with a corneal arcus compared with men in Stockholm (8.5%) ($p < 0.005$).

Blood Pressure

In Edinburgh there were significantly higher systolic and diastolic blood pressures compared with Stockholm men ($p < 0.001$).

Cigarette Smoking

There were more cigarette smokers in Edinburgh (51%) when compared with Stockholm (40%), and in Edinburgh cigarette smokers smoked more cigarettes with 41% smoking more than 15 daily compared with 22% in Stockholm ($p < 0.01$).

Histocompatibility Antigen

There was no significant difference in the number of men with HLA 8 in the two populations.

Table 1

SERUM LIPID AND LIPOPROTEIN CONCENTRATIONS

Serum Concentrations nmol/l	Edinburgh Mean	Edinburgh S.D.	Stockholm Mean	Stockholm S.D.
Cholesterol (a)	5.54	0.90	5.39	0.81
Triglyceride (b)	1.82	1.06	1.28	0.67
VLDL				
Cholesterol (c)	0.71	0.43	0.49	0.33
Triglyceride (c)	1.24	0.94	0.77	0.54
LDL				
Cholesterol (a)	3.55	0.79	3.44	0.76
Triglyceride (d)	0.39	0.16	0.33	0.16
HDL				
Cholesterol (d)	1.25	0.25	1.37	0.40
Triglyceride (e)	0.16	0.05	0.14	0.04
K_2 (IVFTT)%/min	0.44	0.20	0.49	0.21

Significance:
a) Means and Distribution, not significant
b) Means, $p<0.001$; distribution, $p<0.005$
c) Means, $p<0.001$; distribution, $p<0.01$
d) Means, $p<0.025$; distribution, not significant
e) Means, $p<0.005$; distribution, $p<0.001$

Electrocardiographic Findings

Both, at rest, during and after exercise Edinburgh men showed more ECG abnormalities. Fewer men in Edinburgh were able to complete a standardized ergometric load.

Table 2

SERUM LIPID AND LIPOPROTEIN CONCENTRATIONS
TESTS FOR SIGNIFICANCE

Serum Concentrations nmol/l	High Cut-Off		Low Cut-Off	
	10% Limit	Significance	10% Limit	Significance
Cholesterol	> 6.50	$p < 0.025$	< 4.50	n.s.
Triglyceride	> 2.50	n.s.	< 0.60	$p < 0.005$
VLDL				
Cholesterol	> 1.00	$p < 0.05$	< 0.30	$p < 0.001$
Triglyceride	> 2.50	$p < 0.025$	< 0.75	$p < 0.001$
LDL				
Cholesterol	> 4.50	n.s.	< 2.75	n.s.
Triglyceride	> 0.60	n.s.	< 0.20	n.s.
HDL				
Cholesterol	> 1.70	$p < 0.01$	< 1.00	n.s.
Triglyceride	> 0.22	n.s.	< 0.10	n.s.
K_2 (IVFTT)%/min	> 0.70	n.s.	< 0.30	n.s.

Table 3

PERCENT OF LINOLEIC ACID (18:2) IN PLASMA LIPID AND ADIPOSE TISSUE
WITH ADIPOSE TISSUE P/S RATIO*

Measurement**	Edinburgh		Stockholm	
	Mean	S.D.	Mean	S.D.
Plasma Cholesterol Esters 18:2%	48.4	6.53	56.4	5.96
Plasma Triglycerides 18:2%	10.8	3.8	18.2	4.5
Adipose Tissue 18:2%	7.3	1.5	11.8	2.1
Adipose Tissue P/S Ratio	0.30	0.07	0.44	0.11

* The P/S Ratio and 18.2% showed entirely different distribution in the two cities.

** Means and distribution of all measurements significant at $p < 0.001$.

Serum Lipids and Lipoproteins

The serum cholesterol and low density lipoprotein (LDL) cholesterol concentrations were the same in Edinburgh and Stockholm men. Serum triglyceride and very low density lipoprotein (VLDL) triglyceride concentrations were significantly higher in Edinburgh men. Fewer Edinburgh men had high concentrations of high density lipoprotein (HDL) cholesterol. These and other lipid measurements are illustrated in Tables 1 and 2.

There was a significant difference in the means and frequency distribution of serum cholesterol linoleic acid and serum triglyceride linoleic acid concentrations between the two cities (Table 3).

Adipose Tissue Biopsy

There was a striking difference in the polyunsaturated/saturated (P/S) ratio in adipose tissue biopsies in Edinburgh men compared with Stockholm men with the latter showing higher ratios (Table 3). This difference was even more striking when the percent of linoleic acid (18:2%) in adipose tissue was compared for the two cities. There were significant correlations in both cities between adipose tissue 18:2% and plasma cholesterol 18:2% (E=r0.58; S=r0.52; $p<0.01$) and serum triglyceride (E=r0.57; S=r0.70; $p<0.01$).

Intravenous Fat Tolerance Test

There were no differences in the k_2 values (%/min) between the two cities (Table 3). In both, there were significant correlations between k_2 and log triglyceride (E=r-0.57; S=r-0.75; $p<0.001$) and also log VLDL TG (E=r-0.48; S=r-0.57; $p<0.001$).

Glucose Tolerance Test

There were no significant differences between the two cities in the glucose response to a standardized glucose tolerance test with regard to the peak concentration of glucose and the total amount of glucose (area under the curve), but the peak concentration of glucose occurred earlier in Edinburgh men ($p<0.05$). There was a striking difference in the insulin secretion with

Edinburgh men producing a higher peak insulin concentration ($p<0.001$). This peak occurred earlier ($p<0.005$). The total release of insulin (area under the curve) was greater in Edinburgh when compared with Stockholm men ($p<0.025$). The release of insulin during the first 60 minutes was also more in Edinburgh men ($p<0.001$). Plasma FFA and FG response (areas under the curves) to the glucose tolerance test were also strikingly different for the two populations with Edinburgh men showing significantly less inhibition of lipolysis in response to a glucose load.

Dietary Constituents

These have not yet been analyzed in detail. Information is available, however, concerning alcohol intake and it is clear that Edinburgh men consume significantly more alcohol in a given week compared with Stockholm men.

An extensive analysis is currently being undertaken of total calories, saturated and unsaturated fat, cholesterol, carbohydrate and protein in the diets in the two populations. An attempt will also be made to analyze the dietary concentration of linoleic acid consumed.

COMMENT

This is a unique geographic study of contrasting disease rates, metabolism and environment. It has been complex to carry out. It gives new leads concerning the cause of CHD in the country with the highest overall attack rate in the world, namely Scotland. It is suggested that the excess CHD mortality in Edinburgh compared with Stockholm is a result of several concurrent increases in risk.

The main difference in lipids between the cities was in serum VLDL TG, TG and CE 18:2% and adipose tissue 18:2%. Serum cholesterol and LDL cholesterol were similar in both cities. TG clearance (k_2) was similar in the cities and this suggests an increased liver secretion of VLDL TG in Edinburgh men. The difference in response to oral glucose in FFA may be important in this respect, since relatively more FFA are available in Edinburgh men for incorporation into VLDL TG. The excess alcohol intake in Edinburgh could lead to greater TG production.

The lower linoleic acid present in plasma TG and CE and in adipose tissue are almost certainly due to Edinburgh men eating relatively less polyunsaturated than saturated fat compared with Stockholm men and this is currently being studied.

The excess intake of alcohol and of cigarette smoking suggests a lack of awareness of the deleterious effects of these habits. The physical inactivity and higher frequency of electrocardiographic abnormalities also reflects an alarming lack of fitness in the apparently normal young-middle age male population in Edinburgh.

REFERENCES

1. Armstrong, A., Duncan, B., Oliver, M.F., Julian, D.G., Donald, K.W., Fulton, M., Lutz, W., and Morrison, S.L. Brit. Heart J. 34: 67 (1972)
2. Wikland, B. Acta Med. Scand. Suppl. 524 (1969)
3. World Health Statistics Annual I, (1972)
4. Oliver, M.F., Nimmo, I.A., Cooke, M., Carlson, L.A., Olsson, A.G. Europ. J. Clin. Invest. 5: 507 (1975)

THE HIGH DENSITY LIPOPROTEINS

Stephen B. Hulley, M.D., M.P.H.

Departments of International Health and Epidemiology, and of Medicine, University of California, San Francisco, California, U.S.A.

AN EPIDEMIOLOGICAL REVIEW

HDL and CHD: An Epidemiological Review

Attention has recently been focused on the association between plasma high density lipoprotein (HDL) concentration and the risk of coronary heart disease (CHD) (1-6). Unlike most of the conventional risk factors that confer increased risk of disease, plasma HDL appears to be a risk-lowering factor. This is an important statement, and its basis requires careful examination.

Epidemiologic criteria for risk factors*. A risk factor is a characteristic of an individual that conveys predictive information about the probability of his developing a disease. In other words, a statistical association exists between the variable and the disease. However, not all such associations represent risk factors of any relevance to the practice of preventive medicine. Among the categories shown in Table 1, only associations that are biologic and causal are of primary importance as risk factors.

How does one identify associations that have a causal basis? This is a critical question for epidemiologists,

---

*The logic for examining a risk-lowering factor such as HDL is the same as that for the conventional risk factors (that might more properly be termed "risk-raising" factors).

Table 1

Categories of statistical associations between a variable and a disease:

A. Spurious
The variable and the disease are related through bias or artifact

B. Biologic
(1) Non-causal
(a) the variable is (in part) a consequence of the disease
(b) both the variable and the disease are (in part) consequences of some other variable

(2) Causal
The disease is (in part) a consequence of the variable

and has led to the establishment of the following criteria [modified from Hill (7)]:

1. The association should have a graded response pattern, reflecting a biologic gradient. (U-shaped curves and discontinuities make it more likely that the association is confounded or spurious.)
2. The association should be strong, accounting for a substantial risk differential.
3. The association should be independent of other known risk factors, reducing the possibility that both the variable and the disease are a consequence of some third variable.
4. The association should be consistent, a term that includes reproducibility among studies and generality for different manifestations of disease, and among various age, sex, and race groups.
5. The time sequence should be such that the variable is a precursor, rather than a consequence, of the disease.

Examination of whether the inverse HDL-CHD association meets the risk factor criteria. The inverse association between HDL and CHD can be examined for these characteristics in the Cooperative Lipoprotein Phenotyping Study (CLPS) (4). 6,859 men and women of black, Japanese and white ancestry and over 40 years of age were examined in this case-control study of populations in Albany,

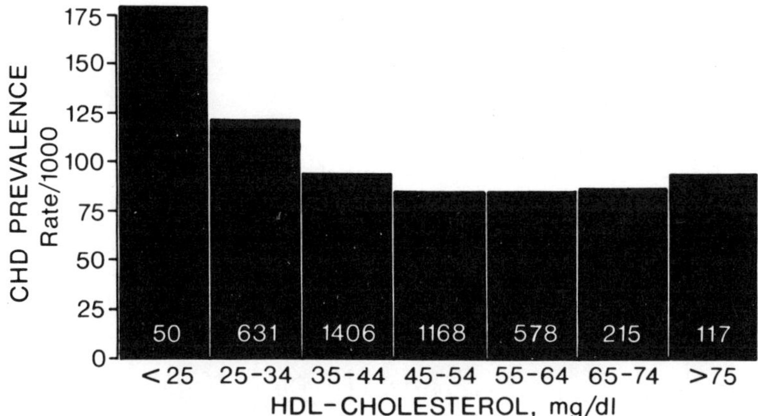

Figure 1: CHD prevalence according to plasma level of HDL-cholesterol, redrawn from the Cooperative Lipoprotein Phenotyping Study (4). The data are for men aged 50-69 in all population samples pooled; the number of subjects is shown in each bar.

Framingham, Evans County, Honolulu and San Francisco. HDL was estimated by measuring the cholesterol content of plasma drawn after an overnight fast and subjected to heparin precipitation. CHD prevalence was based on evidence of prior myocardial infarction (assessed by electrocardiogram or questionnaire) or angina pectoris (assessed by Rose questionnaire).

Figure 1 shows that the inverse association between HDL-cholesterol and CHD prevalence meets the first two risk factor criteria. There is a graded response (at least among subjects with low to moderate HDL-cholesterol levels) and the association accounts for a two-fold risk differential.

The independence criterion is a particular concern because of the correlations that exist among the plasma fractions. HDL-cholesterol is inversely correlated with the levels of triglyceride (r ranging from -.28 to -.44 in the various CLPS populations) and LDL-cholesterol (r -.01 to -.30), so the greater rates of CHD among subjects with low HDL might be due to the higher mean triglyceride and LDL-cholesterol levels in such subjects. However, multivariate analyses in this (4) and other (5,6) studies demonstrates that the inverse HDL-CHD

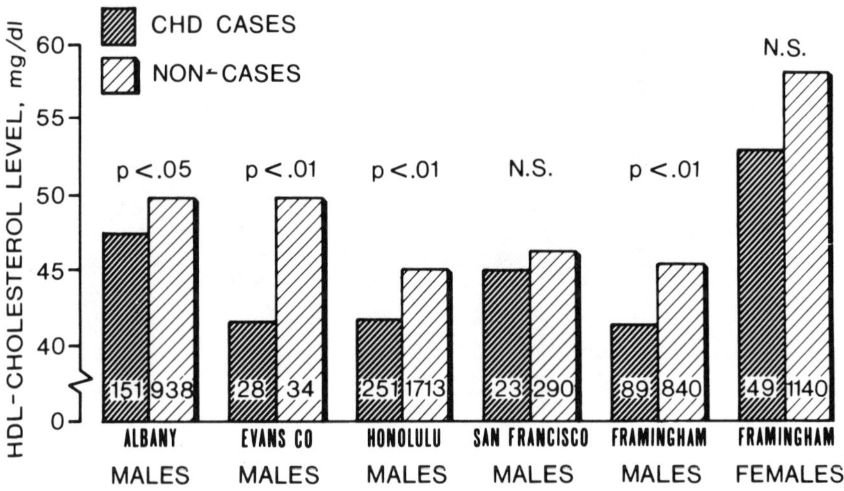

Figure 2: Mean plasma HDL-cholesterol by presence or absence of prior CHD and by population sample, redrawn from the Cooperative Lipoprotein Phenotyping Study (4). Statistical significance is shown for each comparison between cases and non-cases.

association persists after adjusting for the other lipids.

The fourth risk factor criterion, consistency, can be examined in Figure 2. In every population sample the mean HDL-cholesterol among CHD cases is lower than that among persons without disease. The magnitude of the difference is small (about 4 mg/dl) but the similarity of the pattern among the various populations is striking. Figure 2 also demonstrates that HDL-cholesterol levels are higher in women than in man, an observation that fits with their lower rates of CHD. So the inverse HDL-CHD association was reproducibly found in the several studies that make up the CLPS, and has generality among population samples that differ in race, sex and geographic location. Additional analyses showed the association to also be consistent for two categories of CHD (angina pectoris and myocardial infarction) and within each of the age groups 40-49, 50-59, 60-69, and $\geq$ 70 years (4).

Cross-sectional studies such as the CLPS leave open the possibility that the HDL levels may be a consequence of heart disease rather than a precursor. However there are several prospective studies (5,6,8,9) that demonstrate this not to be the case. In the Framingham study for example (5), HDL-cholesterol concentration was inversely related to the subsequent incidence of CHD in both women and men. The other risk factor criteria were also present; a graded response pattern (which in this study extended over the whole range of HDL-cholesterol values) and independence from other risk factors tested; these included LDL-cholesterol and triglyceride levels, systolic blood pressure, left ventricular hypertrophy, relative weight and diabetes, but not smoking or physical activity. Of particular interest in this study, likelihood ratio calculations revealed the association of HDL with CHD to be stronger than that of any other risk factor.

Historical notes. These clear-cut findings lead to the question: why has HDL received so little attention until recently? Lipoproteins have been studied for more than three decades, and the inverse HDL-CHD association was observed in many early studies (10-18). Nor was this finding ignored; Barr wrote in 1951 that "The outstanding fact in our observations is the relative and absolute reduction in alpha-lipoprotein in atherosclerosis." (10)

One can only speculate on the basis for the dormancy of interest. The difference in mean HDL levels between cases and controls is quite small, and a confounding influence of VLDL (triglyceride) was suspected by Gofman (8) and others. But my guess is that the main barrier was analogous to that confronting Galileo: a reluctance of the human mind to pursue an observation that did not seem to make sense. What was needed to open the mind was a plausible mechanism.

In 1975 Miller and Miller accomplished this by suggesting that HDL may serve to transport cholesterol from the arterial wall cells to the liver for excretion (1). It is beyond the scope of this discussion to review the evidence for this hypothesis, nor that for the promising alternative (discussed earlier in this symposium), that HDL inhibits the uptake of LDL by the arterial wall cell (19). For the purpose of this epidemiological analysis it is sufficient to note that possible mechanisms do exist (19-21).

Additional characteristics that would support the causal hypothesis. In sum, evidence has been presented that HDL is a risk-lowering factor with many of the characteristics of major risk factors. As a result, there is a temptation to draw the exciting inference that the HDL-CHD association has a causal basis, i.e. that HDL is a protective factor.

However, such a conclusion is premature. For one thing the epidemiologic observations have not yet stood the test of time, and the weathering of criticism and scientific debate. For example, physical activity may confound the association; sedentary life style has been associated with low levels of HDL (22) and with high rates of CHD (23), but the relationship among all three variables (HDL, physical activity, and CHD) has not yet been examined in a single study. A similar case could be made for cigarette smoking, and there may well be other as yet unidentified covariables.

A more fundamental reservation stems from the difficulty in drawing causal inferences from observational epidemiology. Final proof is generally elusive, but further lines of evidence may be helpful. These approaches are numbered 6-8 below because they may also be considered to be additional criteria for major (i.e. causal) risk factors. [Items (6) and (7) taken together with the epidemiologic criteria, are sometimes combined under the heading "coherence."]

6. As has been mentioned, the causal hypothesis should be biologically plausible. Further work is needed to expand our knowledge of the mechanisms by which HDL might prevent CHD.

7. There should be support for causality from tests of analogous hypotheses in animals. It appears that work in this important area is limited to early experiments on the relationship of gonadal hormones to lipoproteins and disease (24,25).

8. Experimental epidemiology in humans will perhaps provide the strongest basis for causal inference; the demonstration that raising HDL levels leads to a lowered incidence of CHD.*

---

*One such trial may have already been carried out serendipitously, with negative results; exogenous estrogens did not prevent recurrence of myocardial infarction among men in the Coronary Drug Project (26). However, there were no direct measurements of plasma HDL in this trial, and the presumption that estrogens raised HDL-cholesterol levels of the participants is open to question.

It should be clear from these remarks that intervention directed at plasma HDL in the general practice of preventive medicine would be premature at this time. On the other hand, it is timely to begin examining the factors that may influence HDL. In the next section of this paper I will discuss some early experiences in the MRFIT that contribute to our knowledge, as yet quite rudimentary, of the determinants of circulating HDL level.

PRELIMINARY FINDINGS IN THE MRFIT*

The Multiple Risk Factor Intervention Trial (MRFIT) is a randomized collaborative study to test the hypothesis that a six-year program for lowering coronary risk factors will reduce mortality from coronary heart disease (CHD) (27). Beginning four years ago, 12,866 men aged 35-57 were recruited in 22 centers during a two-year intake period. All were initially free of overt CHD but judged at high risk because they had one or more of the three major risk factors: hypercholesterolemia, hypertension and the cigarette smoking habit. Participants in the special intervention group were advised to follow a fat-controlled eating pattern designed to lower serum cholesterol concentration; hypertensive subjects entered a stepped-care program of weight loss and medication; and cigarette smokers were counseled in cessation efforts. Participants in the control group were referred to their usual source of care for preventive medical advice. This paper is a preliminary examination of an aspect of the data peripheral to the main objectives -- the HDL findings.

HDL-Cholesterol Levels

The participants described herein are a cohort of men who have completed two years of participation in the trial. HDL-cholesterol levels were measured following heparin precipitation of EDTA plasma drawn after an overnight fast; specimens were shipped at +4°C to a central laboratory that is continuously monitored by the CDC Lipid Standardization Laboratory.

---

*On behalf of the MRFIT Research Group (a roster of collaborating investigators follows the text).

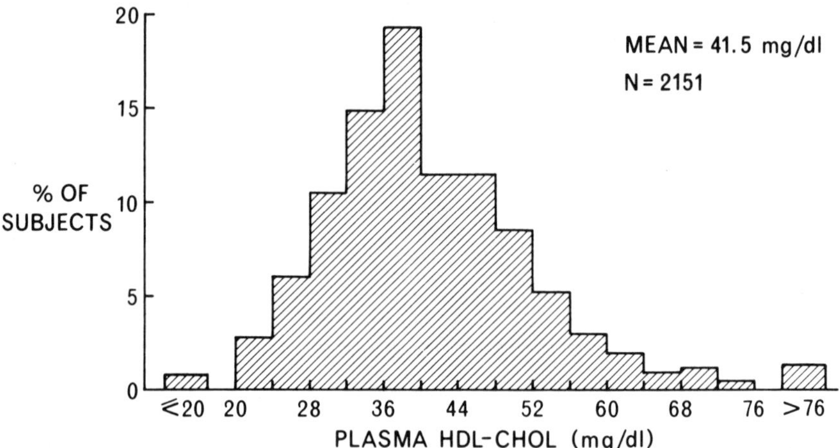

Figure 3: Percent frequency distribution of plasma HDL-cholesterol levels at baseline in a cohort of MRFIT participants who have subsequently completed two years in the study (at the time of this presentation).

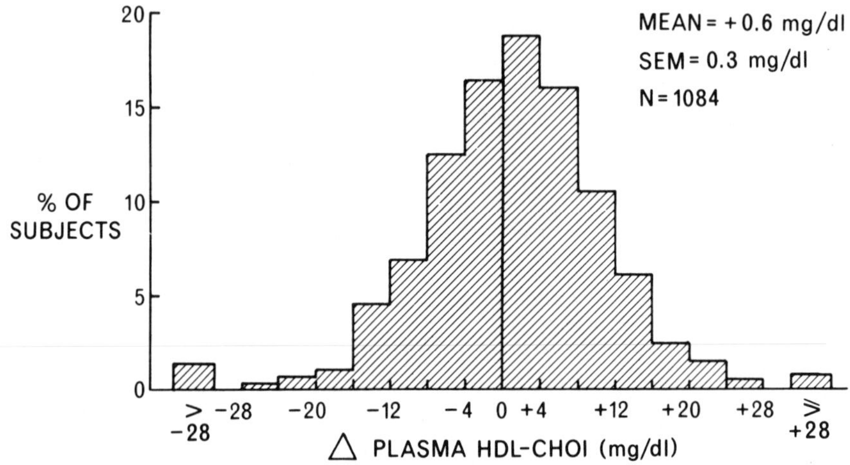

Figure 4: Percent frequency distribution of change in plasma HDL-cholesterol levels between baseline and the second annual examination for the special intervention group of the cohort in Figure 3.

Figure 3 shows the frequency distribution of HDL-cholesterol levels at baseline. The mean level in this sample of participants is 41.5 mg/dl and the distribution is roughly normal with a slight skew toward higher levels.

The epidemiologic finding that HDL-cholesterol may be an independent CHD risk-lowering factor gives rise to an important question: might the MRFIT intervention efforts, and especially the dietary recommendations designed to lower total plasma cholesterol concentration also cause a decrease in the level of HDL-cholesterol? Such an event might increase CHD incidence and diminish the preventive impact of the MRFIT.

Figure 4 shows the frequency distribution of the individual values for change in HDL-cholesterol level between baseline and second annual examination among participants in the special intervention program. The mean change, +0.6 mg/dl, is not significantly different from zero. So the first and perhaps most important conclusion is that multifactor coronary prevention programs directed at conventional risk factors are not likely to have an adverse influence on HDL-cholesterol levels.

An interesting feature of Figure 4 is the degree of spread in the distribution of values for change in HDL-cholesterol level. Although the average change for the cohort over the two years was near zero, there were major deviations from baseline, both upwards and downwards, in many individuals. This large variance - the standard deviation of the change was 10 mg/dl - was probably not due to laboratory variation alone; the reproducibility of determinations on a single specimen is relatively high and has a standard deviation in our laboratory of 3 mg/dl. We infer that biologic sources of variance probably had an influence on the plasma HDL-cholesterol levels of some individuals. The quest for these determinants will constitute the remaining portion of this paper, an enlargement on the findings in a smaller cohort studied over a shorter period (one year) in the San Francisco MRFIT clinic (28).

Body Weight and HDL

Previous studies have implicated an inverse relationship between body weight and HDL (3,22,29). Figure 5 shows plasma HDL-cholesterol level according to body mass index at baseline in the MRFIT. There is a graded

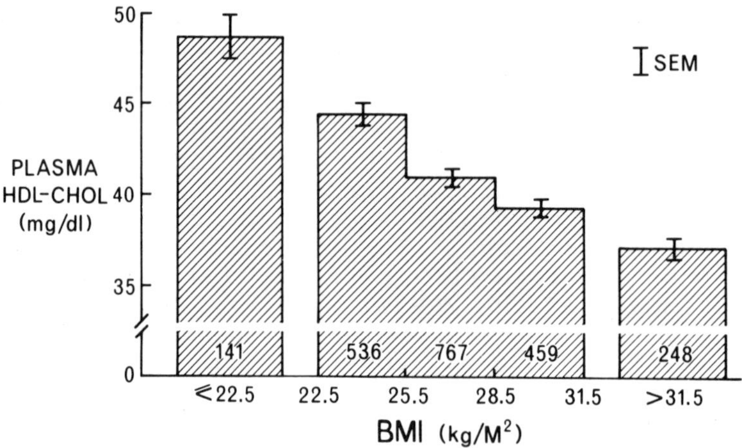

Figure 5: Mean plasma HDL-cholesterol level (±SEM) according to body mass index (BMI) at baseline for the same cohort as Figure 1.

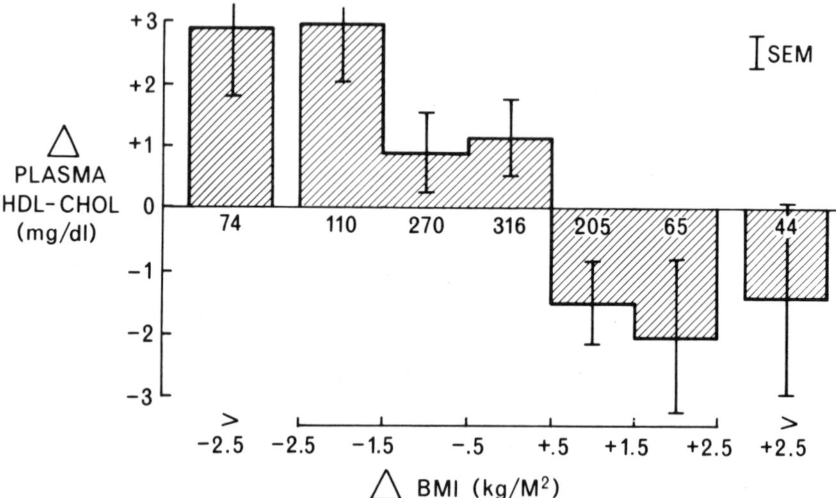

Figure 6: Mean change in plasma HDL-cholesterol (±SEM) according to change in body mass index between baseline and the second annual examination for the same cohort as Figure 1.

response pattern, obese individuals having lower levels of HDL-cholesterol. This is a graphic representation of a statistical association, and as was true in our earlier discussion, the problem is to discover whether the association has a causal basis. That is, does obesity cause the HDL-cholesterol level to decrease?

The data in Figure 5 do not provide a reliable answer to this question because cross-sectional associations are quite likely to be confounded. For example, obese persons are often less active than their slim counterparts, and it may be the habitual level of physical activity, rather than the obesity *per se*, that influences the HDL levels.

The *longitudinal* findings in the MRFIT contain additional information that bears on causal inference. If the relationship between change in HDL-cholesterol level and change in body weight over the two years of the study jibes with the cross-sectional findings at baseline, it becomes less likely that the association is confounded. Figure 6 shows that this is in fact the case in the MRFIT, subjects who lost weight having an increase in HDL cholesterol level and vice-versa. Although the magnitude of the mean HDL-cholesterol change is small, there is a clear graded response pattern. The case for body weight being a determinant of circulating HDL is strengthened, but (as in the first part of this paper) confirmation will depend on (1) accumulating evidence for biologic plausability, (2) demonstrating the validity of analogous hypotheses in animals, and (3) experimental verification in humans.

Habitual Alcohol Intake and HDL

Prior studies have implicated a direct association between reported habitual alcohol intake and plasma HDL-cholesterol levels (3,29-32). Figure 7 shows data from the Cooperative Lipoprotein Phenotyping Study (31). The reproducibility of the graded response pattern is remarkable when one considers the inherent unreliability of the questionnaire approach to assessing alcohol habits.

The findings at baseline in the MRFIT are similar (Table 2).

The association between reported alcohol intake and HDL-cholesterol level has a correlation coefficient of

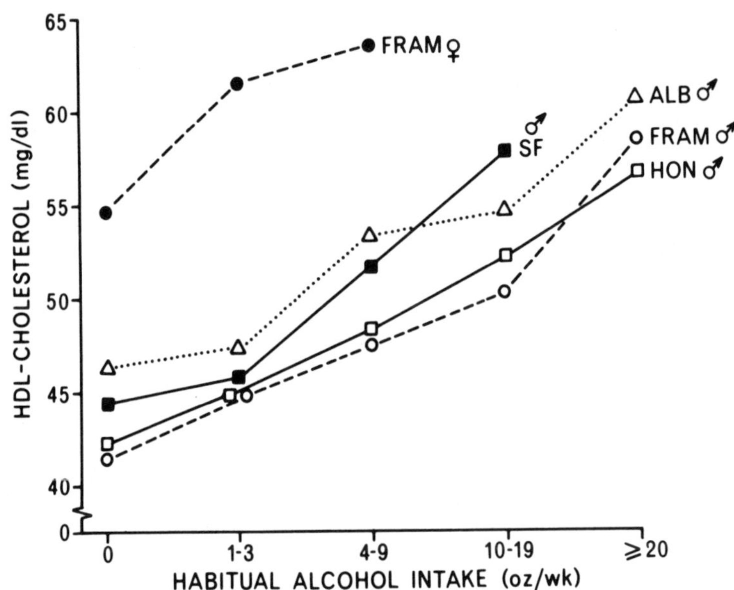

Figure 7: Mean plasma HDL-cholesterol level by reported habitual alcohol consumption and by population sample, redrawn from the Cooperative Lipoprotein Phenotyping Study (31).

.26 at baseline, slightly stronger than the inverse correlation between body mass index and HDL-cholesterol levels (r=-.24). However, causal inference (i.e. that drinking alcohol causes HDL-levels to increase) is not appropriate here because of the longitudinal findings; change in alcohol intake was not related to change in HDL levels in the MRFIT.

Other Variables and HDL

One approach to the key epidemiologic question concerning the independence of each of these associations has been noted: to compare the longitudinal findings with those at baseline. A second approach is the use of multivariate analyses. In table 2 the multivariate coefficient for each of the independent variables listed is a measure of its association with HDL when all the other variables are held constant. Standardizing the

Table 2

REGRESSIONS OF SELECTED VARIABLES ON PLASMA HDL-CHOLESTEROL LEVEL IN THE MRFIT (N=2151)

	STANDARDIZED REGRESSION COEFFICIENTS			
	Cross-Sectional		Longitudinal[b]	
Independent Variable	Univariate[a]	Multivariate	Univariate[a]	Multivariate
Body mass index	-.24[c]	-.22[c]	-.09[c]	-.14[c]
Habitual alcohol intake	.26[c]	.21[c]	.01	.02
Habitual cigarette frequency	-.09[c]	-.17[c]	-.07	-.10[c]
Diastolic blood pressure	.09[c]	.06[d]	.09	.11[c]
Adherence to fat-controlled diet			-.01	.00

[a] Univariate standardized regression coefficients are mathematically identical to Pearson correlation coefficients

[b] Change in HDL-cholesterol and in the independent variable over first two years of the trial

[c] $p < .001$

[d] $p < .01$

multivariate coefficients, (i.e. multiplying by the standard deviation of the independent variable) allows the relative importance of the associations to be estimated. It is evident from Table 2 that neither body mass index nor habitual alcohol intake depend on the other variables studied for their associations with HDL-cholesterol.

Among the other associations in Table 2, the inverse correlation between reported cigarette smoking frequency and plasma HDL-cholesterol level may be important. Non-smokers tend to have higher levels of HDL than smokers (at baseline), and the inference that smoking may cause HDL levels to decrease is supported by the significant association in the longitudinal analysis. The finding, which has also been observed in Framingham (33), may contribute to our understanding of the link between smoking and CHD.

The implications of the direct association between HDL-cholesterol level and diastolic blood pressure in both cross-sectional and longitudinal analyses are uncertain. Other variables of interest, particularly the relationship between physical activity and HDL levels, and associations among the various lipids and lipoproteins, are currently under study.

Diet and HDL

All participants in the MRFIT are counseled in a fat-controlled diet that includes reduction of dietary cholesterol and saturated fats, and a moderate increase in polyunsaturated fats. The bottom line of Table 2 is an important preliminary finding - there does not appear to be an association between the degree of adherence to the MRFIT diet (judged by interview) and the mean change in HDL-cholesterol level. A more thorough and sophisticated exploration for a potential influence of dietary constituents (34-36) is currently in progress.

Conclusions

The preliminary MRFIT experience reveals several variables to be independently associated with high levels of HDL-cholesterol at baseline: low body mass index, high alcohol intake, avoidance of cigarettes and high diastolic blood pressure. Except in the case of alcohol, causal inference (that these variables have a role in controlling HDL levels) is strengthened by the longitudinal analyses over the first two years of the Trial. Of considerable importance, the overall mean plasma HDL-cholesterol level does not appear to be effected by this general risk factor reduction program.

Acknowledgement

Special thanks are due to Glenn Bartsch, Sc.D. and Steve Broste at the MRFIT Coordinating Center.

REFERENCES

1. Miller, G.J. and Miller, N.E.
   Lancet I: 16 (1975)
2. Leading Article: Lancet II: 131 (1976)
3. Rhoads, G.G., Gulbrandsen, C.L., and Kagan, A.
   New England J. Med. 294: 293 (1976)
4. Castelli, W.P., Doyle, J.T., Gordon, T., Hames, C., Hjortland, M.C., Hulley, S.B., Kagan, A., and Zukel, W.J.
   Circulation 55: 766 (1977)
5. Gordon, T., Castelli, W.P., Hjortland, M.J., Kannel, W.B.,
   Amer. J. Med. 62: 707 (1977)
6. Miller, N.E., Thelle, D.S., Forde, O.H., Mjos, O.D.
   Lancet I: 965 (1977)
7. Hill, A.B.
   Principles of Medical Statistics, Oxford U. Press, New York, 1971, p. 309
8. Gofman, J.W., Young, W. and Tandy, R.
   Circulation 34: 679 (1966)
9. Medalie, J.H., Kahn, H.A., Neufeld, H.N., Riss, E. and Gouldbourt, U.
   J. Chron. Dis. 26: 329 (1973)
10. Barr, D.P., Russ, E.M., and Eder, H.A.
    Am. J. Med. 11: 480 (1951)
11. Nikkila, E.
    Scand. J. Clin. Lab. Invest. 5: Suppl.8: 1 (1953)
12. Oliver, M.F. and Boyd, G.S.
    Brit. Heart J. 17: 299 (1955)
13. Jencks, W.P., Hyatt, M.R., Jetton, M.R., Mattingly, T.W., and Durrum, E.L.
    J. Clin. Invest. 9: 980 (1956)
14. Dodds, C. and Mills, G.L.
    Lancet I: 1160 (1959)

15. Brunner, D. and Lobl, K.
Ann. Int. Med. 49: 732 (1958)
16. Keys, A. and Fidanza, F.
Circulation 22: 1091 (1960)
17. Carlson, L.A.
Acta Med. Scand. 167: 399 (1960)
18. Mills, G.L. and Wilkinson, P.A.
Brit. Heart J. 28: 638 (1966)
19. Carew, T.W., Koschinsky, T., Hayes, S.B. and Steinberg, D.
Lancet I: 1315 (1976)
20. Hamilton, R.L., Williams, M.D., Fielding, C.J. and Havel, R.J.
J. Clin. Invest. 58: 667 (1976)
21. Small, D.M.
New Engl. J. Med. 297: 873 (1977)
22. Wood, P.D., Haskell, W., Klein, H., Lewis, S., Stern, M.P., and Farquhar, J.W.
Metabolism 25: 1249 (1976)
23. Paffenbarager, R.S., Hale, W.E., Beard, R.J., and Hyde, R.T.
Am. J. Epidemiol. 105: 200 (1977)
24. Stamler, J., Lewis, L.A., Page, I.H., Berkson, D.M., Kaplan, B.M., Katz, L.N., Pick, R., and Century, D.
In: Cardiovascular Drug Therapy, J.H. Moyer and A.N. Brest, editors, Grune & Stratton, New York, 1965, p. 353
25. Stamler, J.
In: Treatment of the Hyperlipidemic State, H.R. Casdorph, editor, Charles C. Thomas, Springfield, Ill., 1971, p. 310
26. The Coronary Drug Project Research Group,
J.Am.Med.Assoc. 226: 652 (1973)
27. MRFIT Investigators
J.Am.Med.Assoc. 235: 825 (1976)
28. Hulley, S.B., Cohen, R. and Widdowson, G.
J.Am.Med.Assoc. 238: 2269 (1977)
29. Berg, B. and Johansson, B.G.
Acta Med.Scand.Suppl. 552: 13 (1973)
30. Johansson, B. and Medjus, A.
Acta Med. Scand. 195: 273 (1974)
31. Castelli, W.P., Doyle, J.T., Gordon, T., Hames, C.G., Hjortland, M.C., Hulley, S.B., Kagan, A., and Zukel, W.J.
Lancet II: 153 (1977)
32. Yano, K., Rhoads, G.G., and Kagan, A.
New Engl.J.Med. 297: 405 (1977)
33. Garrison, R.J., Kannel, W.B., Feinleib, M., Castelli, W.P., McNamara, P.M., and Padgett, S.J.
Circulation 56: III-44 (1977)

34. Hulley, S.B., Wilson, W.S., Burrows, M.I., and Nichaman, M.Z.
Lancet II: 551 (1972)
35. Sachs, F.M., Castelli, W.P., Conner, A., and Kass, E.H.
New Engl.J.Med. 292: 1148 (1975)
36. Schonfeld, G., Wideman, S.W., Witztum, J.L., and Bowen, R.M.
Metabolism 25: 261 (1976)

MRFIT PROGRAM PARTICIPANTS
MASTER ROSTER

American Health Foundation

C.B. Arnold, M.D., Principal Investigator
E.L. Wynder, M.D.
D. Burton, M.S.
R.Ames, M.D.
S. Goldstein, B.S.
R. Manariota, M.S.

Boston University

T.R. Dawber, M.D. - Principal Investigator
H.E. Thomas, Jr., M.D. - Co-Principal Investigator
F.N. Brand, M.D., M.P.H.
L.K. Smith, M.D.
C. Ford, M.S.
H. Lewis, Ph.D.

Cox Heart Institute

P. Kezdi, M.D. - Principal Investigator
E.L. Stanley, M.D.
F.A. Ernst, Ph.D.
W.L. Black, M.D.

Dade County Department of Public Health

G. Christakis, M.D., M.P.H. - Principal Investigator
J. Burr, M.D. - Co-Principal Investigator
T. Gerace, Ph.D.
M.E. Wilcox, R.D., M.Ed.

Dalhousie University

P.M. Rautaharju, M.D., Ph.D. - Principal Investigator
H. Wolf, Ph.D.

Harvard University

R. Benfari, Ph.D. - Principal Investigator
K. McIntyre, M.D.
J. Ockene, M.A.
D. Kousch, R.N.
J. Hewitt, Ed.D.
P. Remmell, R.D.

Kaiser Foundation Research Institute (Portland)

J.B. Wild, M.D. - Principal Investigator
M. Greenlick, Ph.D.
J. Grover, M.D.

Lankenau Hospital

W. Holmes, Ph.D. - Principal Investigator
J.E. Pickering, M.D.
G. Rubel, M.S.
A. Goldberg, M.S.
B. Feinstein, M.S.
A. Shellenberger, R.N.

National Center for Disease Control

G.R. Cooper, Ph.D., M.D. - Principal Investigator
M. Kuchmak, Ph.D.

New Jersey Medical School (Newark)

N. Lasser, M.D., Ph.D. - Principal Investigator
N. Hymowitz, Ph.D. - Co-Principal Investigator
E.D. Munves, Ph.D.
K.C. Mezey, M.D.

Northwestern University

J. Stamler, M.D. - Principal Investigator
O. Paul, M.D. - Co-Principal Investigator
L. Mojonnier, Ph.D. (Retired)
V. Persky, M.D.
D. Moss, M.S.
E. Robinson, M.S.
J. Berkson, M.D.
D. Meyers, M.D.
A. Dyer, Ph.D.
L. VanHorn, M.S.
R. Schupp, Ph.D.
G. Greene, Ph.D.

University of Chicago

S. Oparil, M.D. - Principal Investigator
L.A. Slowie, M.A.

St. Joseph Hospital

D.M. Berkson, M.D. - Principal Investigator
G. Lauger, M.S.
S. Grujic, M.D.
D. Obradovic, M.D.

Institutes of Medical Sciences - University of California at San Francisco and Berkeley

S.B. Hulley, M.D., M.P.H. - Principal Investigator
W.M. Smith, M.D., M.P.H. - Co-Principal Investigator
S.L. Syme, Ph.D. - Co-Principal Investigator
J. Billings, Ph.D., M.P.H.
T.M. Vogt, M.D., M.P.H.
M.J. Jacobs, B.A.
R. Cohen, M.A.
B. Singh, M.A., R.D.
L. Dzvonik, M.A., R.D.
J. Applebaum, M.A.
D. Davies, R.N.
M. Woolley, M.A.

Institutes of Medical Sciences, San Francisco Central Lab

G.M. Widdowson, Ph.D. - Principal Investigator

University of Pittsburgh

L. Kuller, M.D. - Principal Investigator
R. McDonald, M.D.
B. Coniff, M.S.
A. Caggiula, M.S.
L. Falvo, M.P.H.

University of South Carolina

W.K. Giese, Ph.D. - Principal Investigator
S. Blair, P.E.D. - Co-Principal Investigator
J.F. Martin, M.D. - Co-Principal Investigator

University of Southern California

J. Marmorston, M.D. - Principal Investigator
E. Fishman, M.D.
R. Johnson, R.D.

Policy Advisory Board

J.C. Cassel, M.D. - Chairman
H.P. Dustan, M.D. (Former member)
J. Farquhar, M.D. (Acting Chairman)
W. Insull, Jr., M.D.
C.D. Jenkins, Ph.D.
D.J. Thompson, Ph.D.
P.W. Willis, M.D.
C.M. Young, Ph.D.
W.J. Zukel, M.D. - ex officio

National Heart, Lung and Blood Institute Staff

M. Farrand, R.D.
W. Friedewald, M.D.
L. Friedman, M.D.
E. Furberg, M.D.
T. Gordon
M. Halperin, Ph.D.
C. Kaelber, M.D.
J. Tillotson, R.D.
A. Vargosko, Ph.D.
W.J. Zukel, M.D.

National Heart, Lung, and Blood Institute Staff - cont'd

*Design and Analysis Committee

*Information Exchange Committee

*Intervention Committee

*Publications and Presentations Committee

*Quality Control Committee

* Many of the participants on these committees are included in the roster above

Rush Presbyterian-St. Luke's

J.A. Schoenberger, M.D. - Principal Investigator
R.B. Shekelle, Ph.D.
Y. Hall, M.S.
J. Schoenenberger, Ph.D.
G. Neri, M.D.
T. Dolecek

Rutgers Medical School

H.N. Jacobson, M.D. - Principal Investigator
S.A. Kopel, Ph.D. - Co-Principal Investigator

St. Louis Heart Association

N. Simon, M.D. - Principal Investigator
J.D. Cohen, M.D. - Co-Principal Investigator
H.B. Zimmerman

University of Alabama in Birmingham

H.W. Schnaper, M.D. - Principal Investigator
G.H. Hughes, Ph.D.
A. Oberman, M.D.
C.C. Hill, Ph.D.

University of California at Davis

N.O. Borhani, M.D. - Principal Investigator
D.T. Mason, M.D.
J. Foerster, M.D.

University of Maryland

R. Sherwin, M.D., B. Chir. - Principal Investigator
M.S. McDill, Ph.D. - Co-Principal Investigator
P. Dischinger, Ph.D.

University of Minnesota

H. Blackburn, M.D. - Principal Investigator
H.L. Taylor, Ph.D. - Co-Investigator
D. Jacobs, Jr., Ph.D.
A.S. Leon, M.D.
M. Gouze, Ph.D.

University of Minnesota ECG Coding Center

R.J. Prineas, M.B.B.S., Ph.D. - Director
R. Crow, M.D.

University of Minnesota Coordinating Center

M.O. Kjelsberg, Ph.D. - Principal Investigator
G.E. Bartsch, Sc.D.
J. Neaton, M.S.
P. Ashman, B.A.
A. Reynolds, M.A.
P.V. Grambsch, B.A.

LOW FAT, LOW CHOLESTEROL DIET IN SECONDARY PREVENTION OF CORONARY HEART DISEASE

J.M. Woodhill, A.J. Palmer, B. Leelarthaepin, C. McGilchrist and R.B. Blacket

Department of Medicine, University of New South Wales, Prince Henry Hospital, Little Bay, Australia

SUMMARY

Four hundred fifty-eight men with coronary heart disease participated in a trial of secondary prevention for 2 to 7 years. Overall five year survival was 81%. For those with first heart attacks it was 86%.

From infarct to entry into the trial the majority of men had already made changes in their diet and smoking habit and has lost weight. They were allocated randomly to two dietary groups. In one group the diet consumed derived 9.8% of calories from saturated fatty acids and 15.1% from polyunsaturates. In the second group saturated fatty acids contributed 13.5% and polyunsaturated fatty acids 8.9% of total calories. Survival was slightly better in the second group. Multivariate analysis showed that none of the dietary factors were significantly related to survival. Prognosis was determined largely by the extent of the coronary and myocardial disease as judged by the usual clinical parameters. Recreational physical activity had a strong favourable influence on survival when all other factors were kept constant.

Although body weight and cigarette smoking were not significantly related to survival there are grounds for the belief that relative leanness and low cigarette consumption may have had a favourable influence in both dietary groups.

It is concluded that because of multiple changes in lifestyle men who have had myocardial infarction are not a good choice for testing the lipid hypothesis. Weight loss, reduction in cigarette smoking, increase in physical activity and other readjustments may well have more important beneficial effects than change in dietary lipids.

*****

The Sydney Diet-Heart Study was conceived in 1964. At that time there was a strong belief among epidemiologists and medical scientists that the high dietary intake of saturated fats and cholesterol in the Western nations was a major determinant of premature vascular disease, especially angina pectoris and myocardial infarction. It was thought that differences in diet might explain, at least in part, the five- to ten-fold differences in reported coronary mortality between populations with a Northern European culture and those in the Mediterranean region and in Asia (1). It has also been established that substitution of polyunsaturated fatty acids for saturated fatty acids in the diet lowered serum cholesterol. The American Heart Association had recommended changes in the American diet appropriate to these beliefs. Data from a variety of sources also implicated cigarette smoking and high blood pressure as important risk factors.

The dietary hypothesis had never been submitted to a field test. There was much debate then and now on its relevance to the cardiac problems of Western man. Obesity was given a low rating as a risk factor despite the obvious adiposity of Western man and statistics from life insurance companies showing its unfavourable effects on longevity (2). It was apparent that the lifestyle of Western man must bear on the etiology of vascular disease/ The complexity of the risk factors, known and unknown, and their interactions in people with different genetic make-up was only dimly appreciated.

Feasibility studies in our department had shown that it was possible to modify the diet in properly motivated people along the lines suggested by the American Heart Association. It seemed that application of the new dietary principles to men who had already demonstrated their proclivity to premature coronary disease might so improve their survival that the dietary hypothesis would gain substantial support.

The Sydney Diet-Heart Study was begun in 1966. Four hundred fifty-eight men aged 30-59 with clinical coronary disease were studied for two to seven years. They were accepted into the study not less than eight weeks (mean eleven weeks) after their most recent coronary episode. Three hundred ninety-five men (86%) had experienced myocardial infarction as judged by a typical history, ECG and enzyme changes. Sixty-three men (14%) has recent-onset angina or had experienced acute coronary insufficiency with ECG but without enzyme changes. Two hundred seventy-six (60%) of the 458 men had had no previous cardiac symptoms. One hundred eight-two (40%) had had probable or confirmed angina or myocardial infarction previously.

After work-up the men were allocated by random numbers to one of two dietary regimens. Two hundred thirty-seven men (the P group) were given no specific dietary instruction apart from restriction of calories if thought to be overweight. As a concession to the popular and medical beliefs of the time they were allowed to use polyunsaturated margarine instead of butter if they wished. Two hundred twenty-one men (the F group) were advised and tutored individually to reduce saturated fat intake to approximately 10% of calories and dietary cholesterol to 300 mg or less per day. They were encouraged to use food containing polyunsaturated fatty acids to 15% or more of daily calories. The diets of all participants were assessed by interview and/or food log three times during the first year and twice yearly thereafter, The dietary data were converted to mean daily nutrient intake on a previously established computer programme and utilized in the subsequent analyses of survival.

Table 1 shows some characteristics of the two dietary groups on entry and during follow-up. They were well-matched for age, infarct weight, entry weight, systolic and diastolic blood pressure, serum cholesterol, serum triglyceride and serum urate. They were also well-matched for disability index, cigarette smoking, previous coronary disease, occupation and physical activity. There was no difference in entry characteristics, nor in survival between men whose most recent episode was myocardial infarction and men in whom it was angina or acute coronary insufficiency. The latter have been included with the former in all analyses. There had been appreciable and significant loss of weight in both groups from infarct to entry and further loss occurred during follow-up. Significant changes also occurred in smoking habit. These are discussed later.

Table 1

SOME CHARACTERISTICS OF THE TWO DIETARY GROUPS, P AND F AT ENTRY AND DURING FOLLOW-UP. MEANS ± S.D.*

	Group P N=237	Group F N=221
ENTRY		
Age	49.1±6.5	48.7±6.8
Weight at infarct	75.9±11.4	76.4±10.6
Weight at entry	73.2±9.5	73.1±9.3
Systolic blood pressure	136.9±21.1	136.6±20.1
Diastolic blood pressure	88.5±12.0	88.5±12.5
Serum cholesterol	282.0±55.6	281.3±63.4
Serum triglyceride	185.9±132.9	189.0±199.1
Serum urate	6.7±1.6	6.7±1.6
FOLLOW-UP		
Mean weight	71.3±8.5	71.4±8.6
Systolic blood pressure	137.9±16.1	136.8±16.1
Diastolic blood pressure	88.7±9.6	88.4±9.4
Serum cholesterol	262.3±42.0	250.2±44.7**
Serum triglyceride	154.5±76.5	144.4±80.9

* During follow-up mean weight, serum cholesterol and serum triglyceride were significantly lower in both groups than on entry.

** $p > 0.01$.

Sixty-seven died during follow-up. Sixty deaths were due to coronary disease, three to cerebral vascular disease, two to cancer and two to motor accidents. In one of the latter death was thought due to sudden cardiac death. Twenty-eight deaths occured in the P group and 39 in the F group. Overall 5 year survival of the 458 men was 81% (Figure 1). For the 276 men without hint of previous cardiac symptoms five year survival was 86% giving an attrition rate of approximately 3% per annum. Cumulative percentage survival of the P and F groups is shown in Figure 2. Survival was significantly better in the P group, although the difference was not marked.

Because of the apparent lack of influence of diet on

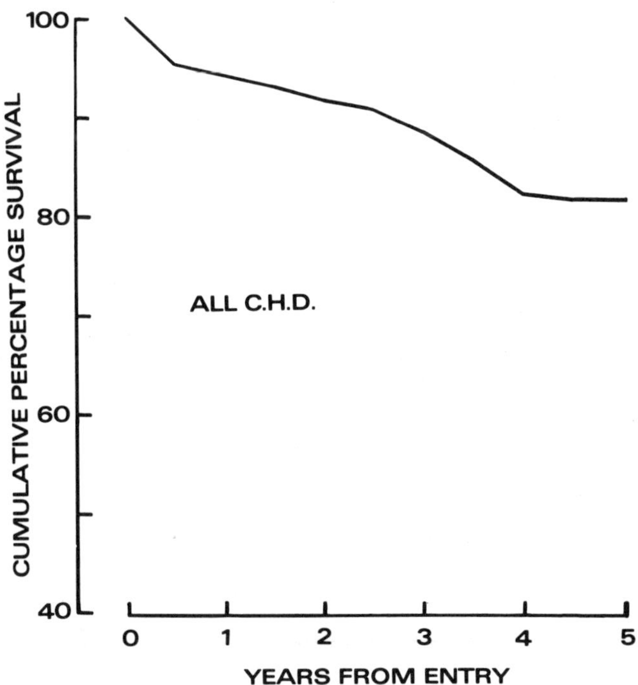

Figure 1: Cumulative percentage survival of 458 men with coronary disease followed over 5 years.

survival univariate analysis of the data of the whole group was done to determine the factors present on entry which might have prognostic significance. The following were unfavourable for survival when each was considered as a single variable; previous coronary disease, severe as opposed to mild or moderate infarction, presence at entry of angina pectoris or unusual dyspnoea on exertion, cardiac enlargment, ST-T and Q wave abnormalities in the ECG, excessive weight, hyperuricemia. Survival according to severity of angina is shown in Figure 3. Age, systolic blood pressure, serum cholesterol, serum triglycerides, glucose tolerance, smoking habit, history of premature coronary disease in first degree relatives and site of infarction by ECG were not related to survival. It was clear that the extent of the coronary disease and the functional performance of the myocardium were the major determinants of the prognosis.

The diets being consumed on entry to the study by

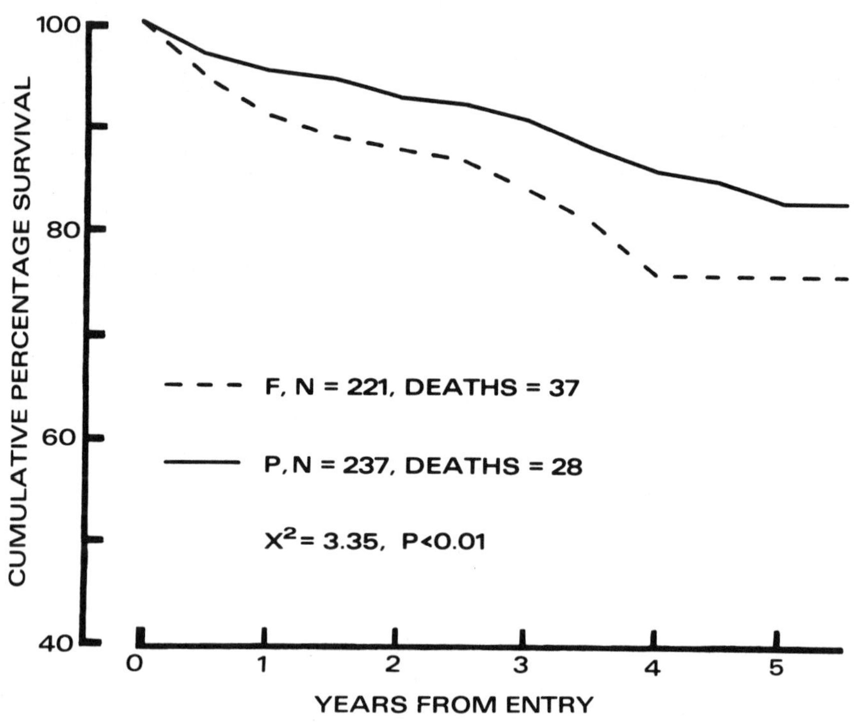

Figure 2: Cumulative percentage survival of the dietary groups P and F during 5 years of follow-up.

the P and F groups are shown in Table 2. The pattern of the nutrients conformed well to that found in normal subjects in Australia (3). However, there were slight but probably important differences. The caloric intake was lower, the saturated fatty acids and cholesterol intake were lower and the polyunsaturated fatty acid intake was higher than in normal healthy men. These changes had been made following infarction and before attending our clinic. There were no significant differences between the diets of the two groups on entry. Our estimate was that mean intake had declined by 500 calories or more per day.

Change in diet after infarct was reflected in body weight on entry. Three hundred seven of the 458 men had

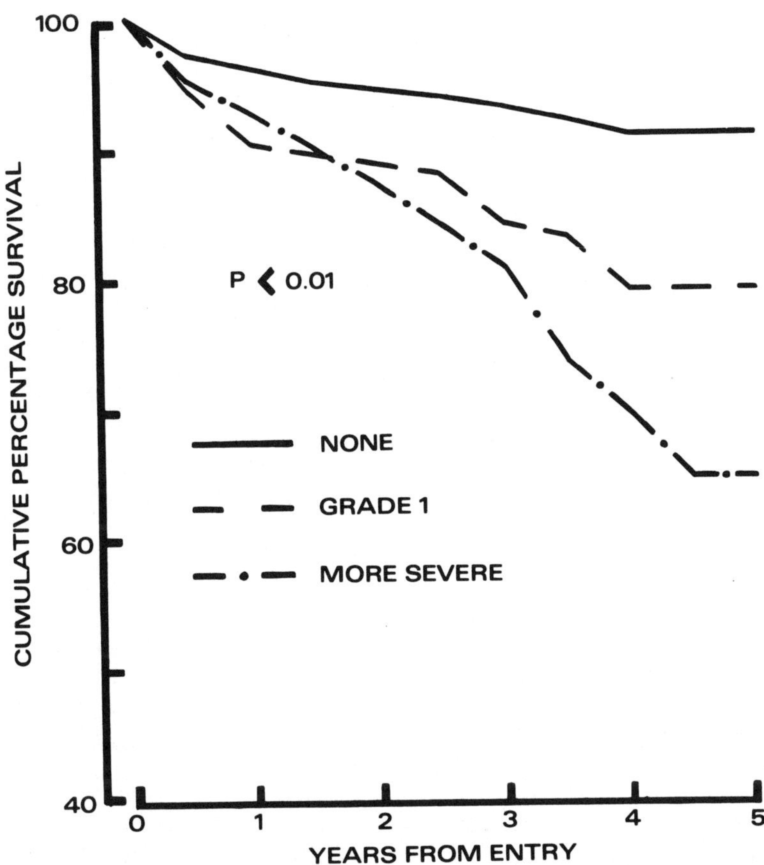

Figure 3: Cumulative percentage survival by grade of angina pectoris on entry.

Grade 1 = angina while hurrying on the level or climbing stairs or hills at normal speed.

Table 2

MEAN COMPOSITION OF THE DIET IN EACH GROUP ON ENTRY*

	GROUP P N=221		GROUP F N=205	
	% CALS.	GRAMS	% CALS.	GRAMS
Protein	14.7±3.8	85±21	14.7±3.0	87±19
Fat	39.4±6.0	105±30	39.9±6.6	108±31
Sats.	15.9±4.2	43±16	16.4±4.1	45±16
Monos	14.9±3.1	40±12	14.9±2.9	40±11
PUFA	6.6±3.8	18±11	6.6±4.1	18±13
Carbohydrate	40.8±6.9	246±75	40.3±8.3	253±101
Alcohol	5.0±6.1	18±25	5.0±6.4	18±26
Cholesterol(mg)		486±214		508±226
Calories		2397±602		2457±645
P/S		0.5±0.4		0.5±0.4

* None of the differences were significant. The data from 16 men in the P group and 16 men in the F group were considered unreliable and have been omitted.

lost a mean of 5.4 kg since infarction; they lost a further 1.4 kg during follow-up. One hundred fifty-one men had gained a mean of 2.3 kg after infarction; they lost a mean of 2.5 kg during follow-up. Both the P and F groups were lighter than they had been at infarction and had already made changes in their diet prior to randomization.

Table 3 shows the dietary patterns of the two groups during follow-up. There was a fall in mean daily intake of approximately 200 calories per day in both groups. The F group showed changes in saturated fat, polyunsaturated oils and dietary cholesterol which, on average, agreed well with the dietary prescription. Unfortunately the P group, thought of as controls, also changed in the same

Table 3

MEAN COMPOSITION OF THE DIET IN EACH GROUP ON FOLLOW-UP[a]

	GROUP P N=221		GROUP F N=205	
	% CALS.	GRAMS	% CALS.	GRAMS
Protein	15.7±3.4	83±17	15.2±2.8	85±16
Fat	38.1±5.4	92±23	38.3±5.9	96±22[b]
Sats.	13.5±3.2	33±11	9.8±2.6[c]	25±8[c]
Monos	13.8±2.5	33±9	11.5±2.1[c]	29±7[c]
PUFA	8.9±3.5	22±10	15.1±4.3[c]	38±13[c]
Carbohydrate	40.3±7.3	226±81	40.9±7.3	240±83
Alcohol	5.7±5.8	19±21	5.4±5.8	18±20
Cholesterol (mg)		342±103		248±75[c]
Calories		2191±549		2289±508
P/S		0.8±0.5		1.7±0.6[c]

[a] Both the percentage composition and the absolute amount of the nutrients were significantly different from those on entry in both groups for nearly all the nutrients at the 0.001 level. Alcohol and percentage carbohydrate were not significantly different.

[b] $p < 0.05$

[c] $p < 0.001$

direction but to a lesser extent. Weight loss was 1.9 kg in the P group and 1.7 kg in the F group. The P group was now 4.6 kg and the F group 4.8 kg lighter than at infarction. Serum cholesterol declined by 19.7 mg/100 ml in the P group and by 31.1 mg/100 ml in the F group (Table 1). There was no significant change in blood pressure from entry to follow-up in either group.

Table 4 shows the profound change that occurred in

Table 4

SMOKING HABIT AT INFARCTION AND ON ENTRY TO THE DIET-HEART STUDY

	AT INFARCTION	ON ENTRY
Non-smokers	137 (30%)	284 (62%)
Smokers	321 (70%)	174 (38%)
Total	458	458

smoking habit. Non-smokers increased from 30% at infarction to 62% on entry. Those who continued to smoke reduced their intake drastically. At infarction 47.1% of the total group were smoking more than 20 cigarettes a day. At entry only 6.1% exceeded that usage.

It is apparent that the difference in diet between P and F groups was smaller than we had hoped. It was unlikely to show significant advantage for the F group in the numbers studied. However there was considerable intra group variation in diet and overlap between the groups. To determine whether those with the higher fat diets did worse than those with a low fat diet multivariate analysis by the method of stepwise regression in life tables was done (4). In this method the diets of subjects who die are compared with the diets of those living at the time of each death. No significant differences were found. Simple comparison of the mean diet of those who died with those who survived also revealed only trivial differences. There was a trend towards better survival of those with the lowest levels of serum cholesterol but this did not quite reach the 5% level of significance. Serum cholesterol level was significant for survival in the control subjects of the Coronary Drug Project (5). However it was low on the list of determinants and very large numbers were needed to show its influence.

Clearly what was planned as a test of the lipid hypothesis became a multifactorial study. Changes in smoking habit, dietary pattern, body weight, lifestyle and physical activity before and after entry to the trial may well have had a significant effect on prognosis. On that background any added effect of further dietary change could not be shown. Both the number of subjects and the duration of the study may have been insufficient. However, the force of strict fat modification must be low if very large numbers are needed to show its benefit in secondary prevention. More drastic restriction of fat and cholesterol to the levels prevailing in Asian countries and elsewhere might yield a positive answer. General acceptance of such change in unlikely.

In an effort to determine the separate influences of the large number of variables, medical, behavioural and dietetic data from infarction to death or the conclusion of the study were submitted to a number of multivariate analyses using the same method of stepwise regression in life tables (4).

Preliminary computer analyses were directed to reduction of the variables to manageable numbers so that only those which had any likelihood of being important were included in the final run. In addition a number of entry variables of interest were included. The final input comprised 26 entry variables plus 10 medical variables and 12 dietary variables during follow-up. By this method of analysis the entry variables which were associated with poor survival were, in order, the use of digitalis, the presence of angina, marital separation or divorce, history of diabetes, Q and ST-T changes in the ECG, left ventricular hypertrophy by ECG and the presence of clinical cerebrovascular disease. Other indicators of myocardial disease found significant by univariate analysis, such as severity of infarction and radiological cardiac enlargement, were accounted for by these variables. The factors which were non-contributory on univariate analysis remained non-contributory on multivariate analysis.

During follow-up serum cholesterol, serum triglycerides, body mass index, blood pressure and smoking habit had no predictive value. Recreational physical activity had a highly favourable effect. The use of diuretics for the first time during follow-up had an unfavourable effect. The development of new angina pectoris, the new use of digitalis and the appearance of any degree of cardiac failure were also unfavourable but added little to the prediction of probability of death. As found previously none of the dietary variables had predictive power. The multivariate analysis confirmed the dominant effect on prognosis of the coronary and myocardial disease present on entry to the study.

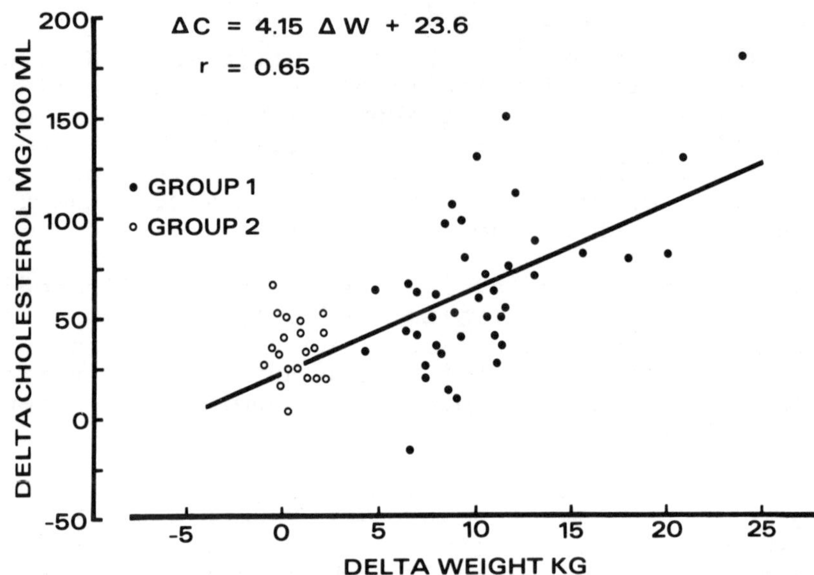

Figure 4: Change in serum cholesterol (Δc) plotted against change in body weight (Δw). Group 1 comprised 41 overweight hypercholesterolemic men who lost weight and Group 2 comprised 20 similar men whose weight did not change significantly during follow-up.

This study has brought home to us the almost insuperable difficulties of conducting intervention studies of this nature in coronary disease. Apart from the difficulties in the diet itself alterations in lifestyle which follow personal reappraisal introduce other variables which may have a greater influence than the dietary variables. It is neither practical nor ethical to advise men with coronary disease to continue to smoke, to ignore overweight and to remain physically inactive. Smoking, obesity and physical inactivity deserve brief comment.

The dramatic reduction in cigarette smoking in the whole cohort made the numbers of heavy smokers so few that the probable harmful effects were not apparent. In Gothenburg Wilhelmsen and his colleagues (6) have confirmed the expectation that continued smoking is unfavourable to survival in men with coronary disease.

The potential importance of weight change was not fully appreciated at the time this work was begun. There is now good evidence that weight loss, particularly when combined with change in dietary lipids, has important favourable effects on both serum cholesterol and blood pressure (7,8,9). This is shown in Figure 4 which illustrates the relationship between weight loss and change in serum cholesterol in men from this study who were both obese and hypercholesterolemic (10). The fall in serum cholesterol in those who lost more than 5 kg in weight during follow-up was slightly more than double that of men whose weight was steady during follow-up. Both the P and F groups lost approximately 5 kg from infarct to the steady state during follow-up; the whole cohort had become lean by modern standards. This may account for the apparent lack of influence of body weight on survival. It may also explain in part the similar survival of the two dietary groups.

Recreational physical activity was shown to have a protective effect against heart disease in a recently reported prospective study of British civil servants (11). The favourable effect of physical activity observed in the present study is consistent with this. It was present after allowing for all other variables. This interesting finding merits further study.

Despite the imperfections of the present study the results are not very different from those reported by Leren (12) and by Dayton et al (13). The Leren study comprised 412 Norwegian men of similar age to our men and was done at a time when a control group could be maintained more easily on a normal western diet. There were a number of important differences in other features of the trial which cannot be discussed here. The dietary group lost 2.5 kg in weight and 52 mg/100 ml in serum cholesterol compared with 0.5 kg in weight and 11 mg/100 ml in serum cholesterol for the controls. Total 5 year cardiovascular mortality was 38 in the 206 dieted subjects and 52 in the controls. Sudden death accounted for 27 deaths in each group. Myocardial infarction caused 10 deaths in the diet group and 23 in the control group ($p<0.03$). The annual death rate from heart and cerebrovascular disease was 3.7% in the diet group and 5.0% in the control group. Thus the possible saving by diet was 1.3 lives per 100 per year. In the Los Angeles study of Dayton *et al* (12) the men were much older and there was no improvement in overall five year survival in the diet group. It must be concluded that the lipid hypothesis has gained little support from secondary intervention studies.

Finally it is important to emphasize the remarkably good survival of unselected patients who have had myocardial infarction. The annual overall attrition rate of 3 to 4% per annum found here was similar to that in the Norwegian study (11), in the Coronary Drug Project (13) and in the Gothenburg study (6). How much this good survival is due merely to the natural history of the disease and how much is due to multiple changes in lifestyle after infarction is an open question.

REFERENCES

1. Report of the Inter-Society Commission for Heart Disease Resources.
Circulation 42, 1970. Revised, 1972.
2. Build and Blood Pressure Studies. Society of Actuaries. Chicago, 1959
3. Woodhill, J.M., A.J. Palmer and R.B. Blacket
Food Technol. Aust. 21: 264 (1969)
4. McGilchrist, C.A., unpublished
5. Coronary Drug Project Research Group
J. Chron. Dis. 27: 267 (1974)
6. Wilhelmsen, L., 1977, unpublished data
7. Ashley, F.W. and Kannel, W.B.
J. Chron. Dis. 27: 103 (1974)
8. Leelarthaepin, B., J.M. Woodhill, A.J. Palmer, and R.B. Blacket
Lancet II: 1217 (1974)
9. Chiang, B.I.Y., L.V. Perlman and F.H. Epstein
Circulation 39: 403 (1969)
10. Blacket, R.B., B. Leelarthaepin, C.A. McGilchrist, A.J. Palmer and J.M. Woodhill
Submitted for publication
11. Morris, J.N., S.P.W. Chave, C. Adam, C. Sirey and L. Epstein
Lancet I: 333 (1973)
12. Leren, P.
Acta Med. Scand. Suppl. 466 (1966)
13. Dayton, S., M.L. Pearce, S. Hashimoto, W.J. Dixon and U. Tomiyasu
Circulation 40: Suppl. II (1969)
14. The Coronary Drug Project Research Group.
J. Am. Med. Assoc. 231: 360 (1975)

A REAPPRAISAL OF THE MECHANISMS OF HYPOCHOLESTEROLEMIC ACTION OF THERAPEUTIC AGENTS

H.S. Sodhi, B.J. Kudchodkar, C. Clifford, N. Borhani, and D.T. Mason

University of California, School of Medicine
Davis, California, U.S.A.

ABSTRACT

The most commonly used methods to study the mechanisms of hypocholesterolemic action of therapeutic agents generally determine the turnover of total (exchangeable) cholesterol pools in the body. This approach is based on the view that whatever increases the total load of cholesterol in the body will increase the levels of plasma cholesterol, and vice versa. Despite the importance of this assumption it has never been tested, and there is no evidence to indicate that it is valid under all conditions.

This "overload" hypothesis dates from the times before the importance of plasma lipoproteins was recognized and their role in the transport of lipids was well understood. However, it is becoming increasingly clear that the levels of plasma cholesterol are determined more directly by the "transport" of cholesterol into and out of plasma compartment by lipoproteins than by the synthesis, absorption and elimination of cholesterol from the total body pools. Any effects that the latter parameters of cholesterol metabolism have on the levels of plasma cholesterol must be mediated through changes in synthesis and the subsequent metabolism of plasma lipoproteins. In other words, in any equation relating changes in the levels of plasma cholesterol to the changes in synthesis, absorption and elimination of cholesterol from the body pools we must consider the "transport" of cholesterol by lipoproteins and their metabolism.

During the last three days you heard that there are factors both in plasma and in arterial wall (1-5) which bear on the problem of atherosclerosis (Table I). However, it is worth emphasizing that the conclusive evidence for association with clinical disease exists only with elevated levels of plasma cholesterol. The protective role of plasma high density lipoproteins was discussed this morning and is also worth noting. The importance of most other factors listed in Table I is yet quite uncertain, and therefore attempts directed to influence those factors, in the current state of our knowledge, cannot be viewed as necessarily therapeutic. However, all these factors should be examined in the hope of elucidating the evolution of atherosclerosis. All we have at this moment is the hope and possibly some evidence suggesting that reducing levels of plasma cholesterol may be helpful.

Means sought to lower plasma cholesterol have generally been directed specifically to decreasing absorption, inhibiting synthesis, and increasing elimination of cholesterol from the body. This traditional approach delineated by Dr. Ahrens this morning has been based on a notion which I have termed the "overload hypothesis" (Figure 1). This has been well defined in one of the papers from Dr. Ahren's laboratories as below (6):

"The total body cholesterol is regulated by a complex dynamic interplay between absorption, synthesis and excretion. Any imbalance among the principal determinants might result in swelling or depletion of the exchangeable body pools of cholesterol, and it might be expected that the size of plasma cholesterol pool would reflect such imbalances."

With all humility to my teachers and my senior colleagues, I would like to suggest that the time has come for us to replace the above hypothesis with a new approach termed here as "transport hypothesis" (Figure 2). The purpose of my talk is to clarify and define the traditional view as well as the other view which has been gradually evolving with the increase in our knowledge of plasma lipoproteins (7). Receptor hypothesis is another view recently formulated by Brown and Goldstein (8), but it is too limited in scope in so far as the development of the new drugs is concerned and therefore I would not talk about it this morning.

Triparanol was the first major drug specifically

Table I

FACTORS IN PLASMA AND IN ARTERIAL WALL
RELEVANT TO ATHEROMATOUS LESIONS

IN PLASMA
Concentration of plasma cholesterol
Concentration of chol-rich remnants of chylomicra
Turnover of plasma LDL
Concentration of plasma HDL
IN ARTERIAL WALL
Receptors for circulating LDL
Factors which precipitate circulating VLDL and LDL
Factors which precipitate circulating cholesterol
Tissue enzymes acting on cholesterol

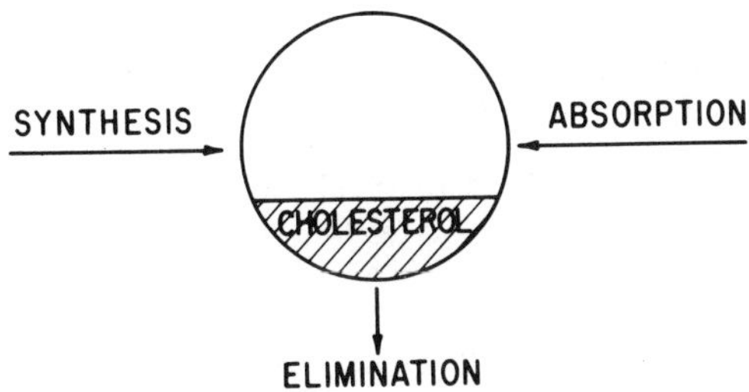

Figure 1. Overload hypothesis

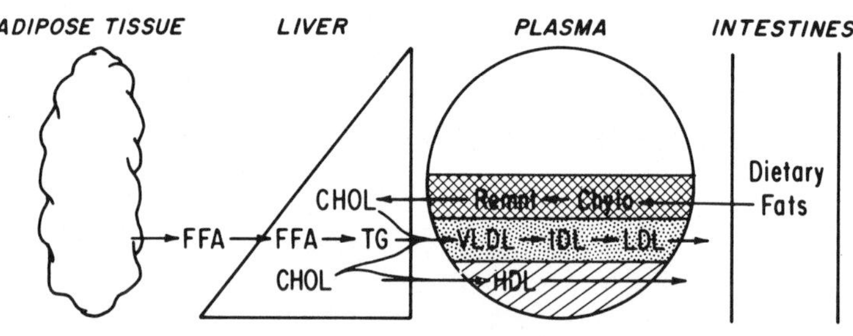

ASSUMPTIONS

Free cholesterol serves as one of the packaging materials for synthesis of Lipoproteins and its esterification in plasma reflects disposal of excess packaging material (surface coat) as the contents of the package are depleted.

Figure 2. Transport hypothesis

developed and introduced as a hypocholesterolemic agent. It inhibited the conversion of desmosterol to cholesterol and it also reduced levels of plasma cholesterol. However, triparanol also caused accumulation of desmosterol in tissues and in plasma causing serious toxic side effects and this sensitized most of us to the potential risks of using inhibitors of cholesterol synthesis.

The physiological control of cholesterol synthesis is exercised at a single step in its synthetic pathway. This is considered to be the ideal site for any drug's action. It is assumed that by acting at such an early step in the biosynthetic pathway the accumulation of undesirable precursors of cholesterol does not occur. A large number of inhibitors of cholesterol synthesis were developed which also did reduce plasma levels of cholesterol, but as immortalized in Dr. Kritchevsky's lyrics they were also "toxic to the rat."

The biosynthesis of cholesterol involves a large series of enzymatic steps and the probability of any one inhibitor affecting only this single step (at the level of HMG-CoA reductase) on entirely random basis would of course be slight. Clofibrate, when first introduced was thought to decrease plasma cholesterol specifically by inhibiting synthesis of cholesterol at this site (9).

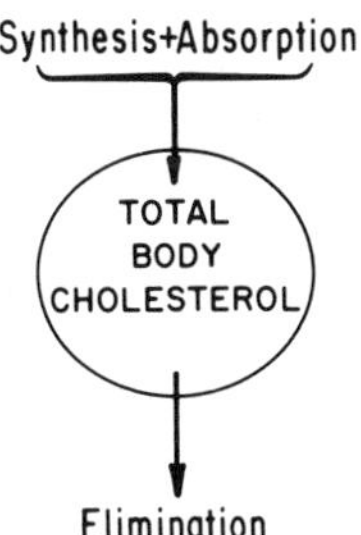

Figure 3. Turnover of total (exchangeable) cholesterol in the body

Studies carried out in many laboratories (10,11), including ours (12-15), suggest that the drug's hypocholesterolemic action can be attributed to its effects on other aspects of lipoprotein metabolism and we think that its inhibitory action on cholesterol synthesis is secondary to such other actions (15).

Cholestyramine was the next major drug introduced especially to reduce plasma cholesterol levels. Since it increased the elimination of cholesterol from the body, as fecal bile acids (16,17), the same action was then considered to be the mechanism of the drug's action (16).

Equally important in the evolution of the traditional view was the development and the introduction of reliable methods for the study of cholesterol metabolism in man. Ahrens, Grundy, Miettinen and their associates (18,19) developed the cholesterol balance methods which rightfully became the "gold" standards for comparing the validity of other methods. Work of Goodman (20), Wilson (21) and Nestel (22) provided a second and simpler method which gave almost equally reliable information.

It is clear that the estimation of absorption, synthesis and elimination of cholesterol from the body determined by these methods gives information about the turnover of total body cholesterol (Figure 3) and as such any changes in these parameters of cholesterol metabolism would directly influence only the levels of total cholesterol in the body and not the levels of plasma cholesterol.

During the past decade there has been considerable interest both in these methods and in the development of hypocholesterolemic agents. Efforts were directed by the pharmaceutical industry to develop agents which were specifically directed to either inhibit synthesis, decrease absorption, or increase elimination of cholesterol from the body. And, if any of the agents also decreased plasma cholesterol, the very characteristic the agent was directed to have, was, then considered to be the mechanism of its action. Thus, in a sense there was a narcisstic relationship between the origin and the mechanism of action attributed to any hypocholesterolemic drug.

Experimental data bearing directly on the critical assumption (6) made in the traditional approach or the overload hypothesis are not available. What little evidence there is in the literature does not support the suggestion that changes in the total body cholesterol are necessarily associated with corresponding changes in the levels of plasma cholesterol.

Earlier studies of Insull and his associates (23), and more recent studies from Dr. Ahren's laboratories, by Crouse and Schriebman (24), failed to reveal any correlation between plasma levels and tissue pools of cholesterol. Additional studies from Dr. Ahren's laboratories showed that when tissue pools of cholesterol are increased by feeding large amounts of cholesterol, they were not necessarily associated with increase in plasma levels of cholesterol (25).

We have analyzed data from 121 subjects reported in the literature in whom levels of plasma cholesterol and approximation of tissue cholesterol (based on two pool models) were available. The levels of plasma cholesterol showed no correlation either with the size of pool B or with the tissue component of pool A (Table II). Similarly in another study from Dr. Goodman's laboratory (26), the pool B calculated on a three pool model failed to show any correlation, although the minimal values of pool C in this study did show significant positive correlation. Recent data published by Miller and Nestel (27) also confirmed the absence of correspondance between tissue and plasma pools of cholesterol.

There are two aspects of any correlation between

Table II

CORRELATIONS BETWEEN PLASMA CHOLESTEROL CONCENTRATIONS AND TISSUE CHOLESTEROL POOLS

	TISSUE COMPONENT			
	Pool A		Pool B	
Group	No.	r	No.	r
Normal	34	0.28	37	0.28
Hypercholesterolemia	38	0.20	40	0.40 *
Hypertriglyceridemia	9	0.16	10	-0.10
Hyperchol. & Hypertrig.	34	0.09	34	-0.06
Total	115	0.09	121	0.13

* Only significant correlation, $p<0.01$.

tissue and plasma pools of cholesterol. The overload hypothesis assumes that a primary increase in tissue cholesterol leads to a secondary increase in plasma cholesterol. In fact, it appears that whatever tissue cholesterol is mobilized into plasma, is, rapidly excreted by the liver and thus it does not significantly influence the levels of cholesterol into plasma (28). The reverse, however, appears to be true, that a primary increase in plasma levels of cholesterol can lead to a secondary increase in tissue pools as suggested by the development of xanthomata in patients with hypercholesterolemia.

Work of Mattson (29), Connor (30) and others showed that increase in intake of cholesterol generally leads to increase in plasma levels of cholesterol. It was generally believed that man does not possess a negative feedback control of endogenous synthesis, therefore increased absorption was assumed to increase the load of new cholesterol entering the body and this increase in the total cholesterol in the body was then reflected as elevation of plasma cholesterol. More recent studies, however, indicate that the man has a fairly efficient system of control of endogenous synthesis by dietary cholesterol (25,31). Thus, the increase in plasma cholesterol on cholesterol-rich diets cannot always be attributed to increase in the load of new cholesterol in the body.

These experimental studies are corroborated by our analysis of the majority of published data on cholesterol balance (32). Synthesis in patients on low cholesterol diets was greater than that in those on high cholesterol intake. The total amounts of new cholesterol derived from absorption, plus, synthesis, were essentially the same in both groups in every class of patients examined, thus suggesting that increased intake may increase plasma cholesterol without necessarily causing an increase in the load of new cholesterol.

During the steady state conditions the fecal elimination of cholesterol and its metabolites about equal the input of new cholesterol from absorption, and synthesis. Immediately after the administration of hypocholesterolemic agents, it is obvious that some cholesterol must leave plasma. It may enter tissue pools or be eliminated from the body. In addition, there is mobilization of tissue cholesterol as levels of plasma cholesterol fall, which also appears to be readily excreted in the feces (28). Although increased fecal elimination is considered to be a mechanism of hypocholesterolemic action of therapeutic action, there is no evidence to suggest that it is a direct effect of any of the hypocholesterolemic agents. Indeed, evidence for mobilization and increased fecal elimination of cholesterol is seen in all conditions associated with fall in plasma cholesterol even when no drug is used, e.g. restriction of caloric intake (33). Furthermore, comparable decrease in plasma cholesterol can occur with or without an increase in the fecal metabolites of endogenous cholesterol (14,15). Whether or not there is an increase in fecal cholesterol depends upon the balance of <u>new</u> turnover rate and cholesterol lost from tissue-plasma pools, as illustrated in the example given in Table III.

Since plasma levels of cholesterol are controlled by the rates of entry into plasma of intestinal and hepatic lipoproteins and the rates of subsequent metabolism (Figure 4), the development of therapeutic agents should

Table III

Control Periods	Hypertrig (mg/day)	Normotrig (mg/day)
Synthesis	1400	700
Absorption dietary cholesterol	300	300
Total turnover rates, or Total fecal metabolites of endogenous cholesterol	1700	1000
After Starting Treatment		
Inhibition of synthesis	(30%)	(30%)
New synthetic rate	980	490
Absorption dietary cholesterol	300	300
Losses from tissue-plasma pools	350	350
Total fecal metabolites of endogenous cholesterol	1630	1140
Changes in total fecal steroids	-70	+140

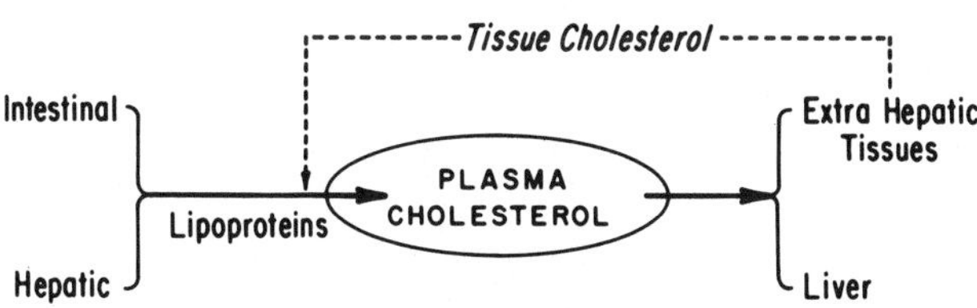

Figure 4: Diagram of pathways involved in turnover of plasma cholesterol.

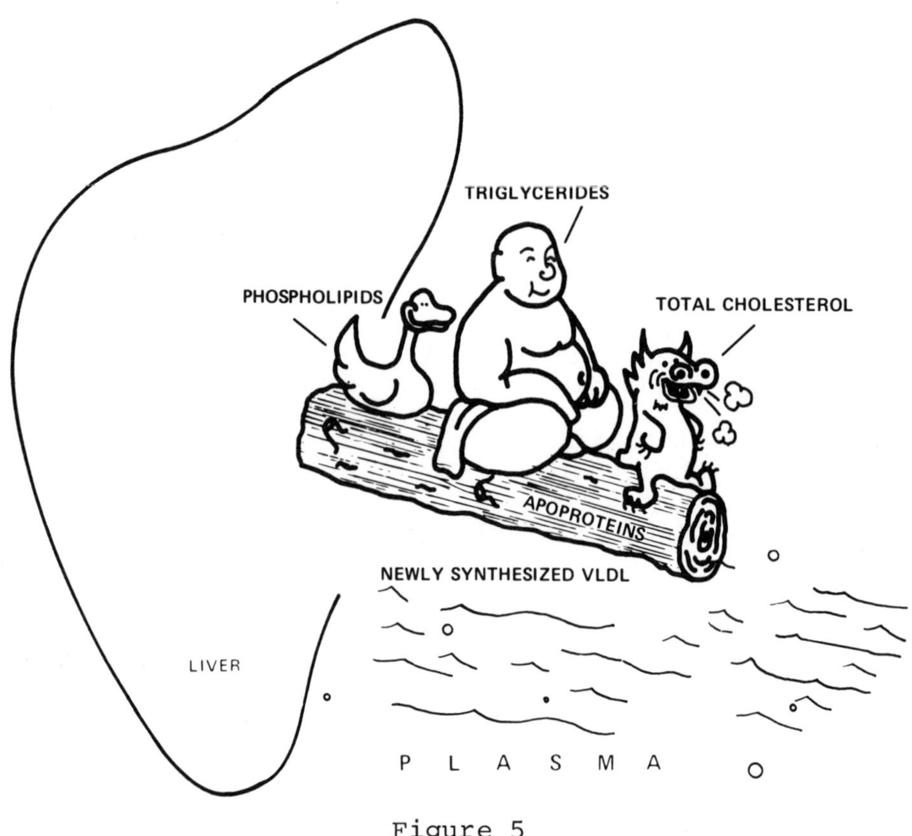
TRIGLYCERIDES
PHOSPHOLIPIDS
TOTAL CHOLESTEROL
APOPROTEINS
NEWLY SYNTHESIZED VLDL
LIVER
P L A S M A

Figure 5

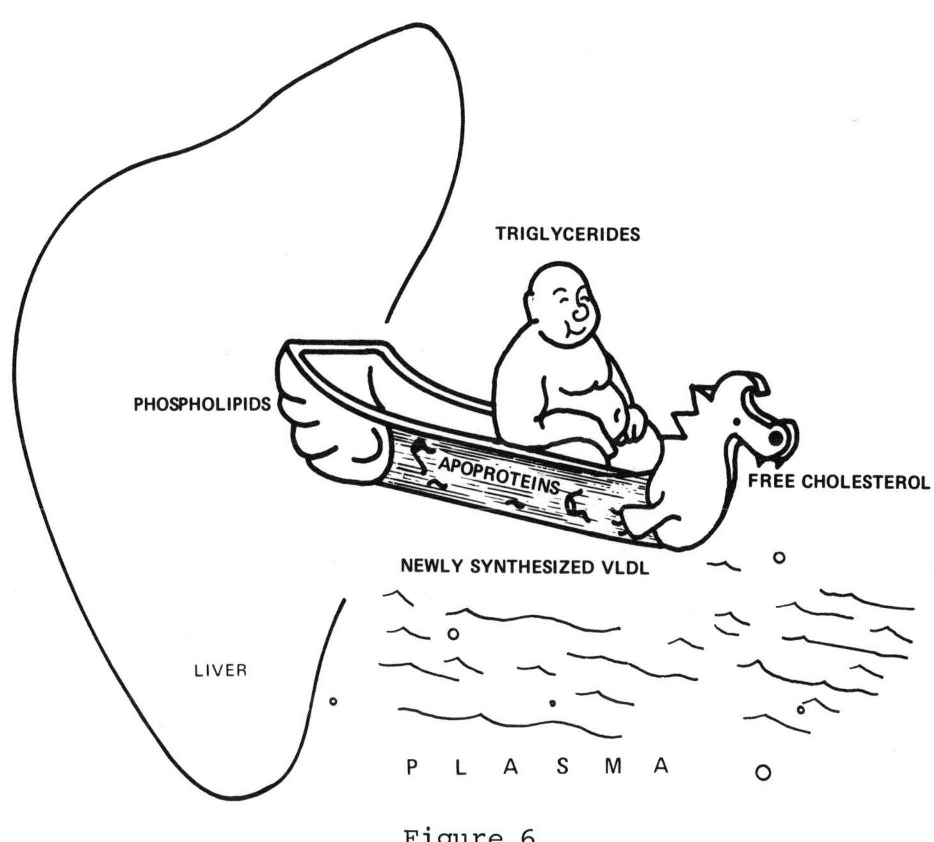
TRIGLYCERIDES
PHOSPHOLIPIDS
APOPROTEINS
FREE CHOLESTEROL
NEWLY SYNTHESIZED VLDL
LIVER
P L A S M A

Figure 6

Table IV

MECHANISMS OF HYPOCHOLESTEROLEMIC ACTION ACCORDING TO

Drug	Literature on cholesterol metabolism or the "Overload Hypothesis"	Lipoproteinologists or the "Transport Hypothesis"
Clofibrate	↓ Biosynthesis of cholesterol	↓ Flux of FFA from adipose tissue ↓ Hepatic secretion of VLDL into plasma ↑ Clearance of circulating VLDL
Nicotinic Acid	↓ Biosynthesis of cholesterol	↓ Mobilization of FFA from adipose tissue ↓ Hepatic secretion of VLDL into plasma ↓ Synthesis of LDL
Cholestyramine	↑ Catabolism of cholesterol	↑ Turnover of VLDL ↑ Rate of clearance of circulating LDL
Polyunsaturated fats	↑ Fecal elimination of cholesterol and its metabolites. Shift of plasma cholesterol into tissues	Possible increased rate of clearance of circulating lipoproteins

not be directed to synthesis, absorption and elimination of cholesterol, but to the metabolism of various plasma lipoproteins to achieve hypocholesterolemia.

The difference between the approaches based on the "overload" and the "transport" hypotheses may be illustrated with the help of some visual aids (Figures 5 and 6). Most of you are perhaps familiar with the representation of a lipoprotein molecule first popularized by the NIH group. Cholesterol, phospholipids, and triglycerides were all shown as passengers in a boat constituted by the apoproteins: which is in accord with the traditional view. I have represented the same concept in Figure 5. More in accord with the "transport" hypothesis is the representation shown in Figure 6, where free cholesterol and phospholipids are represented as parts of the transport system and not as the passengers. Only the triglycerides are the prime passengers in the recently synthesized hepatic very low density lipoproteins. It is further suggested that the metabolism of cholesterol is dictated more by the metabolism of the triglycerides than by the absorption, synthesis and catabolism of cholesterol itself. Cholesterol esters are other passengers in this transport system. However they come abroad later during the sojourn of lipoproteins through the intravascular compartment.

Table IV further distinguishes between the possible mechanisms of action of different therapeutic agents according to the "overload" and the "transport" hypotheses.

REFERENCES

1. Zilversmit, D.B.
Circ. Res. 33: 633 (1973)
2. Kudchodkar, B.J., Sodhi, H.S., Horlick, L., and Nazir, D.J.
Proc. Soc. Exp. Biol. Med. 148: 393 (1975)
3. Tracy, R.D., Dzoga, K.R. and Wissler, R.W.
Proc. Soc. Exp. Biol. Med. 118: 1095 (1965)
4. Iverius, P.H.
Ciba Found. Symp. 12: 185 (1973)
5. Kramsch, D.M. and Hollander, W.
J. Clin. Invest. 52: 236 (1973)
6. Pertsemlidis, D., Kirchman, E.H. and Ahrens, E.H.,Jr.
J. Clin. Invest. 52: 2368 (1973)

7. Sodhi, H.S., Kudchodkar, B.J., Borhani, N. and Mason, D.T.
Artery 3: 120 (1977)

8. Brown, M.S. and Goldstein, J.L.
N. Engl. J. Med. 294: 1386 (1976)

9. Avoy, R.D., Swyryd, E.A. and Gould, R.G.
J. Lipid Res. 6: 369 (1965)

10. Gould, R.G., Swyryd, E.A., Avoy, D. and Coan, B.
Biochem. Pharmacol. 2: 345 (1967)

11. Segal, P., Roheim, P.S. and Eder, H.A.
J. Clin. Invest. 51: 1632 (1972)

12. Sodhi, H.S., Kudchodkar, B.J. and Horlick, L.
Metabolism 20: 309 (1971)

13. Sodhi, H.S., Kudchodkar, B.J., Horlick, L. and Weder, C.
Metabolism 20: 348 (1971)

14. Horlick, L., Kudchodkar, B.J. and Sodhi, H.S.
Circulation 43: 299 (1971)

15. Kudchodkar, B.J., Sodhi, H.S., Horlick, L., and Mason, D.T.
Clin. Phar. Therap. 22: 154 (1977)

16. Grundy, S.M., Ahrens, E.H., Jr., and Salen, G.
J. Lab. Clin. Med. 78: 94 (1971)

17. Nazir, D.J., Horlick, L., Kudchodkar, B.J., and Sodhi, H.S.
Circulation 46: 95 (1972)

18. Grundy, S.M., Ahrens,E.H., Jr., and Miettinen, T.A.
J. Lipid Res. 6: 397 (1965)

19. Miettinen, T.A., Ahrens, E.H., Jr., and Grundy, S.M.
J. Lipid Res. 6: 411 (1965)

20. Goodman, D.S. and Noble, R.P.
J. Clin. Invest. 47: 231 (1968)

21. Wilson, J.D.
J. Clin. Invest. 49: 655 (1970)

22. Nestel, P.J., Whyte, H.M. and Goodman, D.S.
J. Clin. Invest. 48: 982 (1969)

23. Insull, W.M., Si, B.H., and Hoshimura, S.
J. Lab. Clin. Med. 72: 885A (1968)

24. Crouse, J.R. and Schreibman, P.H.
Clin. Res. 23: 317A (1975)

25. Quintao, E., Grundy, S.M. and Ahrens,E.H., Jr.
J. Lipid Res. 12: 233 (1971)

26. Smith, F.R., Dell, R.B., Noble, R.P. and Goodman, D.S.
J. Clin. Invest. 57: 137 (1976)

27. Miller, N.E., Nestel, P.J., and Clifton-Bligh, P.
Atherosclerosis 23: 535 (1976)

28. Sodhi, H.S., Kudchodkar, B.J. and Horlick, L.
Atherosclerosis 17: 1 (1973)

29. Mattson, F.H., Erickson, B.A. and Kligman, A.M. Am. J. Clin. Nutr. 25: 589 (1972)
30. Connor, W.E., Hodges, R.E. and Bleiler, R.E. J. Clin. Invest. 40: 894 (1961)
31. Nestel, P.J. and Poyser, A. Metabolism 25: 1591 (1976)
32. Sodhi, H.S. In Handbook of Experimental Pharmacology, Volume 41, D. Kritchevsky, editor, Springer Verlag, New York, 1975
33. Kudchodkar, B.J., Sodhi, H.S., Mason, D.T. and Borhani, N.O. Am. J. Clin. Nutr. 30: 1135 (1977)

THE TRUE MEANING OF PLAQUE REGRESSION

Robert W. Wissler

Department of Pathology, University of
Chicago, Chicago, Illinois, U.S.A.

Dear Friends, that I've known for many a year,
I want you to know that I'm glad to be here.
But can you imagine the pickle I'm in--
No projector's available for love or a fin!
So though I'm prepared with a talk and new slides,
I'll not be showing them, Bill Holmes confides.
Sadly, no tables or graphs on regression
It's enough to bring on a deep, dark depression.
Unlike Bill, who can give a superb talk on any title
Or Dave, who can sing up a storm and give a recital,
I suddenly felt stranded in this city of Brotherly Love:
I turned, in desperation, to the heavenly muses above.
They said, "Just act natural, at ease, and at home,
And convert your "after-dinner talk" into a poem!"
So that's what I've done for this banquet session,
I'll contrast Healing and Remodeling with Regression.

Some of my friends think I've a magnificent obsession
With this process known as atheromatous plaque regression.
"What is the evidence," they say, "that makes you think,
Than an atherosclerotic plaque can really shrink?"
It starts with studies of populations
With changes in death rates in starving nations.
Well, we must be frank; this evidence is not substantial.
It is retrospective, uncontrolled and largely circum-
stantial.
Epidemiological studies often leave us at sea,
While pathological studies give us something to see.
Are there pathological studies that seem to indicate
That human atheromatous plaques regress; to vindicate
The view that Plaques do decrease in size
And danger, so they will kill fewer gals and guys?

Yes, we find that such studies do exist,
And reports of age- and sex-matched autopsies list
Aschoff's post-World War I observations to support the view;
And Vartiainen's Finnish studies after World War II;
And Wilens studies of wasted New York patients do
Show benefits of decreased fats, to mention a few.

But these, too, can be criticized, according to my friends.
They're retrospective, semi-quantitative and only give us trends.
What we need are prospective, quantitative studies
Of non-selected living patients, to take away the muddies.

And, fortunately, at least two such projects are underway
With sequential arteriograms to show if lesions go or stay.
Dave Blankenhorn has published two papers now
Of primary and secondary intervention to show us how
To quantitate the effects of lowered cholesterol
On lumen size in coronary or femoral
Arteries of patients with early or advanced lesions
And now he is beginning to show us the reasons.
While Buchwald finds that lesions stop progressing or improve
In 85% of those whose cholesterol shows a downward move.
Whereas by arteriography 65% of those who are controls
Show a steady progression of plaque and lumens with small holes.

Added to this encouraging evidence in human beings,
The animal work is making the whole process easier for seeing.
Several models now utilized by epidemiologists
Have remarkable resemblance to the human lesions studied by pathologists.

And monkeys, who often seem related to us in the end,
Now may really turn out to be our very best friend.
Since their advanced plaques look very much like ours
With similar components when studied at all microscopic powers.

With great skill, hard work and real good sense,
Armstrong, Connor and Warner, in several experiments,
Have shown that coronary arteries will open up
From 65% narrowed to 25% their lumen plaques interrupt.

And their chemical results when they came back
Showed that most of the lipids left the plaque.
Lowering the blood lipids brought on this halt--
That's all they did to achieve this result.

This has now been confirmed in Chicago four times
And in Albany more graphically by using swine
And with variations of one kind or another, it's true;
It is also successful in Winston-Salem and at L.S.U.
Now I submit this is really regression
Since lipid comes out of the artery's possession.

But collagen and elastin are really another of the
  puzzle's piece;
They "remodel" more it seems than they really decrease.
As in wounds or fractures they change their alignment
And get smaller in size but denser in confinement.
So they may be increased per unit dry weight
But really they are smaller in the anatomical state.
So "remodeling" appears to be a right proper term
When arterial fiber proteins are becoming more firm.

Of Giorgio Weber's studies using intimal scans,
Plaques lose their "ulcers" when exposed to therapeutic
  plans.
In fact, many of the changes that are called regression
Might better be called "healing" if one makes a confession.
I'm talking of monocytes as reported by Stary,
And Daoud's decrease in cells, it's a term we can "borry,"
For the decrease in calcium that they have observed
If this is confirmed, then "regression's" the word.

Right now I must stop, I think there's no doubt
Because Wissler's regressing; the word will get out.
Remember that "free speech" is part of our way,
And when you hear a "free speech" you don't have to pay.
So thanks for not throwing your tomatoes and eggs
And when next I show slides, your forebearance I beg.
Just remember, my friends, as you go to your homes,
Wissler's lecture with slides outclasses his poems!

Summary and Abstracts

SUMMARY

Hugh Sinclair

International Institute of Human Nutrition,
Oxford, England

Don Zilversmit doubted if this was a City of Brotherly love, but certainly when William Penn founded it he called it Philadelphia, City of Love. There has obviously been no sexual discrimination in the warmth of our welcome here, and we are deeply grateful to William Holmes for yet another superb Symposium and to his wife Phyllis for joining him in gracious hospitality. Dave Kritchevsky not only arranged an admirably blended programme but regaled us with splended music of which perhaps the lipid variations on a theme of Fagin were especially outstanding. Our presence here has been greatly assisted by the generosity of various pharmaceutical companies that are listed. But we cannot be here without filling in forms of application to state our needs, and scientists - although no doubt brilliant lipidologists - are singularly inept at doing this. However, Mr. Hollerorth and particularly the indefatigable Mrs. Hyatt have made good our deficiencies. And as usual the Symposium was rounded off by the presence of the ubiquitous Rodolfo Paoletti who in an extraordinary way combines producing books and journals, organizing and attending congresses and carrying out important original research; some of you may not know that he has recently set up an Italian Nutrition Foundation. To all I have mentioned, and to the others who work so hard behind the scenes, we are deeply grateful for without their tireless efforts the Symposium could not be so remarkably successful.

Paoletti reminded us that the first Symposium was in Milan in 1960. That was in the Dark Ages: Steinberg discussed triparanol, Lynen fluoridated mevalonic acid, and Kritchevsky iodothyronines. I recall that in my

Summary at the end I was a little bitter because some people seemed to think that the ultimate aim in life was to reduce plasma cholesterol as near zero as possible, without noticing that the animal might be dead. Now we have passed from the Dark Ages to molecular and cell biology. We knew little then about lipoproteins. The elucidation of their composition, formation, interaction and catabolism has been a triumph. To select just two events, I recall my naive surprise when four years ago Steinberg and colleagues showed that catabolism of LDL was increased after hepatectomy because I had thought that if I was Jehovah with a tidy mind I would have made Adam's LDL go back to the liver to pick up triglycerides and become VLDL again. Then at our last Symposium in Milan Goldstein elaborated on the work he had described just before at the Berlin Atherosclerosis Congress. Now we can actually see the coated pits with ferritin-LDL in them and the entry of these by endocytosis into the cell before being degraded and regulating in opposite ways cholesterol synthesis and esterification. Various normal cells (such as aortic smooth muscle cells) do this at the same rate, adding up to about a gram per person per day catabolised, except in Type II.

Obviously this catabolism of LDL lowers plasma cholesterol if other things are equal, and it will be raised by VLDL from liver or gut, and by HDL removing cholesterol from tissues. Looked at another way, as Sodhi did just now in the "overload hypothesis", plasma cholesterol will be increased by absorption from the gut or synthesis in tissues especially the liver; and lowered by elimination into the gut of cholesterol or bile acids, and by entry of LDL into cells of tissues. Tissue cholesterol can be increased by this passage from plasma or by local synthesis or diminished removal - Sodhi's "transport hypothesis." Most of us (I hope) believe that our "Western" diet produces plasma LDL levels that are too high (Brown and Goldstein suggest by a factor of five), but we need more information about why these high levels are accompanied by accumulation in aortic smooth muscle cells when culturing these cells in a medium rich in LDL does not cause excessive entry. And we need more information about the removal of cholesterol from cells by HDL (which are rich in linoleic acid). As Paoletti and others pointed out, drugs may lower LDL in plasma or raise HDL or both or neither. We now have a galaxy of drugs: Bencze included about 50 of them in his 15 slides. We also have diet. The Prudent Diet lowers plasma LDL but leaves HDL unchanged. However,

Japanese have (or had until recently) low LDL and high HDL, as have Eskimos whom Schlierf regarded as a red herring; but a herring is sometimes red only if it reflects the blush of confusion of the speaker - caused of course by PGE_1, or uniquely in Ahrens by nicotinamide.

In trying to combat atherosclerosis we need methods of protecting the arterial wall, and Paoletti discussed doing this by modifying prostaglandins. Clearly permeability is important, and Walton showed this. Elspeth Smith has shown that in the first two decades of life esterified cholesterol in the perifibrous lipid of the "normal" intima remains constant and is different in composition from that of plasma, having high C18:1 and C16:0, and low C18:2. After 20 years of age there is a steady increase, LDL can be shown by immuno-electrophoresis to be entering; and C18:2 becomes the most prevalent. She finds that if there is no hypertension, the absolute amount of LDL in the "normal" intima is very highly correlated with the level of serum cholesterol a week before death, and is at the same concentration in intima as in plasma. Hypertension increases the amount in the intima. Atheroma occurs particularly where cells are rapidly dividing, as at branches from the aorta; and dividing cells have increased requirement of EFA for their membranes. Although injury to the endothelium was mentioned in several papers, the curious fact was overlooked that no atheroma occurs where a cervical rib repeatedly injures it.

The best animal to use for the effect of drugs on lipid metabolism is man, but there are limitations. Day made an eloquent plea for the SEA Japanese quail or the cynomolgus monkey. Zilversmit introduced us to the mink which has 250 mg/dl cholesterol in plasma throughout life, mainly in HDL, and no atherosclerosis. No one mentioned the hippopotamus which has been alleged to have a plasma cholesterol of only about 10 mg/dl and extensive atheroma. In these days of genetic engineering we might cross the carnivorous mink with the herbivorous hippopotamus and produce an omnivorous minkopotamus with about our size and habits. We can study diseased humans with great reward, and apart from the lipoproteinemias we did not hear much about them. Since we rightly regard HDL as being so important in removing cholesterol from tissues (and Hulley's interesting findings support this), why does not early IHD, as in homozygous Type II, occur in the few known cases of Tangier disease in which certainly cholesteryl esters accumulate in cells of reticuloendothelial tissue but not with the disastrous results we might expect? In Wolman's disease, in which the acid lipase is missing so that cholesteryl esters accumulate in cells, why is the fatty acid composition of these esters so different from that of the LDL that has entered? Why are children with cystic fibrosis, in which a curious form of EFA-deficiency occurs, completely free of fatty streaks (as was shown by the late Russell Holman); very recently it has been found that in Down's syndrome there is apparently no atheroma whatever although IHD occurs.

We have to distinguish between atherosclerosis and IHD. Morris and the late Margaret Crawford showed that according to the London Hospital records coronary atheroma had not increased in the last half-century, but obliteration of the lumen had increased more than two-fold. The changes in national deaths attributed to IHD in European countries in the 1939-45 war must be dietary for reasons I have discussed before, and occur so quickly that this must be a manifestation of changed thrombotic tendency rather than of a chronic process such as atherosclerosis. We have rightly discussed the very important recent work on drugs that affect platelet aggregation and release, particularly the advances in the prostaglandin field. Vane's prostacyclin is a very interesting development. And prostaglandins are now being modified to prevent their rapid catabolism while preserving biological activity. The balance is interesting between thromboxanes which aggregate platelets and certain prostaglandins which make them unsticky (E_1, D_2, prostacylin), and as no talk is decent without a slide I want to show one although unlike Dr. Smith I have reduced mine to schoolboy simplicity with no formulae. (Figure next page)

Since Ahrens is present I will not say that I speak without fear of contradiction, but I will say that I speak with the certainty of being right when I point out that there are two classes of EFA (as I have maintained for a quarter of a century despite trivial opposition). With Doctors Bang and Dyerberg I have been studying one of the last remaining groups of Eskimos subsisting mainly on their traditional diet of seal and fish, very high in protein and long-chain fatty acids of the linolenic class but very low in all fatty acids of the linoleic class and in linolenic acid itself. They have no dietary fibre but none of the diseases currently attributed to deficiency of this, and no thrombotic diseases such as IHD. Presumably they make

TWO CLASSES OF ESSENTIAL FATTY ACIDS
AND PROSTAGLANDINS

Vitamins F1

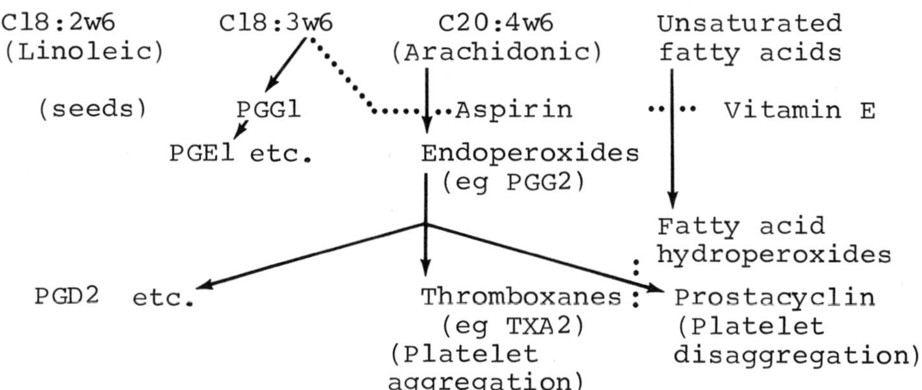

Vitamins F2

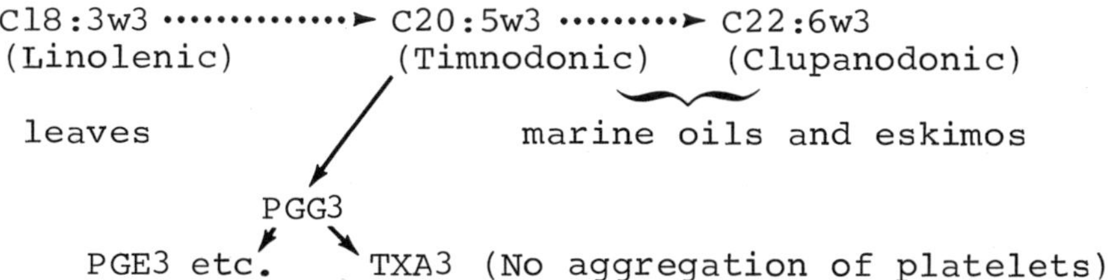

little of the thromboxanes that aggregate platelets and neither make nor need normal amounts of prostacyclin. They have high HDL and low LDL, their plasma cholesterol (which is low) being esterified predominantly with timnodonic acid rather than with linoleic. Timnodonic and clupanodonic acids, in presence of docopherols to prevent peroxidation, may be very important "drugs" affecting lipid metabolism. We urgently need further studies of eskimos and other fast-disappearing fish-eating carnivores.

Another type of epidemiological study was described by Oliver, and this supported the "dietary lipid hypothesis," disliked by Ahrens who criticized Senator McGovern's "Dietary Goals for the United States" and joined the 8% of those against the hypothesis in Norum's questionnaire (a minority that was supported by Hulley, Blackett and Sodhi). Ahrens quoted Bertrand Russell in his support: "When experts are not agreed no opinion can be regarded as certain by non-experts." At the last Symposium held here Irvine Page, chairing the Panel discussion, agreed that we were not in a position to make final recommendations, but "in public health work we cannot always wait for irrefutable proof." In 1933 Sherrington, the greatest biologist since Darwin, expressed the same opinion: "Science, nobly, declines as proof anything but complete proof; but common sense, pressed for time, accepts and acts on acceptance." The modern epidemic of IHD presses us for time, and I might send Senator McGovern a bottle of Scotch whiskey with the compliments of Dr. Hulley. On this theme, perhaps I may end with some stanzas from an Indian saga I heard when recently travelling by dog-sledge in the Arctic hoping to examine the aorta of Eskimo Nell.

Hiawatha's Lipid-Lowering Drug

Should you ask me why this Congress,
On the drugs that lower lipids -
This Symposium on lipids
Which implies we drink together
(So at least thought Hiawatha
With his schoolboy erudition -
"Etymology" he called it),
And results of Dr. Hulley
Show we ought to drink together;
So perhaps it should be christened
A Syrrophium on lipids
Since we swallow pills together,
As the children of the wigwam
Swallow lumps of seal together;
Should you - I repeat the question -
Ask me why these doctors gather
To discuss recondite questions
Of the drugs that lower lipids,
I should answer, I should tell you
Straightway in such words as follows.

Since Milan in 1960,
Every three years in September
Lipidologists foregather
To review the progress in their

Fight against their heart diseases;
As the chieftains in the wigwams
Meet together to conduct their
Fight against some hostile tribesmen,
So these scientists foregather
To prevent their heart infarctions,
To attack their lipoproteins
(LDL the hostile compound),
To reduce their atheroma
Washing out the fat deposits
As the chain on waterclosets
Or the handle on the toilets
Flushes out unwanted refuse,
So new therapeutic practice
Flushes out the atheromas -
Lipoproteins, sterol esters
Sphingomyelin, phospholipids
And a lot of other debris.

William Holmes this Congress summoned,
He no Pennsylvania native
But from Canada he ventured;
From the Lankenau's tall turret -
Like a King or Mandarin or
Gitche Manito the Mighty
(He the maker of all lipids,
Whether phospholipids, sterols,
Or triglycerides or squalene) -
Stood erect and called his colleagues;
From the continents he called them,
Bid them come to Philadelphia -
Philadelphia, Friendship City,
Brothers, sisters - no distinction
(So Don Zilversmit decided) -
To discuss the drugs that lower
Lipids in the furred up vessels,
Vessels that are chocked with lipids
As a beaver's dam obstructs the
Stream and chokes the flow of water;
So the lipid in the vessel
Wall obstructs the flow of blood and
Causes stasis in the bloodstream.
Then the platelets make thromboxanes
From arachidonic acid;
Prostaglandins made from PUFA -
Special PUFA, only EFA -
From arachidonic acid
Going through endoperoxides
(PGG2, PGH2)
Which by aspirin prevented,

Then thromboxanes (TXA2)
(Made by platelet microsomal
Enzymes) caused their aggregation.
And the aggregated platelets
Stick to collagen, to red cells,
Microfibrils, basement membranes;
As the icycles and snowflakes
Stick to Hiawatha's whiskers;
And the aggregated platelets
Then release a lot of compounds:
ADP and amines, proteins,
PF4 and often thrombin,
And a mitogenic factor,
And some lysosomal enzymes;
As the boiling fierce volcano
Spews out larva on the mountain,
So the platelets, stuck together,
Vomit out a lot of compounds
But this sticking is prevented
By an endothelial compound
(Microsomal), prostacyclin,
Which inhibits aggregation;
As the blubber on the snowshoes
Stops the snow from sticking to them,
Prostacyclin stops the platelets
From adhering to each other
With a viscous kiss on meeting.

How does atheroma gather?
Benditt states its monoclonal -
All the atheroma comes from
Only one cell amongst many;
As the Indian tribe throws up a
Criminal with altered genes who
Breeds a race of wanton tribesmen,
So one cell 'neath endothelium
Eats up lipid, reproduces,
Breeds a tribe of fat-filled offspring
(Fat-filled like most US offspring);
Thus arises atheroma
In the mind of Doctor Benditt,
But the Congress just ignored him.
First Dan Steinberg from La Jolla,
Bearded, critical and clever,
Praised the alpha-lipoproteins:
HDL you should have in you
For cholesterol removal,
As a chain pulled in a closet -
I've this simile exhausted
Sterols are flushed out of tissues
By the HDL in plasma.

Next Rodolfo Paoletti
With his kymographic tracings,
Circling round the world so often
From one Congress to another
Like a satellite in orbit,
Hurtling through the cirro-nimbus
Moving round the world so often
Since Symposia come so often.
With his kymograph he traces
Prostaglandin stimulation
(PGY or $Z_{2\alpha}$)
Of the guinea-pig's intestine,
Of the guinea-fowl's cloaca,
On smoked paper tracing tracings
As the smoke above the wigwam
Traces figures in the twilight.

Many authors showed a picture
Of a coated pit that catches
LDL and then engulfs them
By an endocytic process
(Trapped by apoprotein B, or
Else by arginine-rich protein);
As a pit with covered brushwood
Traps the reindeer in the prairies
Which are then engulfed by Indians -
Hiawatha and his colleagues -
And presumably digested
Since the meat is not recovered;
So the lysosomal enzymes
Break trapped LDL in pieces.
If the coated pits are absent
Type II lipoproteinemia
(homozygous, autosomal)
Kills you in your teens or earlier.

Oliver and Carlson showed that
Others die before they ought to:
Scots and Finns get heart infarctions -
Swedes have 3 times less infarctions -
Finns because they live on butter,
Scots since whiskey is expensive
(This the ancient Scottish liquor)
And are truthful in their statements;
Swedes may lie to Doctor Carlson
How much alcohol they swallow.

Drugs that lower lipid levels
In the cynomolgus monkey,
In the mink and quail and rabbit,

In the chimpanzee and ferret,
Were discussed in great profusion.
Michael Oliver prescribes them:
Pills for breakfast in the morning,
Pills again with midday coffee,
Pills for luncheon, pills at teatime
(Though a party held in Boston
Stopped this ancient British custom),
Pills with cocktails, pills with dinner,
And a dozen pills at bedtime -
(Barbara Cartland swallows eighty) -
Till the patient patient rattles
With the pills inside his stomach,
As the pebbles on the seashore
Rattle when the waves break o'er them,
As a pestle in a mortar
Grinds the particles together.

Dave Kritchevsky writes on fibre -
Lignin, pectin, bran and roughage,
But these things were hardly mentioned.
Bencze listed 50 compounds
For the lowering of lipids:
Acetone diaryl ether,
Clofibrate and cyclized compounds,
Gemfibrozil and tibric acid,
Allicin (which comes from garlic),
Metformin and ciprofibrate,
Chenic acid, ursic acid
which is found in polar bear oil
Ursus arcticus excretes it),
Procetophen and lipanthyl,
Bezafibrate, oestradiol,
Nicotinic acid also.
All these drugs and many others
Lowered plasma lipid levels,
But the patients still had in them
Atheromatous aortas.

Hiawatha knew the answer
("Mr Fit" supports his theory
As was told by Dr. Hulley):
Scots when whiskey was much cheaper,
Swedes with slivovitz and lager,
Italy's and France's peasants
Drinking claret by the litre,
Tokay drunk by Dr. Gero
(That is why he's over 70),
Russians swilling down their vodka -
There's one common factor here that

Stops them getting atheroma:
Ethanol's a lipid solvent
And should be prescribed by doctors
As a lipid-lowering potion,
As a panacea for illness,
For longevity and pleasure -
So at least thought Hiawatha
As he staggered from this Congress.

EFFECTS OF CHENODEOXYCHOLIC ACID (CD) TREATMENT ON ENDOGENOUS PLASMA TRIGLYCERIDE (TG) TRANSPORT IN HYPERLIPOPROTEINEMIA (HLP)

B. Angelin, K. Einarsson and B. Leijd

Department of Medicine, Karolinska Institutet at Serafimer-lasarettet, S-112 83 Stockholm, Sweden

CD treatment inhibits hepatic cholesterol and bile acid formation. Preliminary reports suggest a plasma TG-lowering effect. This study was aimed at characterizing the alterations in TG concentration and turnover during CD treatment.

Methods: Twenty-three patients with HLP (7 IIa, 8 IIb, and 8 IV) were studied before and during CD treatment, 3 months, 750 mg/day. Routine tests, plasma cholesterol and TG were determined at intervals of 4 weeks. In 5 IIa and 7 IV patients, endogenous TG synthesis was determined using a ^{3}H-glycerol technique before and after 3 months therapy.

Results: Transient elevation of serum aminotransferases were seen after 4 weeks. Cholesterol concentration was unchanged, while that of TG decreased 33% in type IIb ($p<0.001$), 17% in type IV HLP ($p<0.05$), and 21% in the total series ($p<0.001$). TG formation was reduced from 13.1±1.2 to 7.9±0.5, μmol/kg/h ($p<0.01$) in type IIa and from 23.6±3.7 to 15.5±1.8 ($p<0.02$) in type IV HLP. In both groups the fractional turnover rate of TG decreased during treatment.

Conclusions: CD reduces plasma TG by suppressing its synthesis. This lends further support to the concept of an integrated regulation of lipoprotein and hepatic cholesterol/bile acid metabolism. CD may prove to be a useful adjunct in treatment of HLP, especially considering its bile cholesterol solubilizing capacity.

LIPID TRANSPORT ACROSS THE INTESTINAL EPITHELIAL CELL. EFFECT OF TOLBUTAMIDE

C.A Arreaza-Plaza, M. Otayek and V. Bosch

Instituto de Medicina Experimental, Catedra de Fisiopatologia, U.C.V. Caracas, Venezuela

It has been reported that tolbutamide increases the insulin secretion acting on the microtubular system of the beta cells. Colchicine has an opposite effect. We reported that colchicine blocks the release of chylomicrons to the lymph. Tolbutamide (10 mg), injected into rats one hour after feeding a fat emulsion, produces in 30 minutes a fall in plasma triacylglycerol concentrations: 110±2, control and 50±2, experimental, mean ± Sem. $p<0.001$. Blood glucose was also diminished. However if Triton WR-1339 was injected, together with the fat feeding, a rise in triacylglycerol was observed after the treatment with tolbutamide: 345±30 and 490±10 $p=0.001$. In alloxan diabetic rats, similarly treated, triacylglycerol concentrations also rise: 481±36 and 1095±69 $p<0.001$. The results obtained in normal rats was probably due to chylomicron hydrolysis by lipoprotein lipases activated by insulin When the action of the enzyme is impaired by the detergent or the insulin secretion was suppressed, a rise in triacylglycerol follows after the injection of tolbutamide.

We propose that tolbutamide probably acts by increasing the polymerization of the microtubular system of the intestinal epithelial cell, resembling its action on the pancreas.

Supported by grant from CONICIT N°31-26-SI-0696. "HOECHST" - Venezuela provide "Rastinon" Technical Assistance: Mrs. Marta de Rodriguez.

EFFECT OF A NEW NIACIN-DERIVATIVE ON SERUM LIPIDS IN MAN

P. Avogaro, G. Bittolo-Bon, M. Pais and G.C. Taroni

Ospedale Regionale, 30100 Venezia, Italy

Ninety-seven H.L. patients (37 IIa; 40 IIb; 20 IV) received a niacin-derivative (nicotinic hexaester of D-glucytol) providing 375 mg of N.A. four times daily for two months after two months of dietary treatment. Thirty patients were given the drug for one year. In type IIa, a normalization of plasma C was obtained in 18.9% of the subjects after two months and in 45% after 6 months. A significant reduction (from 10 to 30%) was obtained in 32.4% after 2 months and in 15% after 6 or 12 months. In type IIb a normalization of C was greater with the drug (30%) than after diet (22.5) while the lowering of TG was the same (35%) both after diet or 2 months therapy. In the long-term treatment the normalization was recorded up to 50% for C and up to 66% for TG. A significant lowering was recorded in the long-term treatment only for TG (33.2%). In type IV the decrease of TG was 20% after the dietary period; 40% after 2 months of treatment and 75% after 12 months of treatment.

U.C. LIPOPROTEIN CLASS VARIATIONS INDUCED BY AN EXTRACTIVE MYOCARDIAL PHOSPHOLIPID

P. Avogaro, G. Bittolo-Bon, G. Cazzolato and G.B. Quinci

Unit for Atherosclerosis, Regional General Hospital, Venice, Italy

Seven patients affected by IIa or IV H.L. were given 200 mg i.v. daily of an emulsion of an extractive myocardial phospholipid for 20 days. Total C and mostly LDL-C were significantly reduced while no variations have been observed in total-TG, VLDL-C and HDL-C. Electroimmunoassay revealed a decrease of tot. apo-B and of LDL-apo-B while VLDL-apo-B and apo-A_I remained unchanged.

CHENODEOXYCHOLIC ACID THERAPY FOR HYPERTRIGLYCERIDEMIA

M.C. Bateson and I.A.D. Bouchier

Department of Medicine, Ninewells Hospital and Medical School, Dundee, DD1 9SY, Scotland

Ten patients with hypertriglyceridemia (5.06 S.D. 2.28 mM) not completely controlled by a diet low in carbohydrate (3.27 S.D. 0.45 mM) received chenodeoxycholic acid 500-750 mg daily for 6 months. On this treatment serum triglycerides fell further to 2.73 S.D. 0.36 mM ($p < 0.01$). In 9 of these patients treated for a further month on placebo capsules values returned to diet-treated levels, and fell again over 6 months on clofibrate 2G daily to 2.67 S.D. 0.94 mM ($p < 0.05$). Duodenal bile was sampled in hypertriglyceridemic patients with normal gallbladders. In 5 patients on chenodeoxycholic acid 750 mg daily cholesterol content fell in every case after 6 months' therapy (from 13.04 S.D. 3.12 to 6.58 S.D. 0.72 moles %, $p < 0.005$). By contrast biliary cholesterol showed a rise in 5 out of 6 patients receiving clofibrate 2G daily for at least 6 months (from 12.77 S.D. 4.04 to 17.11 S.D. 2.84 moles%). The degree to which bile was saturated with cholesterol was highly significantly less on chenodeoxycholic acid than on clofibrate. In one patient on clofibrate therapy for 2 years the increased cholesterol content of bile was associated with the development and growth of radiolucent gallstones.

Conclusion: (1) Chenodeoxycholic acid is as effective as clofibrate in hypertriglyceridemia not completely responsive to diet. (2) Clofibrate enhances cholesterol content of bile and causes gallstones. Chenodeoxycholic acid therapy diminishes cholesterol content and protects from gallstones.

CONTROL OF PLASMA AND HEPATIC CHOLESTEROL LEVELS IN CHOLESTEROL-FED RATS BY SULFONATE ESTERS OF FATTY ALCOHOLS

F.P. Bell and F W. Quackenbush

The Upjohn Company, Kalamazoo, Michigan 49001, and Purdue University, Department of Biochemistry, West Lafayette, Indiana 47907, U.S.A.

A number of sulfonate esters of fatty alcohols have been found to possess potent hypocholesterolemic activity. Linoleyl-p-toluene sulfonate (LPTS) is one of the most active sulfonate esters tested. LPTS exerts a cholesterol-lowering effect in plasma and liver of cholesterol-fed rats. In rats fed a diet containing 1% hydrogenated coconut oil, 1% cholesterol, and 0.5% cholic acid (HC-diet), LPTS was effective prophylactically in controlling plasma and hepatic cholesterol levels when fed at a level of 0.15% in the diet. In 4 week trials with LPTS feeding, plasma total cholesterol and hepatic total cholesterol were 70 mg% and 10 mg/g wet weight, respectively, as compared to 250 mg% and 42 mg/g in rats not receiving LPTS. In rats with hypercholesterolemia established during 4 weeks on the HC-diet, addition of 0.15% LPTS to the HC-diet for an additional 4 weeksresulted in reduction of plasma and hepatic cholesterol to levels similar to those observed when LPTS was given prophylactically in the HC-diet. Preliminary studies suggest that LPTS acts by increasing bile acid production and inhibiting intestinal absorption of cholesterol.

EFFECT OF PROCETOFEN ON HEPATIC UPTAKE OF CHOLESTEROL AND BILIARY SECRETION BY THE ISOLATED PERFUSED LIVER

C. Bentzen, C. Tourne and E. Wulfert

Centre de Recherches, Laboratoires Fournier, 21300 Chenove, France

Acute administration of Procetofen has a profound activity in lowering plasma cholesterol levels in the rat, 30% in 4-7 hours. The isolated perfused liver system was chosen to investigate the possible involvement of the liver in this acute hypocholesterolemic activity. Procetofen treatment dramatically increased the initial rate of hepatic ^{14}C-cholesterol uptake from the circulating perfusion media and resulted in a more efficient clearing of radioactivity over time, 93 ± 2.6% compared to 76.2 ± 3.1% for control livers. Concomitantly, biliary secretion of radioactivity was 2.05 times in the presence of the compound indicating a rapid mobilization of ^{14}C into bile. In both groups, more than 90% radioactivity was found as bile acids. Fasted and fed rats were also studied with regard to cholesterol uptake and secretion. Although liver weights varied, ^{14}C-cholesterol uptake per gram liver was not altered. However, biliary secretion of radioactivity was correspondingly enhanced depending upon duration of fasting. Hepatic uptake of ^{14}C acetate appeared enhanced (17%) in the presence of procetofenic acid in contrast to a 71% inhibition of radioactivity secreted as biliary sterols. These data indicate that the compound induces a rapid uptake of cholesterol and possibly alters the metabolic state of the liver, which results in an increased biliary secretion of cholesterol, as also seen in the fasted state.

ACTIVATION OF LIPOPROTEINLIPASE BY SERUM AFTER TREATMENT WITH STEROID CONTRACEPTIVE DRUGS (SCD)

A. Bizzi, S. Garattini, A.M. Tacconi and E. Veneroni

Istituto di Ricerche Farmacologiche "M.Negri", 20157 Milan, Italy

When lipoproteinlipase from normal rats was challenged against a substrate of a) exogenous triglyceride and serum from normal rats, and b) exogenous triglyceride and serum from SCD treated rats, it was observed that lipoproteinlipase activity was decreased by the presence of serum from SCD-rats.

Similar results were observed when the serum was deprived of VLDL. Lipoproteinlipase was also challenged against chylomicrones either from normal or SCD treated rats; chylomicrones from normal rats proved better substrates than those from SCD-rats. SCD treatment seems to alter the availability of both the exogenous and the endogenous substrate to lipoproteinlipase activity. This effect might be responsible for altered clearance and hypertriglyceridemia observed in some SCD users. These results will be discussed in the light of possible alterations in the apoprotein pattern.

ENDOTHELIAL INJURY AND PLAQUE GROWTH IN MODERATE HYPERLIPOPROTEINEMIA

S. Bjorkerud, G. Bondjers, R. Brattsand and A. Bylock

University of Gothenburg, Department of Medicine I, S-413 45 Gothenburg, and Astra Pharmaceuticals, S-151 85 Sodertalje, Sweden

The distribution of injured cells in aortic endothelium in rabbits with dietarily induced moderate hyperlipoproteinemia was studied light microscopically after supravital dye exclusion test for cellular injury and with scanning electron microscopy (SEM).

Injured endothelium was predominantly found in the periphery of atherosclerotic plaques, i.e. in the junctional zone between plaque and unthickened wall. In addition to apparently injured endothelial cells spindle-formed cells, possibly related to endothelial restitution, were also found in this zone. The presence of endothelial defects after defined experimental mechanical injury invariably leads to intimal thickening. In analogy, we propose that spreading and extension of arterial plaques in hyperlipoproteinemia may be an effect of selective damage to endothelium in the junctional zone between plaque and non-thickened wall. Conceivable factors for selective endothelial injury in this zone are hemodynamic changes related to the presence of a plaque or abrupt changes in the junctional zone of the mechanical properties of the wall itself.

ENDOTHELIAL INTEGRITY AND MODERATE HYPERLIPOPROTEINEMIA - EFFECTS ON CHOLESTEROL DEPOSITION IN NON-ATHEROSCLEROTIC ARTERIAL TISSUE

S. Bjorkerud, G. Bondjers, R Brattsand and G.K. Hansson

Department of Medicine I, University of Gothenburg, S-413 45 Gothenburg, and Astra Pharmaceuticals, S-151 85 Sodertalje, Sweden

Hyperlipoproteinemia as well as endothelial injury may lead to cholesterol deposition in arterial tissue. The relative significance of these factors may be disputed. Therefore, the effects of different serum lipoprotein fractions and endothelial integrity on cholesterol deposition in non-atherosclerotic arterial tissue were investigated in rabbits with serum cholesterol from 40 to 500 mg%. Hypercholesterolemia was induced with 0.1-0.3% cholesterol in the diet. The transfer of radioactive cholesterol was lower into tissue with intact endothelium than into tissue with defective endothelium in normo-lipoproteinemic rabbits. However, it increased with increasing serum LDL in both types of tissue. The extent of this increase was approximately the same in both types of tissue. Nevertheless, the concentration of cholesterol increased 20-fold more in tissue with defective endothelium than in tissue with intact endothelium. This suggests that the intact arterial endothelium may protect the underlying tissue from cholesterol deposition in moderate hyperlipoproteinemia, although the protection from increased permeability to cholesterol is small. Consequently, the results suggest that deposition of cholesterol is avoided by enhanced elimination in arterial tissue with intact endothelium, as serum lipoprotein concentrations increase. Therefore, an intact arterial endothelium may be one pre-requisite for efficient elimination of cholesterol.

INHIBITION OF TRIACYLGLYCEROL SYNTHESIS BY BENFLUOREX

D.N. Brindley

Department of Biochemistry, University Hospital and Medical School, Nottingham NG7 2UH, United Kingdom

Benfluorex, 1-(3-trifluoromethylphenyl)-2-[N-(2-benzoyloxyethyl)amino] propane or S-780, decreases the synthesis of triacylglycerols *in vitro* by inhibiting phosphatidate phosphohydrolase. The ability to control phosphatidate phosphohydrolase activity is an important property since this enzyme is regulatory in glycerolipid synthesis. Daily administration of 50 mg of benfluorex/kg of body weight to rats decreases the rate of hepatic triacylglycerol synthesis *in vivo*. This is observed if glucose is fed before the experiments, but is more pronounced after ethanol feeding. Ethanol (5 g/kg body weight) increases the rate of hepatic triacylglycerol synthesis by 2.3-fold and the hepatic activity of phosphatidate phosphohydrolase by 4.7-fold. Pretreatment of the rats with benfluorex significantly decreases the ethanol-induced stimulation to both of these parameters. The hypolipidemic effects, which are observed during the clinical use of benfluorex, can be partly explained by an interference with phosphatidate metabolism leading to a decreased synthesis of triacylglycerol.

AGGREGATION OF TRIGLYCERIDE-RICH LIPOPROTEINS BY SYNTHETIC ANIONIC DETERGENTS IN THE PRESENCE OF B2 GLYCOPROTEIN 1

M. Burstein and P. Legmann

Centre National de Transfusion Sanguine, 75015 Paris, France

We have shown previously that with appropriate concentration of sodium lauryl sulfate (SLS) or of sodium decyl sulfate (SDS) very low density lipoproteins (VLDL) and chylomicrons are selectively precipitated from human serum at 35°C. This precipitation requires the presence of a serum factor; in fact, isolated VLDL and chylomicrons are precipitated by SLS and SDS when they are suspended in serum but not in buffered saline.

We were able to isolate the serum factor in the following way: SDS was added to lipemic plasma and the mixture was incubated at 35°C; after two hours, the precipitated chylomicrons plus VLDL were separated by centrifugation (the lipoprotein-detergent complex floats and forms a creamy layer on the top) delipidated by ethanol-diethyl ether and partially solubilized in buffered saline.

This solution was fractionated by ammonium sulfate precipitation, and the serum factor was found in the 40-50% saturation fraction: indeed, addition of this fraction to SDS containing saline elicits precipitation of the lipoproteins.

Using specific antisera it was shown that this fraction is identical with B2 glycoprotein 1 isolated by Schultze (1961). We were able to show that in the very few sera where this factor is absent there is an excess of VLDL.

SYNERGISTIC OR SUMMATION ACTION OF HYPOLIPOPROTEINEMIC DRUGS

A.M. Aparicio, E. Boyle, and F.L. Canosa

Miami Heart Institute, Miami Beach, Florida 33140, U.S.A.

Study, begun January 9, 1974, is designed to establish the effect of a specific diet and a combined drug therapy according to the subject's phenotype. Fifty subjects, type II-A phenotype, and fifty type II-B phenotype were enrolled in this study. The medications used in this study are Probucol (trade name is "Lorelco", The Dow Chemical Company), Cholestyramine, Atromid-S and Niacin. On entering the study, each subject is placed on a specific diet for two months. Probucol is then prescribed for the next four months, at the end of which, subject is randomly assigned to Probucol with either Niacin, Atromid-S or Cholestyramine, for periods of five months each. At the end of the periods of combined therapy, subject is given Probucol only for one month for a washout period. Consequently, all drugs are combined to Probucol in the same fashion, followed by a placebo phase at the end of the study. Results: Probucol alone produced a serum cholesterol reduction from 311 to 267 mg% ($P<.001$), serum beta lipoproteins by the K-Agar Delta Method ($P<.0024$). The addition of a second drug induced additional decreases in serum lipids. Some of these combinations demonstrated a highly significant reduction in their lipid values.

EFFECTS OF CLOFIBRATE - NICOTINIC ACID COMBINATION IN RATS

M.N. Cayen, D. Dvornik and W.T. Robinson

Department of Biochemistry, Ayerst Research Laboratories, Montreal, Quebec, Canada, H3C 3J1

The effect of combined oral administration of clofibrate and nicotinic acid (NA) on the serum lipid levels and pharmacokinetics of the drugs was investigated in rats. Male albino rats were given by gavage various doses of clofibrate and NA, both alone and in combination, daily, for 1 week. In normal animals the combinations produced greater decreases in serum lipids, notably triglycerides (TG), than either drug alone. Greater decreases in serum TG were also observed in rats rendered hypertriglyceridemic with fructose when treated simultaneously with both drugs. The area under the serum NA concentration/time curve (AUC) was twice as large for NA when given with clofibrate than when given alone. The serum half-life of NA after i.v. injection was longer (78 min) in rats pretreated for 1 week with clofibrate than in appropriate controls (30 min). In contrast, pretreatment for 1 week with NA had no statistically significant effect on the half-life and AUC of clofibric acid injected i.v. The presence of NA in rat serum did not affect the protein-binding of CPIB. The results show a combined hypolipidemic effect in rats treated simultaneously with clofibrate and NA; the effect was associated with a decrease in the rate of NA elimination.

COLESTIPOL HYDROCHLORIDE, A NEW HYPOLIPIDEMIC DRUG: A TWO-YEAR STUDY

E.E. Cooper and A.M. Michel

505 Howard Street, San Antonio, Texas 78212, U.S.A.

Colestipol hydrochloride is an insoluble, nonabsorbable copolymer with bile-acid-binding capacity. It prevents reabsorption of cholates from the intestinal tract into the enterohepatic circulation causing a net loss of bile acids, and therefore of cholesterol. Sixty subjects with cholesterol levels over 250 mg/100 ml were studied for 104 weeks. Patients with normal phenotypes, types 2,3, and 4, were given 5 gm three times daily and experienced an average drop of 40 mg/100 ml (14%). While patients with types 2,3 and 4 hyperlipidemia responded effectively, cholesterol levels in type 2 patients dropped earliest and most consistently with an average decrease of 50 mg/100 ml (19%). A comparable group of patients with hyperlipidemia taking placebo showed on average no change in serum cholesterol. Serum triglyceride values were not altered significantly. The resin is not absorbed from the gastrointestinal tract and produced a slight increase in fecal volume. Results of chemistries, enzyme assays, prothrombin times, hematology, and urinalysis and body weights were unaltered. There was no evidence of lithogenic bile production. Colestipol is a tasteless and odorless copolymer with high acceptability. Side effects were limited to occasional bloating, gas and constipation. The drug is a safe, effective, palatable hypolipidemic agent.

THE EFFECT OF INHIBITION OF PROSTAGLANDIN SYNTHESIS ON HUMAN PLATELET-COLLAGEN INTERACTION

D.H. Cowan, A.L. Robertson, Jr., P. Giroski, and P. Shook

Departments of Medicine and Pathology, Case Western Reserve University, School of Medicine, Cleveland, Ohio, U.S.A.

Factors affecting the alteration by aspirin (ASA) and indomethacin (IND) of platelet adherence to collagen and the release reaction were evaluated by affinity chromatography. Platelets were anticoagulated with EDTA or sodium citrate. Aggregation was inhibited by EDTA and/or the ADP-removing enzyme system, creatine phosphate-creatine phosphokinase (CP-CPK).

The adherence and release of untreated, ASA- and IND-treated EDTA platelets were 67 ± 6% (1 SD) and 33 ± 5%, 44 ± 5% and 12 ± 6%, and 39% and 25%, respectively. Removal of ADP using CP-CPK or addition of exogenous ADP (10μM) did not alter the adherence or release of EDTA-platelets. The adherence and release of untreated, ASA-, and IND-treated citrated platelets were 68 ± 4% and 44 ± 3%, 38% and 31%, and 38% and 30%, respectively. The adherence of EDTA and citrated platelets treated with ASA or IND was normal in the presence of 0.5 mM $MgCl_2$. The decrease in release of drug-treated platelets incubated with 0.5 mM $MgCl_2$ was one-half that seen in the absence of $MgCl_2$. Correction of the drug-related reductions in adherence and release was less with $CaCl_2$ than with $MgCl_2$. Scanning electron microscopy confirmed the presence of shape change with EDTA, the differences in adherence observed with ASA and IND, and the absence of platelet aggregation. The results suggest that the adherence of platelets to collagen and the release reaction occur independently of shape change and are dependent on prostaglandin synthesis. The influence of prostaglandin synthesis on platelet-collagen interaction is moderated by divalent cations, particularly Mg^{++}, but is not affected by shape change or availability of ADP.

LONG TERM TOLERANCE STUDY OF DAILY CLOFIBRATE THERAPY IN 132 PRIMARY HYPERLIPIDEMIAS

J.L. de Gennes, J.C. Piette and A.M. Piette

Hopital de la Pitie, 75013 Paris, France

Long term tolerance of Clofibrate (1, 5 or 2 g daily) was reviewed in 132 primary hyperlipidemias (HL) (44 women and 88 men) divided into: 21 type IIa with xanthomas; 29 type IIa without xanthomas; 67 minor mixed HL; 15 major hypertriglyceridemias (7 type II and 8 type IV HL). The mean total cholesterol level decreased 27.3% during the first year (from a control value of 388 mg%) and continued at that level. The mean triglyceride level decreased 64.4% in hyperglyceridemic patients during the first year (from a control value of 337 mg%) and also continued at that level. These results reflect both the high initial level of HL, and the unquestionable biologic efficacity of Clofibrate. The mean duration of treatment was 4.5 to 12 years in some cases, for a total survey of 600 years. Regarding C.D.P. results, the incidence of thromboembolism phenomena was markedly less frequent (2%) so it was with myocardial infarction (7% of the 45 patients with initial coronary disease). No cases of enlarged spleen or liver was mentioned. Liver function tests were studied in 80 patients, showing slight increase of SGPT in 12 cases, and mild retention of BSP in 20 cases. These abnormalities, usually transient and not correlated with duration of treatment, never justified withdrawal of Clofibrate. Nine patients exhibited some symptoms suggestive of cholelithiasis (without major complications such as acute pancreatitis or angiocholitis). Each of them had been receiving Clofibrate for at least 3 years. Major side effects of Clofibrate therapy were: 10 bleeding incidents in 39 patients on anticoagulants; decreased potency, 3 cases; muscular syndrome, 1 case. The following side effects were also registered: 5 leukopenia (without any infection); 5 minor soreness, 4 skin allergic reactions; 2 mild and transient alopecia. In conclusion, Clofibrate may be administered continuously for many years without any decrease in its potent hypolipidemic effectiveness. Despite interference with oral anticoagulant therapy, side effects occurred infrequently and seemed less important than those registered in C.D.P. The relation between Clofibrate therapy and cholelithiasis might only be suggested but the respective contribution of spontaneous lithiasis of parallel long term use of polyunsaturated fats in diet, and of Clofibrate have to be carefully discussed.

ADVANTAGES OF HYPOLIPIDEMIC EFFECTS OF PROCETOFENE OVER CLOFIBRATE THERAPY

J.L. de Gennes and J. Truffert

Hopital de la Pitie, 75013 Paris, France

Procetofene, a new hypolipidemic drug was administered to 250 primary hyperlipidemic patients who were previously treated with clofibrate. There were 10 dropouts but the remaining 240 patients have been on procetofene (300-400 mg/day) for over a year without any reports of major clinical disturbances. In mixed hyperlipidemias (110 M and 21 F) with mean basal cholesterol (TC) and triglyceride (TG) levels of 353 and 310 mg/dl respectively, procetofene caused a mean decrease in TC of 27% and in TG of 50%.

Decrease while on clofibrate were 11% for TC and 39% for TG. The normalization rate on procetofene was 65% after the sixth month of therapy. In 63 type IIa patients with xanthoma tendinosum (31 M, 32 F) mean baseline levels for TC and TG were 430 and 101 mg/dl, respectively. On procetofene TC levels decreased by 33% and TG by 27% whereas on clofibrate therapy decreases were -19% for TC and -14% for TG. In almost 50% of the cases TC levels fell below 260 mg/dl. After one year of procetofene treatment manifest regression of xanthomata was observed in 10 patients. In 66 other type IIa patients (24 M, 42 F) mean baseline levels were: TC - 380 mg/dl and TG 96 mg/dl. Procetofene therapy caused drops of 28% in TC and 23% in TG whereas clofibrate therapy had reduced TC by 20% and TG by 12%. Myocardial infarcts (one first, two recurrent) were observed in 3 patients on procetofene therapy, occurring after 6, 6 and 10 months of therapy respectively. Rises in SGPT were observed in 10% of patients with mixed hyperlipidemias and 20% of those with type IIa hyperlipidemia.

EFFECTS OF CHOLESTYRAMINE ON SERUM CHOLESTEROL, FECAL BILE ACID EXCRETION, AND PLAQUE REGRESSION IN RHESUS MONKEYS

R.G. DePalma, E.M. Bellon, S.Koletsky, L. Klein, and D.L Schneider

2065 Adelbert Road, Cleveland, Ohio 44106, U.S.A.

We observed the effects of cholestyramine (CST) added to an atherogenic diet, and measured its effect on serum cholesterol, fecal bile acid excretion and lesion regression. Ten Rhesus monkeys were observed for 36 months by sequential angiography, surgical exploration, biopsy, and autopsy. After a baseline control period, lesions were produced by feeding a .5% cholesterol/sucrose diet to all animals. When lesions were established after 24 months of feeding, regression was initiated by adding 4 gm of CST to the diet for a period of 10 months. The chemical results are summarized:

Experimental Manipulations	Serum Cholesterol mg/100 ml			Fecal Bile Acid Excretion μ moles daily		
	Experimental		Control	Experimental		Control
	Avg.	Range	Avg.	Avg.	Range	Avg.
1 month, normal diet	141	115-170	150	51.5	34-65	43.5
23 months, atherogenic diet	395	262-545	388	36.9	18-43	43.6
11 months, atherogenic diet + cholestyramine	235	173-325	384	281	158-436	24

Morphologically, the two control animals exhibited fibrofatty plaques in contrast to 8 animals fed CST. Six experimental animals showed regression of plaques at the inferior mesenteric artery, lumbar arteries, and aorta. One showed no change. One demonstrated regression in the lumbar aorta and progression of a plaque in the internal carotid artery. It is noteworthy that the most severe cholesterolemia was attained in this animal during atherogenesis (avg. 575 mg/100 ml) and that it also exhibited the poorest response to CST feeding (325 mg/100 ml). This animal is under current observation on 8 gm. CST daily to determine its effect on the carotid plaque. Cholestyramine is effective in inducing plaque regression by decreasing serum cholesterol as a result of increased fecal bile acid excretion.

EFFECT OF NICOTINIC ACID AND CLOFIBRATE ON LIPOLYSIS OF ISOLATED FAT CELLS IN MAN AND RAT

H.H. Ditschuneit, H.U Klor and H. Ditschuneit

Department Inner Medizin der Universitat Ulm, 7900 Ulm, West Germany

Inhibition of FFA release from adipose tissue is one of the few known ways of action of nicotinic acid (NA) and clofibrate (CPIB). In the rat isoproterenol (0.01 μg/ml) stimulated lipolysis could be inhibited by 10% in the presence of 5 μg NA/ml, while in man the same effect was already obtained by 5-10 ng/ml. A complete inhibition of lipolysis was observed in the presence of 5 μg/ml. In man and rat theophyllin (100 μg/ml) induced lipolysis was reduced by 10% with 5-10 ng/ml, while 1 μg/ml caused a complete inhibition of stimulated lipolysis in both species. Concentrations of NA which caused almost complete inhibition in the theophyllin stimulated lipolysis turned out to be ineffective when lipolysis was stimulated by ACTH (0.1 μg/ml), glucagon (0.01 μg/ml) and dB-cAMP (100 μg/ml). When NA (5-20 ng/ml) and insulin (5-100 μU/ml) were both present a more than additive inhibition of theophyllin induced lipolysis was observed. Clofibrate (100 μg/ml) caused a 15% reduction of both isoproterenol and theophyllin stimulated lipolysis. When adding NA (5-20 ng/ml) an additional antilipolytic effect was observed.

Our results show that even ng amounts of NA are potent inhibitors of stimulated lipolysis of isolated human fat cells. The effect is even more pronounced when small amounts of insulin are present. The addition of almost physiological concentrations of NA to therapeutic concentrations of CPIB results in additional antilipolysis.

EVIDENCE FOR A DIRECT RELATIONSHIP BETWEEN THE HYPOCHOLESTEROLEMIC ACTIVITY AND PLASMA LEVELS OF PROCETOFEN IN TYPE IIA PATIENTS ON CHRONIC MEDICATION

P. Drouin, L. Mejean, C. Tourne, and E. Wülfert

Centre Hospitalier Regional de Nancy, Service de Medecine Generale "G" oriente vers les Maladies Metaboliques et les Maladies de la Nutrition, Hopital Jeanne-D'Arc, Donmartin-les-Toul, 54201 Toul Cedex, France

Patients affected by type IIa, H.L.P., were treated with Procetofen for 3-14 months (200-400 mg daily). Baseline levels of blood cholesterol were determined on the basis of at least 3 determinations during a dietary pretreatment period of 3 months. Diet therapy was maintained throughout the study. The level of blood cholesterol and of circulating drug were determined concomitantly on a monthly basis during the active drug trial. On the basis of 130 observations, it could be demonstrated that the hypocholessterolemic effect of the drug (Δ cholesterol expressed in mg%) was directly correlated to the amount of Procetofen in plasma. The relationship followed a typical Michaelis Menten curve. The half maximal hypocholesterolemic effect was observed with plasma levels of 4,5 mg/l ($K = 1{,}2.10^{-5}$M). No accumulation of drug in the plasma could be observed throughout the study. The clinical and biochemical consequences of these findings will be discussed.

IN VIVO AND *IN VITRO* ANIMAL STUDIES WITH B-DF 184, A NEW HYPOLIPEMIC DRUG

B. Eisele, G. Griss and A. Zimmer

Department of Biochemistry and Department of Chemistry, Dr. Karl Thomae GmbH, D7950 Biberach/Riss, Germany

B-DF 184 (4[2-methoxybenzamido)ethyl]biphenyl-4-oxy(2)isobutyric acid) was shown to be 10-30 times as potent as clofibrate in normo- and hyper-lipemic animals (20% reduction of rat plasma cholesterol levels at 0.6 mg/kg). The fat clearance as measured by the intravenous fat tolerance test is enhanced. In *in vitro* studies the compound was shown to be anti-lipolytic and antilipogenic in rat fat cells. It inhibits the HMG-CoA-reductase and the acyl-CoA-synthetase from rat liver microsomes. It is very strongly bound to human serum albumin (over 99%) the binding constants at 37°C assuming two independent binding sites were determined (n_1=2.2, n_2=9.4, K_1=1.8 · 10^5 M^{-1}, K_2=2.9 ·10^3 M^{-1}). After oral absorption in rats the compound is eliminated predominantly via the bile, the biological half-life being about 10 hours. In animal experiments B-DF 184 is less toxic than clofibrate.

EFFECTS OF ML-236B, A COMPETITIVE INHIBITOR OF 3-HYDROXY-3-METHYLGLUTARYL (HMG)-CoA REDUCTASE, ON CHOLESTEROL METABOLISM

A. Endo, N. Kitano and S. Fujii

Research Laboratories, Sankyo Co., Ltd., Shinagawa, Tokyo 140, and Institute of Protein Research, Osaka University, Osaka 565, Japan

ML-236B is a competitive inhibitor of HMG-CoA reductase (Ki=10 nM) with low toxicity (LD_{50} > 5 g/kg, mouse, p.o.) isolated from cultures of *Penicillium citrinum* (A. Endo, M. Kuroda and Y. Tsujita, J.Antibiotics 29: 1346, 1976; A. Endo, M. Kuroda and K. Tanzawa, FEBS Letters 72: 323, 1976). The compound inhibited sterol synthesis in cultured human skin fibroblasts from normal subjects and patients with familial hypercholesterolemia 50% at 0.1 μM, and its inhibitory effects on the growth of cultured cells were effectively counteracted by mevalonate. Experiments with rats showed that ML-236B was readily adsorbed into liver and preferentially inhibited sterol synthesis in this organ, and that it caused no hepatomegaly when given p.o. at 2 g/kg/day (p.o.) for over 2 weeks. Hypocholesterolemic effects of ML-236B were shown in adult rats, hens, dogs and monkeys at doses of 10-50 mg/kg/day (p.o.) without affecting food consumption and body weight gain.

MODE OF ACTION OF A NOVEL HYPOCHOLESTEROLEMIC Δ^8-DIHYDROABIETAMIDE DERIVATIVE IN RATS

H. Enomoto, Y. Yoshikuni, T. Ozaki, R. Zschocke and K. Ohata

Research Laboratories, Nippon Shinyaku Co., Ltd., Kyoto, Japan, and Klinge Pharma GmbH & Co., Munich, Germany

N-(2,6-dimethylphenyl)- Δ^8-dihydroabietamide, THD-341, at a dietary dose of 0.0003% significantly reduces serum cholesterol (C), triglycerides (TG), and phospholipids as well as liver C and TG in C-fed rats. Its hypocholesterolemic activity is comparable to that of D-thyroxine and 400, 1300, and 4700 times greater than that of clofibrate, β-sitosterol, and cholestyramine, respectively. Also THD-341 effectively reduces serum and liver C in cholate and thiouracil hypercholesterolemic rats and reduces liver C in normal rats.

By the dual-isotope ratio method of Zilversmit THD-341 is found to significantly inhibit C absorption and to possibly accelerate catabolism and/or excretion of endogenous C. Analysis of fecal steroids in C-fed rats after oral pulsing with C^{14}-C and subsequent change to normal and C-diets containing THD-341 at a level of 0.03% again suggests that THD-341 stimulates fecal excretion of endogenous neutral steroids. Comparative views on its mode of action with other known hypocholesterolemic agents will be presented.

LIPID LOWERING DRUGS AND GLUCOSE TOLERANCE

E.B. Feldman, F.B. Gluck and A.C. Carter

Medical College of Georgia, Augusta, Georgia 30901, U.S.A.

Halofenate, a triglyceride and uric acid-lowering drug, potentiated the effect of oral hypoglycemics. Its effect on serial glucose tolerance was evaluated in ten patients with hypertriglyceridemia without overt diabetes. Six hour oral glucose tolerance tests (GTT) were done during a control period and every 24 weeks over two years of halofenate treatment. Abnormal glucose tolerance (chemical diabetes) was observed during the control period in 6 of 10 patients. The number of abnormal tests gradually decreased to none by 48 weeks. Plasma glucose, insulin and FFA values during the GTT were reduced significantly. Halofenate induced significant serum uric acid reduction. No significant regressions were observed among levels of lipids, hormones, glucose or uric acid, or with body weight. Clofibrate was given to ten other hypertriglyceridemic patients. Chemical diabetes in 5 decreased to 3 abnormal tests at 48 weeks. Plasma glucose, but not insulin, was reduced significantly with 40% triglyceride lowering. The sites, interrelations and mechanisms of lipid lowering drug effects on lipid, glucose and purine metabolism are as yet unclear.

THE VARIATION OF 7α-HYDROXYLASE ACTIVITY IN RANDOMLY SELECTED AND LITTERMATE GROUPS OF MALE RATS

L. Flanders and N. Nicholson

Searle Laboratories, 4901 Searle Parkway, Skokie, Illinois 60076 U.S.A.

We attempted to develop a screening assay for regulators of 7α-hydroxylase activity *in vivo*. The basic design involved intragastric administration of drug to male rats fed *ad libitum* followed by an assay of liver 7α-hydroxylase *in vitro* by measuring [4-^{14}C] 7α-hydroxycholesterol as described by Bjorkhem and Danielsson (Eur.J.Biochem. 53: 63-70, 1975). We obtained specific activities (2.7 pmoles/mg protein/min) for 7α-hydroxylase comparable to those of Bjorkhem and Danielsson. However, with time, a wide range of control values was obtained for randomly selected groups of rats (0.9 to 2.7 pmoles/mg protein/min). An analysis of the data revealed that the assay precision was satisfactory (coefficient of variation < 0.02) but the animal variation was quite large (coefficient of variation ranging from 0.11 to 0.35). The 7α-hydroxylase activity for littermates was measured either using groups composed of brothers or using paired comparisons of brothers assigned to different groups. In the latter case, the coefficient of variation for the different groups was equivalent to those values found for randomly selected groups of non-littermate rats (0.24 - 0.34). The data for the littermate groups produced lower coefficients of variation (0.08 to 0.18) for the individual groups but the range of 7α-hydroxylase specific activities between the groups was still large (0.9 to 1.7 pmoles/mg protein/min). Because of this variation then, we felt an accurate screening assay based on this methodology was not practical.

EFFECT OF DIURETICS UPON PLATELET FUNCTION IN HYPERTENSIVE ADULTS

A.I. Fleischman, M.L. Bierenbaum and A. Stier

Division of Community Health Services, New Jersey State Department of Health, Montclair, New Jersey 07042, U.S.A.

Platelet aggregation tendency was determined by theFiltragometer procedure in the presence of all formed elements of the blood in 105 normotensives, 75 hypertensives on diuretic therapy and 37 untreated hypertensives. Mean systolic blood pressures were 124±1.3, 153±2.5, and 162±2.6 mmHg respectively, each different from the other at $p<0.01$, while mean diastolic blood pressures were 76±0.8, 89±1.4 and 91±1.9 mmHg respectively, $p<0.01$. Mean aggregation times were 368±21.6, 331±25.3 and 245±26.6 seconds respectively. Both the normotensives and the diuretic treated hypertensives exhibited a longer aggregation time than the untreated hypertensives, $p<0.01$. The difference between normotensives and treated hypertensives was not statistically significant. Twenty-one percent of untreated hypertensives and 11 percent of normotensives failed to disaggregate, $p<0.05$. No significant difference was found between normotensives and treated hypertensives. The data indicate that treatment of hypertensives with diuretics significantly decreased the aggregation tendency of platelets. (Supported in part by The Charles Edison Fund)

STUDIES ON THE HYPOCHOLESTEROLEMIC EFFECT OF PARTIAL ILEAL BYPASS IN RABBITS

C. Fragiacomo, M.R. Lovati, U. Fox, G. Maione, and C.R. Sirtori

Center E. Grossi Paoletti and III Institute of Surgical Pathology, University of Milan, Milan, Italy

Partial ileal bypass (Buchwald, H., Surgery 58: 22, 1965) markedly reduces cholesterolemia in cholesterol-fed rabbits, even when cholesterol administration is continued after surgery. The composition and metabolism of lipoproteins, particularly of density less than 1.019, from cholesterol-fed (HC) rabbits before and after bypass (BP), is markedly modified by the procedure. D$<$1.019 lipoproteins contain, in fact, a decreased amount of cholesterol and sphingomyelin, increased triglycerides and show significant changes in the apoprotein composition. In particular, the arg-rich protein is decreased, C-proteins are increased and several protein bands, not identifiable with previously described apoproteins, become evident.

Turnover of d$<$1.019 BP lipoproteins after ^{125}I labelling is increased, as compared to HC lipoproteins, and the uptake by the arterial wall is significantly reduced. Immunological analysis of the apoprotein composition of d$<$1.019 and d 1.019-1.063 lipoprotein fractions reveals a significant reduction of the B apoprotein content after bypass.

It is suggested that partial ileal bypass may alter the synthetic pathway of VLDL, IDL and LDL, decreasing their apo B content and causing physico-chemical changes, favoring catabolism and reducing atherogenicity.

OXANDROLONE'S EFFECT ON RAT SERUM LIPOPROTEINS

M.W. Freeman, E. Spring-Mills and A.L. Jones

Cell Biology Section, Veterans Administration Hospital, San Francisco, California 94121, U.S.A.

Oxandrolone, a potent cholesterol-lowering steroid, was given orally to male, retired breeder rats for 21 days. The serum lipoproteins of both the drug treated animals and a control group of rats were isolated by ultra-centrifugation. The experimental animals had 50% less cholesterol in their low density lipoprotein fraction than did the controls; and, a 25% reduction in high density lipoprotein (HDL) cholesterol was noted in the oxandrolone treated group. Very low density lipoproteins (VLDL) were unaffected. LDL and HDL phospholipid, triglyceride, and protein moieties were also altered by the drug. However, these changes differed from those seen in cholesterol and thus indicate an alteration in the composition of the lipoproteins. The biochemical changes wrought by oxandrolone were corroborated by electron micrographs showing no change in VLDL size and decreases in the size of LDL's and HDL's. Preliminary studies on age-matched virgin rats showed that the LDL cholesterol is about 50% less than retired breeders' and is not significantly affected by oxandrolone. The age-matched virgin carries the same amount of cholesterol in the HDL fraction as does the retired breeder and this cholesterol is similarly lowered by the drug.

ADRENERGIC INTERACTION WITH FAT CELLS: POSSIBLE ROLE FOR CALCIUM AND CYCLIC GMP

R.M. Gaion and G. Krishna

Laboratory of Chemical Pharmacology, National Heart, Lung, and Blood Institute, Bethesda, Maryland 20014, U.S.A.

Epinephrine (E) induces lipolysis in fat cells by increasing cAMP. E (1 μM) also causes a marked increase of cGMP accumulation in fat cells in two distinct phases. The cGMP level is increased within seconds, reaching a peak of 400% of the basal value between 15-30 seconds and then declines to about 70% of the peak level in 1 minute. E also induces a parallel increase in calcium efflux within seconds; the rate of efflux reaches a maximum within 15 seconds and declines to the basal efflux rate in about 1 minute. E causes a second, slow phase of increase in cGMP after 2 minutes, that reaches a maximum of about 500% over basal level in 15 minutes. In the presence of E, cAMP reaches its peak level of 5-fold of the basal value in about 6 minutes. Theophylline (T) (0.3 mM) induces only a slow phase of cGMP increase which peaks at about 2 minutes. The absence of the first phase of cGMP accumulation corresponds with the lack of effect of T on calcium efflux. The methyl xanthine increases cAMP level and its time-response curve is similar to that obtained with E. The β-adrenergic blocking agent, propranolol (20 μM), completely inhibits E-induced cAMP and cGMP accumulation, calcium efflux and lipolysis. Phentolamine (20 μM), an α-adrenergic blocking agent, partially inhibits cAMP accumulation and lipolysis, but has no effect either on E-induced cGMP accumulation or calcium efflux. These data suggest that cGMP accumulation is closely related to calcium efflux in fat cells and these messengers could play an unidentified role in the early intracellular modulation and transmission of the adrenergic response.

STIMULATION OF CHOLESTEROL 7α-HYDROXYLASE ACTIVITY BY THE PORPHYROGENIC CHEMICAL ALLYLISOPROPYLACETAMIDE

G. Galli[1], M. Galli-Kienle[2], and A. Sanghvi[3]

[1]Institute of Pharmacology and Pharmacognosy, [2]Institute of Chemistry, University of Milan, 20129 Milan, Italy, [3]Department of Pathology, University of Pittsburgh, Pittsburgh, Pennsylvania 15213, U.S.A.

It has been shown by Sanghvi and Parikh and by Taddeini _et al_ that the activity of rat liver HMG-CoA reductase and the rate of hepatic cholesterol synthesis both are enhanced in animals given a single dose of allylisopropyl-acetamide (AIA). We report here that a single dose of AIA also stimulates the activity of rat liver microsomal cholesterol-7α-hydroxylase, the rate limiting enzyme of the bile acid biosynthetic pathway. The magnitude of increase in cholesterol-7α-hydroxylase activity in treated animals compares with that observed for HMG-CoA reductase activity.

This stimulation could not be attributed to any change in the liver microsomal cholesterol pool. Our finding has possible significance since it has been reported by Javitt _et al_ that 3α,7α-dihydroxy- and 3α,7α,12α-trihydroxy-coprostanes, intermediates in bile acid synthesis, when added to chick embryo liver cells increase the rate of porphyrin synthesis by stimulating the activity of δ -amino-levulinic acid synthetase.

IMMUNOLOGICAL FACTORS IN VASCULAR DISEASES

S. Gero, E. Szondy, M. Horvath, G. Fust, and J. Szekely

Arteriosclerosis Research Group of the Ministry of Health, Budapest, Hungary

1. To investigate the antigenic properties of human arterial and venous wall, an extraction-fractionation procedure was applied to the vascular tissues. The obtained fractions (soluble protein-polysaccharides, soluble tropocollagen, structural glycoproteins, elastin, kappa-elastin) were characterized by electrophoretical, thermoanalytical and immunological methods.

2. The production of antibodies against the various aortic fractions was studied by immunodiffusion methods and by the passive haemagglutination test in the sera of patients with various manifestations of arteriosclerosis. The presence of antibodies was found in 50% of the cases when using the protein-polysaccharide fraction, The presence of anti-vena antibodies in 70% of patients with phlebothrombosis could be demonstrated.

3. In myocardial infarction, arteriosclerosis obliterans and thrombophlebitis a significant cell-mediated immune response could be observed *in vitro* using human vascular antigens, whereas in control persons any cellular reaction could not be detected.

4. Circulating immune complexes were found in 38% of the patients with various vascular diseases. The correlation between the level of the lipid components and that of the immune complexes has also been investigated.

HYPOLIPIDEMIC EFFECT AND SIDE EFFECTS OF XANTINOL-NICOTINATE IN CHRONIC TREATMENT OF PRIMARY HYPERLIPOPROTEINEMIAS

H. Haacke, M.R. Parwaresch and Ch. Mader

II. Medizinische Universitatsklinik, 23 Kiel 1, West Germany

Treatment of primary hyperlipoproteinemia requires chronic application of the hypolipidemic drugs and sets, thus high standards to a critical evaluation of the side effects.

Nicotinic acid derivatives are known as potent lipid lowering drugs. Systematic studies of their side effects under the conditions of chronic application have not been performed so far. We studied 65 cases of primary hyperlipoproteinemias (types IIa, IIb, IV and V) put on Xantinol-nicotinate for six months with monthly controlled nicotinic acid levels in the blood. In addition to measurement of serum lipids (phospholipids, triglycerides, cholesterol, non-esterified fatty acids), different lipoproteins (chylomicrons, VLDL, LDL and HDL) were separated and subjected to lipid analyses covering about 20 parameters. Side effects were studied considering hepatic and renal function tests, as well as uric acid and carbohydrate metabolism and haematological parameters. Lipid lowering effect was clearly detectable in 46 cases. Major side effects, especially any alteration of the 14 parameters studied, could not be observed in all cases followed up.

LONG TERM EFFECTS OF CLOFIBRATE THERAPY ON CARBOHYDRATE TOLERANCE, INSULIN AND LIPID CONCENTRATIONS IN HYPERLIPOPROTEINEMIA (HLP)

H. Haller, W. Bruns, D. Michaelis, J. Schulze, M. Hanefeld and W. Leonhardt

Medical Academy Dresden and Central Institute of Diabetes, Karlsburg, G.D.R.

The prevalence of diabetes is five-fold higher in HLP than in normolipemia (Dresden Study). Therefore, the long term antidiabetic effect of clofibrate is of great interest, but not certain up to now. We examined 86 patients with HLP of types IIa to V. Carbohydrate tolerance was characterized by oral and, in part, i.v. glucose load. The therapy with 1.5 g clofibrate and a carbohydrate and fat restricted diet lasted up to 5 years. Before and thereafter, blood glucose, insulin, triglycerides and cholesterol were measured. As a general result, lipid concentrations leveled down mainly in the first year. In the patients with pathologic carbohydrate tolerance, blood sugar and insulin concentrations after glucose load were lowered three weeks after the beginning of the therapy. The best long-term therapeutic effect of clofibrate is achieved in connection with reduction of overweight and of hyperinsulinemia. Clofibrate therapy is indicated on the basis of body weight reduction and diet in patients with primary HLP and pathologic glucose tolerance. A long-term antidiabetic effect could not be detected with certainty.

LONG-TERM EFFECT OF CLOFIBRATE (CPIB) ON SUBSTRATES AND ULTRASTRUCTURE OF THE HUMAN LIVER

M. Hanefeld, C. Kemmer, G. Roschlau, W. Leonhardt, W. Jaross, and H. Haller

Medical Academy, 8019 Dresden, G.D.R.

With respect to the hepatic actions of CPIB, follow-up studies to elucidate the effects of long-term treatment are of importance. Therefore we performed liver biopsies in 38 patients with primary hypertriglyceridemia before and after three months to 6 years on CPIB. The following questions were analyzed:

1. effect on triglyceride, glycogen and trace element concentrations,
2. effect on glycerol-1-phosphatedehydrogenese and enzymes of glycogen metabolism (by histochemistry), and
3. changes of organelles (by electron microscopy).

Liver glycogen and manganese content decreased significantly whereas triglyceride, copper and zinc concentrations remained constant. Characteristic changes were observed in the mitochondria. Their numbers increased significantly. In 3 patients treated more than 3 years with CPIB, mitochondria contained multilayered circular structures as first described by Lee _et al_. in swine after administration of clofibrate (Exp. Molecular Pathol. 20: 387, 1974). Smooth endoplasmic reticulum and microbodies increased only moderately. Our results support a hypothesis that the elevated content of mitochondria plays a central role in the mode of hepatic action of CPIB.

THE EFFECT OF UNAVAILABLE CARBOHYDRATE ON LIPID AND GLUCOSE ABSORPTION IN NORMAL SUBJECTS

T.M. Hayes, A.W. Jones, J. Munn and R. Mottram

Department of Medicine, Welsh National School of Medicine, University Hospital of Wales, Cardiff, Wales, United Kingdom

Plasma total triglyceride, chylomicron triglyceride, glucose and insulin levels were measured in 5 normal subjects after a standard breakfast and after the same breakfast proceeded by either methylcellulose tablets (5 gm), bran tablets (10 gm), guar gum (10 gm) or pectin (10 gm). The 5 meals in each subject were carried out in random order. Each standard meal contained 78 gm carbohydrate, 60 gm protein and 19 gm fat and the peak triglyceride levels were reached 3 hours after the meal. The levels had fallen by 6 hours but were still 23% above basal. The blood glucose reached a peak at 30 min and after the control meal had returned to basal by 60 min.

The increment in chylomicron triglyceride was reduced by both methylcellulose (from 0.72±0.21 to 0.34±0.12 mmol/L, $p<0.05$) and guar gum (from 0.72±0.21 to 0.41±0.08 mmol/L, $p<0.05$). The total triglyceride increment was reduced by methylcellulose, guar and bran but these reductions only reached significance at the 10% level. Pectin has no significant effect on plasma triglyceride responses but was the most effective of all the preparations in reducing the glucose peak (22% reduction compared with control levels, $p<0.05$). Although the peak levels were reduced the area under the glucose curves was not reduced by any of the preparations and bran increased the area 10% above control values ($p<0.01$). All the preparations decreased the speed with which the blood glucose returned to basal levels. The plasma insulin peak was also reduced most markedly by pectin.

COMPARATIVE ANTI-ATHEROSCLEROTIC EFFECTS OF ANTIPLATELET, ANTICALCIFYING AND ANTILIPEMIC DRUGS WITH SPECIAL REFERENCE TO SODIUM P-HEXADECYLAMINO-BENZOATE (PHB)

W. Hollander, S. Prusty, S. Nagraj, B. Kirkpatrick, J. Paddock, and M. Colombo

Boston University Medical Center, Boston, Massachusetts

The effects of three different groups of drugs on the development of dietary induced atherosclerosis in the cynomolgus monkey was studied over a period of 6 months. The test agents included (1) the antiplatelet drugs, aspirin - 120 mg/kg + dipyridamole - 10 mg/kg; (2) the anticalcifying drugs, ethane-hydroxy-diphosphonate (EHDP) - 5 mg/kg and dichloro-methylene-diphosphonate)Cl_2MDP) - 5 mg/kg and (3) the inhibitor of cholesterol and cholesteryl ester biosynthesis (PHB) - 100 mg/kg. When compared to the findings in untreated control animals, the antiplatelet and anticalcifying drugs had no significant effect on the extent and severity of atherosclerosis of the coronary, aortic and peripheral arteries as revealed by macroscopic, microscopic and chemical analyses of the vessels. In contrast, PHB had a significant inhibitory effect on the extent and severity of atherosclerosis with coronary disease being suppressed by about 50%.

Coronary Luminal Narrowing (%)

	LCOA	LAD	CIRCUM	RCOA
Control	49 ± 8	48 ± 10	62 ± 8	65 ± 9
PHB	25 ± 6	19 ± 8	33 ± 8	34 ± 7

The anti-atherosclerotic effect of PHB was associated with significant reduction in serum and arterial concentrations of cholesterol and cholesterol ester. Conclusion The findings suggest further investigation of PHB as an anti-atherosclerotic drug.

CLINICAL EVALUATION OF GEMFIBROZIL, A NEW HYPOLIPEMIC AGENT

A.N. Howard and P. Ghosh

Department of Medicine, University of Cambridge, Addenbrooke's Hospital, Cambridge CB2 2QQ, England

Gemfibrozil (2,2-dimethyl-5-(2,5-xylyloxy) valeric acid, Parke-Davis) has a pronounced ability to decrease serum triglycerides in rats, mice and monkeys, after oral administration but has no effect on serum cholesterol. The present study examined the effect of the compound in nine type IIa and 14 type IIb/IV hyperlipoproteinemic patients for six months. A dose of 800 mg/day produced the following decreases: serum cholesterol 13%; triglycerides 42%; VLDL 33%; LDL 21%. In one type V subject triglycerides were markedly decreased in both chylomicrons and LDL. A further 12 type IIb/IV patients were treated for two months with either 1.2 g/day gemfibrozil (G) or 2.0 g/day clofibrate (C). Following two months placebo, the drugs were crossed over. The following decreases in serum were obtained: cholesterol; G 12%, C 8%, triglycerides; G 42%, C 21%, VLDL; G 31%, C 23%. Gemfibrozil increased serum HDL cholesterol by 31%; there was no change with clofibrate. It is concluded that gemfibrozil is a very effective hypotriglyceridemic agent, with a moderate action in decreasing serum cholesterol. The development of new compounds with similar hypolipemic properties to clofibrate is worthwhile in view of the adverse effects of the latter on the lithogenic index in bile and the incidence of gallstones.

ACTIVATION OF LIPOPROTEIN LIPASE BY SYNTHETIC FRAGMENTS OF APOLIPOPROTEIN C-II (ApoC-II)

R.L. Jackson, P.K.J. Kinnunen, L.C. Smith, A.M. Gotto, Jr., and J.T. Sparrow

Baylor College of Medicine and The Methodist Hospital, Houston, Texas 77030, U.S.A.

Lipoprotein lipase (LPL) catalyzes the hydrolysis of triglycerides of chylomicrons and very low density lipoproteins and requires apoC-II for maximal activity. ApoC-II contains 78 amino acid residues of known sequence. Cleavage of apoC-II with cyanogen bromide yields 3 fragments with 9, 50 and 19 residues. The cyanogen bromide (CNBr) fragments were tested for their ability to activate homogeneous bovine milk LPL with 3.1 mM tri([1-^{14}C]-oleoyl)glycerol. The carboxyl-terminal CNBr fragment (residues 60-78) at

4.8 μM enhanced release of fatty acid 4.8-fold compared to 6.3-fold for the same concentration of intact apoC-II. A synthetic peptide corresponding to residues 60-78 enhanced the lipolysis to the same extent. However, a synthetic peptide corresponding to residues 66-78 gave no activation. These studies suggest that the activation of LPL by apoC-II requires a minimal amino acid sequence and that residues 60-65 are part of this requirement.

EFFECT OF THREE UNSATURATED OILS ON THE FATTY ACID COMPOSITION OF SERUM AND AORTA OF RATS FED DURING ONE YEAR ON A LOW-FAT DIET

B. Jacotot, M. Girardet and J.L. Beaumont

Unite de Recherches sur l'Atherosclerose, Hopital Henri Mondor, 94010 Creteil, France

Fatty acid composition of rat serum and aorta lipids (cholesterol (CE), triglycerides (TG), phospholipids (PL) and FFA) were determined by GLC, after one year of equilibrated diet using 5% of one of the following oils: sunflower, arachid, Primor (French variety of rapeseed oil with very small amounts of erucic and gadoleic acids).*

Discriminant analysis of serum and aorta FA levels showed:

in serum, the diet did not effect the FA composition of the lipids; with all diets, PL were rich in C18:0, FFA in C16:0, CE in C24:0. The linoleic level was not significantly higher in lipids of animals fed with sunflower oil (it did rise in experiments with hyperlipidic diet containing 40% fat).

in aorta, the diet had also little influence on FA composition which was similar to that observed in serum lipids for FFA and TG. Indeed PL had a high level of C24:0 and C18:0. CE were rich in C14:0, C16:1 and especially in C12:0 in contradistinction to serum CE, which had a high level of C24:0.

We propose the hypothesis that cholesterol laurate accumulation in aorta is due to the lack of dietary saturated FA.

* Oil composition: 1) Sunflower: linoleic acid, 57%; oleic, 27%; palmitic, 7.5%; stearic, 5%.

2) Arachid: oleic, 38%; linoleic, 33%; palmitic, 13%.

3) Primor: oleic, 56%; linoleic, 19%; linolenic, 10%; palmitic, 4.6%.

DETERMINATION OF NICOTINIC ACID BY HPLC-METHODOLOGY AND PLASMA LEVELS OF DIFFERENT PREPARATIONS

H. Jaeger, J.G. Wechsler, H.U. Klor and H. Ditschuneit

Department of Medicine, Division of Metabolism and Nutrition, University of Ulm, Ulm, West Germany

A highly sensitive method has been developed in order to compare plasma and tissue levels of nicotinic acid with its lipid-lowering effect.

Extraction of nicotinic acid was performed with hexane, isopropanol and water. After phase separation the recovery of nicotinic acid was 89% in the aqueous phase. After further precipitation of non-alcohol soluble substances with ethanol the water phase was washed several times with ethyl-acetate. Up to this point the recovery attained 80%. The extract was evaporated to dryness and 1 ml of the solvent chloroform:methanol:acetic acid·water (350:7·1:1 v/v) added and subsequently injected into the high performance liquid chromatograph. The lowest detectable concentration of nicotinic acid was 10 ng/ml as determined by absorption at 254 nm. Isonicotinic acid was used as internal standard.

Plasma levels varied considerably after application of the drug in different preparations such as inositol nicotinate, xantinole nicotinate and β-pyridyl-carbinole. They could also be correlated to the respective pharmacological effects. After application of β-pyridyl-carbinole we found the highest, after inositole nicotinate somewhat lower and after xantinole nicotinate the lowest plasma levels.

USE OF MICROORGANISMS AS CELL MODELS FOR TESTING HYPOLIPIDEMIC DRUGS

J.J. Kabara and R. Vrable

Department of Biomechanics, Michigan State University, East Lansing, Michigan 48824, U.S.A.

Most *in vitro* attempts to screen for hypolipidemic agents or to search for mechanisms of drug action involve the use of eukaryotic cells or organelles from such cells. The elucidation of drug mechanism is, therefore, a function of the particular biological system used. In order to demonstrate the vagaries of such *in vitro* approaches, our own investigation has centered on the use of three simple systems - mitochondrial, bacterial, and yeast. While these simple systems cannot be used as predictors of *in vivo* drug activity, they can be made useful by identifying the most potent member in a chemical series. Results from studies on imidazole compounds will be presented as an example of this approach. Besides its utility as a primary screening method for hypolipidemic agents, some interesting antimicrobial and particularly fungal agents can be discovered. Hypolipidemic properties of drugs may also be relevant to their insecticidal properties. The global aspects of hypolipidemic agent uses will be discussed.

A STUDY ON THE EFFECTS OF SOME HYPOLIPEMIC AGENTS FROM THE VIEWPOINTS OF BOTH LIPIDS AND GLYCOPROTEINS

T. Kanazawa, T. Terata, T. Komatsu, M. Izawa, H. Mori, Y. Oike, H. Metoki*, K. Onodera*, H. Ito*, S. Izumiyama* and T. Matsui**

Second Department of Internal Medicine, Hirosaki University School of Medicine, *Reimeikyo Rehabilitation Hospital, **Health Administration Center of Hirosaki University, Hirosaki, Japan

Such hypolipemic agents such as nicomol, 1-1-bis-[4'-(1"-carboxy-1"-methylpropoxy)phenyl] cyclohexane (S-8527) and oxandrolone were administered for 16 weeks to 56 outpatients with mild hypertension and/or mild diabetes mellitus. The blood was taken 2 weeks before and just before the treatment, and 2,4,8,12 and 16 weeks after the beginning of the treatment.

EFFECT ON SERUM LIPIDS

Drugs	Nicomol	S-8527	Oxandrolone
Cholesterol	↘	↘	↓
Triglyceride	→	↓	↓
Phospholipid	→	→	↓↓
β-Lipoprotein	↓	↓	↓
Free Fatty Acid	↓↓	→	→

EFFECT ON SERUM GLYCOPROTEINS

Total Protein bound to hexose	↓↓	↓↓	↑↑
Mucoprotein bound to hexose	↓↓	↓↓	↑↑

→ = not significant, ↘ = 0.10>p>0.05, ↓ = 0.05>p>0.01, ↓↓ ↑↑ =0.01>p

There can be particular hypolipemic agents, as oxandrolone, which decrease serum lipids but increase serum glycoproteins at the same time, both being regarded as similar factors relating to atherosclerosis.

Therefore, in using hypolipemic agents for the treatment of atherosclerosis, the fact that there hypolipemic agents with particular properties must be kept in mind.

EFFECTS OF VARIOUS TYPES OF PROSTAGLANDINS ON THE HUMAN FAT CELL ADENYLATE CYCLASE

H. Kather and B. Simon

Medizinische Universitatsklinik Heidelberg, D-6900 Heidelberg, Germany

Administration of prostaglandin E1 has been reported to cause an enhancement of the release of glycerol and free fatty acids in human beings *in vivo*, but to inhibit the lipolytic response towards catecholamines in human adipose tissue *in vitro*. Since no direct effects of prostaglandins on the human fat cell adenylate cyclase have been reported, we studied the effects of various prostaglandins on this key enzyme in hormone activated lipolysis. Adenylate cyclase activity was assayed according to Salomon *et al* (Anal. Biochem. 58: 541, 1974).

Of the prostaglandins tested the E- and F-type hormones caused a dose dependent increase of enzyme activity. Saturating concentrations of PG E1 and PG E2 (each 0.5mM) increased enzyme activity by about 300%. The F-prostaglandins were considerably less effective in activating the enzyme (1.3-1.5-fold stimulation). Prostaglandin A2 (0.05-0.5mM) had no stimulatory effect. This compound, however, was found to be a potent inhibitor of PG E1-induced stimulation. At a PG A2 concentration of 0.1mM the PG E1-

induced increase of enzyme activity was decreased by about 70%. The results suggest that prostaglandins may act as modulators of free fatty acid release in human beings. The actual effects appear to depend on the relative concentrations of different types of prostaglandins.

EFFECTS OF BETA-ADRENERGIC AGENTS UPON THE HUMAN FAT CELL ADENYLATE CYCLASE

H. Kather and B. Simon

Medizinische Universitatsklinik Heidelberg, D-6900 Heidelberg, Germany

Most recently a catecholamine-sensitive adenylate cyclase could be demonstrated in human fat cell ghosts. Direct studies on the action of different adrenergic agents upon the enzyme system can now be performed. We tested, therefore, the effects of beta-adrenergic agonists and antagonists on the enzyme system.

Adenylate cyclase activity was assayed according to Salomon _et al_ (Anal. Biochem. 58: 541, 1974).

Isoproterenol by causing an about 4-5-fold increase of enzyme activity was more potent than epinephrine and norepinephrine (2.5-3.0-fold stimulation). The beta$_2$-adrenergic agonists salbutamol, terbutalin and fenoterol were considerably less effective than the naturally occurring catecholamines (1.2-1.7-fold stimulation).

Beta-blocking agents caused a competitive inhibition of catecholamine stimulation. The order of potency was bupranolol > propranolol > alprenolol > prindolol > methypranol > atenolol. Half maximal inhibition of enzyme activity occurred at 4×10^{-7}M (bupranolol), 7×10^{-7}M (propranolol), 3×10^{-6}M (prindolol), 1×10^{-6}M (alprenolol) and 5×10^{-5}M (methypranol). The concentration of atenolol required to produce half maximal inhibition (1 mM) exceeded that of propranolol by about 3 order of magnitude.

Our results raise the possibility to use the human adenylate cyclase system in estimating the metabolic effects of new beta-adrenergic substances of potential therapeutic values.

EFFECT OF TOCOPHEROL-PYRIDOXINE COMBINATION ON LIPID METABOLISM

N.N. Kipshidze

Research Institute of Therapy, Tbilisi 380059, U.S.S.R.

Intramuscular administration of combination of tocopherol and pyridoxine was studied in patients and experimental animals with cholesterol atherosclerosis. A long-term observation of more than 500 patients with a pronounced lipid metabolism disturbance showed that an intramuscular administration of the suggested combination resulted in normalization of lipid metabolism within 15-30 days. Animal experiments using cholesterol atherosclerosis model showed a marked inhibition of atherosclerotic process. Comparison with antilipolytic drugs, such as ateroid and atromid, shows that under the suggested combination normalization of lipid metabolism occurs earlier and persists after the therapy has been discontinued.

ACCELERATION AND ENHANCEMENT OF EXPERIMENTAL ATHEROSCLEROSIS IN RABBITS BY THE ADMINISTRATION OF HIGH DOSES OF ARGININE

A.N. Klimov, S.I. Sonina, G.V. Titova, and V.A. Nagornev

Institute of Experimental Medicine, Leningrad, 197022, U.S.S.R.

One group of rabbits received cholesterol (250 mg/kg of weight, daily) for 90 days. Another group received the same dose of cholesterol for the same period of time and in addition intramuscular administration of arginine hydrochloride in a daily dose of 140 mg/kg of weight for the last 60 days. The extent of the atherosclerotic lesions in the aortas of animals receiving arginine and cholesterol was 84%, whereas in animals receiving only cholesterol it was 43%. The aortas of rabbits which received arginine and cholesterol expressed massive, fused multilayer fibrous plaques containing lipids both within the foam cells and diffusely spread throughout surrounding connective tissue. Cholesterol and arginine concentrations in serum did not differ significantly, but the arginine content of VLDL in animals receiving arginine was two times higher. In addition polyacrilamide gel electrophoresis of VLDL delipidated by TMU revealed more intense bands of arginine-rich apoprotein in this group of rabbits. Although not excluding the possible effect of high concentrations of arginine on permeability of endothelium for lipoproteins or fibrinolysis our data show that the acceleration and enhancement of atherosclerosis in rabbits receiving arginine may be connected with the increased formation of the arginine-rich apoprotein.

EFFECT OF A NOVEL ANTI-LIPIDEMIC OXAZOLE DERIVATIVE ON LIPOPROTEIN PATTERN OF EXPERIMENTAL HYPERLIPIDEMIA

T. Kobayakawa, K. Osuga and H. Yasuda

Research and Development Division, Yoshitomi Pharma. Ind. Ltd., Osaka, Japan

Lipoprotein pattern observed by disc-electrophoresis in normal rats consists mainly of α-lipoprotein and differs from that of humans and monkeys. By feeding 1% cholesterol, 0.2% sodium cholate and 5% olive oil mixed in diet and 0.02% of 6-propyl-2-thiouracil mixed in drinking water, rats developed hyper-β-lipoproteinemia which resembles that of human hyperlipidemia (Type II). Clofibrate was found not effective to reduce serum β-lipoprotein in this model, while it lowered lipid levels in normal rats. A newly synthesized compound, Y-9738 (ethyl 2-p-chlorophenyl-5-ethoxy-4-oxazoleacetate) showed a potent lipid-lowering effect in both normal and hyperlipidemic rats. Y-9738 was 5-10 times more potent than clofibrate in reducing serum cholesterol, triglycerides and phospholipids in normal rats. In the above mentioned model, Y-9738 improved β/α ratio and reduced serum cholesterol and phospholipid levels prophylactically and therapeutically. Similar effect was also observed in rhesus monkeys. The mechanisms of action will be discussed.

STUDIES ON THE COMPLEX FORMATION OF CATECHOLAMINE WITH LECITHIN, WITH SPECIAL REFERENCE TO CONTRACTION OF SMOOTH MUSCLE IN RABBIT AORTAE BY NORADRENALINE

F. Kuzuya and N. Yoshimine

The 3rd Department of Internal Medicine, Nagoya University School of Medicine, Nagoya, Japan

We have reported that adrenaline combines with phospholipid (lecithin) on THE SAISHIN IGAKU 29: 585, 1974, and in the 15th Annual Meeting of Japanese Geriatrics Society in November, 1973, and that in human plasma platelet aggregation was inhibited with incubation of catecholamine and lecithin *in vitro*, while it was induced by catecholamine, in (Jap. Circul. J. 38: 579, 1974). In this paper, authors observed that lecithin combined not only with adrenaline, but also with noradrenaline or dopamine *in vitro*: The radioactivity of ^{14}C-noradrenaline and ^{14}C-dopamine was detected on phospholipid area on thin layer chromatography (Silica-Gel) while no radioactive areas were detected on the others (cholesterol, cholesterol-ester, triglyceride or free fatty acid). Furthermore, we observed that the contraction of smooth muscle in rabbit aortae was inhibited perfectly by preincubation of noradrenaline and lecithin for one hour at 37°C, whereas it occurred in noradrenaline solution. This inhibitory effect of lecithin did not result from destruction of noradrenaline, because the contraction of aortae again occurred in noradrenaline solution incubating for one hour at 37°C. It was concluded that noradrenaline and/or dopamine combined with lecithin *in vitro* as adrenaline did, and that the contraction of smooth muscle in aortae of rabbit induced by noradrenaline was inhibited by preincubation of noradrenaline and lecithin.

LIPIDIC LIVER CHANGES INDUCED BY PERHEXILINE MALEATE

A. Lageron

I.N.S.E.R.M. U 9 - 184, rue du Faubourg Saint-Antoine, Paris XII, France

The histological, histochemical and biochemical studies of 13 livers from 11 subjects treated by perhexiline maleate show numerous changes with various degrees. Hepatocytes are enlarged and filled with lamellar or microvesicular material like Gaucher or Niemann-Pick cells. Steatosis made of triglycerides (red oil, Adams' reaction) is present in many cases; often, nuclei contain invaginated cytoplasm with lipid blots. Some hepatocytes contain free fatty acids (holczinger's reaction) which involve eosinophilic necrosis. Phospholipids (Baker-, O.T.A.N. reactions) are increased in hepatocytes particularly in pericanalicular area. In some livers there are granules whose inner part is formed by triglycerides and outer part by phospholipids. Gangliosides (Dische's reaction) are increased also; in some livers they are located in scattered cytoplasmic vacuoles but, in others they outlined biliary canalicule. This increase is also found by thin layer chromatographic method. Beside lipidic changes these livers present glycogen variations, increase of succino deshydrogenase-, monoamino oxidase activities but β-glucuronidase is deficient. Pexid relations with these complex liver changes are discussed.

PHARMACOKINETICS AND METABOLISM OF BEZAFIBRATE, A NEW LIPID LOWERING DRUG

P.D. Lang, W. Bablok, R. Endele, K. Koch, H. Stork, and H.A.E. Schmidt

Boehringer Mannheim GmbH, 6800 Mannheim 31, and Bethesda Hospital, 4100 Duisburg, West Germany

Bezafibrate in daily doses of 450 to 600 mg has been shown to be more active than standard doses of clofibrate in lowering cholesterol and triglycerides in patients with various types of hyperlipoproteinemia.

The pharmacokinetics and metabolism of bezafibrate were studied in two independent experiments on healthy volunteers with single oral doses of 300 mg, the first using tablets containing unlabelled substance and the second using C_{14}-labelled substance in solution.

With tablets peak levels of bezafibrate were reached within 1.5 to 2.0 hours in the first study on 10 subjects. The half-life of elimination varied from 1.9 to 3.4 hours (median 2.1 hours). Bezafibrate concentrations were determined by a specific gas liquid chromatographic method.

In the second study on 5 volunteers, 94% of the activity given was recovered within 24 hours in the urine, 49% as bezafibrate, 20% as glucuronide and the rest in the form of metabolites. These results agreed well with those obtained with unlabelled drug, showing 54% of unchanged bezafibrate in the urine. 2% of the activity administered was detected in the feces.

The results indicate almost complete absorption of bezafibrate after oral administration.

THREE HYPOLIPIDEMIC DRUGS INCREASE HEPATIC FATTY ACID OXIDATION 1,000 - 2,000 PERCENT

P.B. Lazarow

The Rockefeller University, New York, New York 10021, U.S.A.

Clofibrate, tibric acid and Wy-14,643 were administered to male rats for one week in ground lab chow at dosages of 0.5, 0.1 and 1.0%, respectively. The livers were homogenized and were assayed for their ability to oxidize palmitoyl-CoA bv two independent methods. The rate of palmitoyl-CoA oxidation was found to be 8 to 12 times faster in the homogenates of the drug-treated animals than in the controls. Multiplication of these values by the increases in liver weight gives rates of palmitoyl-CoA oxidation per total liver that are 11 to 18 times greater in the drug treated animals than in the controls (Lazarow, Science, in press).

Differential and equilibrium density analytical cell fractionation experiments were performed to investigate whether these increases occurred in the mitochondrial system of fatty acid oxidation or in the recently described peroxisomal system (Lazarow and de Duve, Proc. Nat. Acad. Sci. 73: 2043, 1976). A large fraction of the increased activities were found in the peroxisomes.

These results strongly suggest that the mechanism of action of hypolipidemic drugs involves an increase in the peroxisomal system of fatty acid oxidation.

BILIARY LIPID COMPOSITION DURING TREATMENT WITH HYPOLIPIDEMIC DRUGS

B. Leijd, B. Angelin and K. Einarsson

Department of Medicine, Serafimerlasarettet, S-112 83 Stockholm, Sweden

Treatment with hypolipidemic drugs often becomes lifelong. It is therefore of importance to consider possible side effects. Recently it was reported that clofibrate increases the incidence of gallstone disease and accordingly other reports have shown that clofibrate increases the saturation of bile with cholesterol.

The aim of the present study was to compare the effect of two other hypolipidemic drugs on the cholesterol saturation of bile with that of clofibrate.

Methods. Altogether 34 patients with primary hyperlipoproteinemia and functioning gallbladder were studied before and after minimum one month of treatment with clofibrate (2 g/d; n=9), nicotinic acid (3 g/d; n=12) or cholestyramine (12 g/d; n=13). During dietary standardized conditions fasting duodenal bile was collected via a duodenal tube after administration of cholecystokinin in order to get concentrated gallbladder bile. The bile samples were analyzed for the molar composition of cholesterol, bile acids and phospholipids.

Results. Clofibrate increased the saturation of cholesterol (9.0 ± 0.7 to 11.4 ± 1.0 molar%, means$\pm$SEM, $p<0.001$). A slight increase of the bile cholesterol was also noted during nicotinic acid treatment (8.7 ± 0.7 to 9.7 ± 0.9 molar%, $p<0.05$). On the other hand, cholestyramine decreased the level of bile cholesterol (8.8 ± 0.6 to 7.3 ± 0.2 molar%, $p<0.005$).

Conclusion. Nicotinic acid increases the cholesterol saturation of bile whereas cholestyramine treatment results in a less saturated bile. An increased risk to develop gallstone during nicotinic therapy should be considered.

CONTENT OF PLASMA LDL IN NORMAL AND INJURED RABBIT ARTERIES

H. Lengsfeld, P. Brand, H.R. Baumgartner, K. Reber, and M. Vecchi

F. Hoffmann-La Roche & Co. Ltd., Grenzacherstrasse 124, Department F/P III, CH-4002 Basel, Switzerland

LDL in normal and deendothelialized rabbit arteries were determined by immunoelectrophoresis (IE). Selective arterial deendothelialization (DE) was performed by the balloon catheter. Antiserum against normal rabbit LDL was raised in guinea pigs. Experiment A: In normal arteries no LDL were found by IE. Three hours to 5 days after DE 1 mg fresh artery contained an LDL plasma volume of 0.06 μl. Concomitantly to formation of a neointima (NI) arterial LDL content increased 3 x. Maximum: 2-4 weeks after DE. Six months after DE arterial LDL were absent, no NI regression was observed. Experiment B: NI thickness 21 days after DE did not differ in normal and cholesterol fed (0.1% for 22 days) rabbits. Plasma and arterial LDL and arterial cholesterol increased severalfold in cholesterol fed rabbits. Conclusion: Normal rabbit arteries do not contain electrophoretically mobile immunoreactive plasma LDL. After DE arterial LDL content varies according to the development of the lesion. After DE NI-formation does not and arterial cholesterol does parallel plasma LDL concentration.

INCREASE OF LIPOPROTEIN LIPASE ACTIVITY IN HUMAN SKELETAL MUSCLE TISSUE AFTER CLOFIBRATE TREATMENT

H. Lithell, J. Boberg, K. Hellsing, G. Lundqvist, and B. Vessby

Department of Geriatrics, University of Uppsala, Uppsala, Sweden

The lipoprotein-lipase activity (LPLA) was determined in tissue from the skeletal muscle of the leg and the subcutaneous, adipose tissue of the abdomen in 14 patients before and after 1 month of clofibrate administration. Clofibrate administration was associated with an average increase of the skeletal-muscle-tissue LPLA of 50% ($p<0.005$). There was a significant correlation between the percentage changes of skeletal-muscle-tissue LPLA and those of the serum-triglyceride (S-TG) concentrations and the K_2-values in an i.v. fat tolerance test during the clofibrate treatment. The adipose-tissue LPLA did not change significantly. One patient with type-I hyperlipoproteinemia HLP had very low values of skeletal-muscle-tissue LPLA and moderately low, adipose-tissue LPLA. In this patient, neither the tissue LPLAs nor the S-TG concentration changed during clofibrate therapy. The fasting S-insulin concentrations decreased significantly during the clofibrate administration and the percentage decrease of the fS-insulin concentration was significantly correlated to the percentage increase of skeletal-muscle LPLA. It is suggested that the lowering of the S-insulin level is a possible mechanism through which the glucagon activity is enhanced, which may produce an increase of the skeletal-muscle-tissue LPLA.

EFFECTS OF COMBINED LIPID LOWERING THERAPY WITH DIET, CLOFIBRATE AND NICERITROL ON CARBOHYDRATE METABOLISM

H. Lithell, B. Vessby, J. Boberg and K. Hellsing

Department of Geriatrics, University of Uppsala, Uppsala, Sweden

One hundred six patients with atherosclerotic cardiovascular disease were treated during six months. During the first two months only diet was prescribed. During the ensuing two months either clofibrate (2 g daily) or niceritrol (3 g daily) was added in a randomized order. During the last two months the second drug was added. Clofibrate was well tolerated. Thirty-seven percent of the patients took less than 3 g daily of niceritrol because of side effects.

When added to diet clofibrate caused an increase of the K-value at intravenous glucose tolerance test (IVGTT) by 27% ($p<0.001$) from 1.30 to 1.65. After addition of niceritrol the K-value decreased again to 1.23 ($p<0.001$). When niceritrol was added to diet only, the K-value decreased by 28% ($p<0.001$) from 1.36 to 0.98 which after addition of clofibrate increased to 1.29 ($p<0.001$).

Fasting blood glucose concentrations (fB-glucose), fasting serum insulin concentrations and the late serum insulin response to intravenous glucose decreased significantly by clofibrate and was increased by niceritrol.

Thus, because of the opposite effects of the two drugs no significant changes were found between the mean values before and after the combined therapy regarding fB-glucose, serum insulin concentrations or K-value at the IVGTT.

THE THERAPEUTIC EFFECT OF CARNITINE ON HYPERLIPEMIA

M. Maebashi, N. Kawamura, M. Sato and A. Imamura

The Second Department of Internal Medicine, Tohoku University School of Medicine, Sendai 980, Japan

On the basis of the observations that carnitine is essential for the oxidation of long-chain fatty acids and that its serum content or urinary excretion correlates inversely with serum triglycerides concentration, the therapeutic effect of carnitine was expected in hyperlipemic patients with types IIa, IIb, III and IV. After oral administration of DL-carnitine chloride, 900 mg/day, for 8 weeks, serum triglyceride concentration was reduced by 42.4%, while total cholesterol concentration showed no significant change. Intravenous infusion of carnitine showed the same effects. The contributory effects were more marked in the patients receiving a newly synthesized carnitine-nicotinic acid complex (nicotinoylcarnitine ethylester chloride, Tanabe Seiyaku). The administration of the drug, 600 mg/day, showed rapid and significant decreases in serum lipid concentrations, 43.2% in triglycerides, 23.3% in total cholesterol and 22.8% in β-lipoprotein. The prolonged administration of the drug kept the serum lipid concentrations lower than the starting values without any side effect. The drug also showed significant lipemia-improving effects in animals. The results suggest that carnitine and its complex are of value in the therapy of certain types of hyperlipemia.

EFFECT OF PLANT GLYCOSIDES ON INTESTINAL ABSORPTION OF CHOLESTEROL

M.R. Malinow, P. McLaughlin, C. Stafford, G.O. Kohler, and A.L. Livingston

Oregon Regional Primate Research Center, Beaverton, Oregon 97005, U.S.A.

Intestinal absorption of cholesterol (C) was studied in rats receiving 2 mg of [^{14}C-4]-C intragastrically and [1,2]-^{3}H-C intravenously. Labeled neutral sterols excreted the ensuing 72 hr were measured and intestinal absorption was calculated from the difference between ingested and excreted sterols. Experimental animals received saponins (S) from the following sources: alfalfa root (AR), alfalfa tops (AT), ladino clover (LC), yucca plant (YP) and foxglove (digitonin, D). S were tested before and after mild acid hydrolysis. Nonhydrolyzed ATS and D decreased cholesterol intestinal absorption. Hydrolysis enhanced the inhibition of cholesterol absorption of ARS and ATS and decreased the activity of D. YPS and LCS - with and without hydrolysis - did not modify cholesterol absorption.

CHENIC ACID, URSIC ACID AND HYPERLIPIDEMIA

E. Marmo, C. Vacca, L. Giordano, A. Schettino, R. Petrarca, and F. Del Vecchio

II Chair of Pharmacology, I Faculty of Medicine, University of Naples, 80121 Naples, Italy

In animals chenic acid and ursic acid presented significant hypolipidemic properties in various forms of hyperdislipidemias (hyperdislipidemia by Triton, by margarine, by diet rich in cholesterol, by olive oil, by cholestane-3 beta, 5 alpha, 6 beta-triol and by ethanol). Comparative activities with dehydrocholic acid, nicotinic acid, tibric acid, clofibrate, clofibrinic acid, clofinol, and beta-sitosterol are also presented.

PLATELET ADHESION - AN INITIAL EVENT IN ATHEROGENESIS?

M. Marshall, H. Hess and J.F.B. de Quiros

Med. Poliklinik der Universitat, Angiologie, D-8000 Munchen 2, West Germany

Some time ago we showed by scanning electron microscopy mainly on rabbits that local irritation with ice or epinephrine as well as cholesterol rich diets always lead to pronounced adhesions of platelets in viscous metamorphosis to the intact appearing arterial endothelium. In recent experiments on minipigs we could demonstrate that beside the irritations mentioned above, cigarette smoke, carbon monoxide inhalation, hypertension and diabetes mellitus lead to similar typical platelet adhesions. Simultaneously in some of these experiments an increased tendency of platelets to aggregate was found. Continued application of these "risk factors" often produced a distinct intimal thickening. In rabbits the continuation of cholesterol feeding for six weeks had caused a progression from the simple platelet adhesions to mixed microparietal thrombi.

Our results are compatible with the hypothesis that a disturbed interaction between flowing blood and arterial wall is a most important mechanism also in the early atherogenesis. In this interaction the adhesion of platelets to the endothelium seems to play a key role.

LONG-TERM COLESTIPOL THERAPY IN DIET-RESISTANT TYPE II HYPERLIPOPROTENEMIA (HLP)

M.A. Mishkel and S.M. Crowther

H.G.H.-McMaster Lipid Research Clinic, Hamilton, Ontario, Canada

Colestipol, a bile acid sequestering resin was an effective hypocholesterolemic agent in 51 diet-resistant patients with Type II HLP. The results in 23 patients followed for 2 years, including 9 followed for 3 years, are given. 15-30 g/day was well accepted, the average drug compliance being above 90%. Initial bloating and constipation were common, but were severe in only 2 of 51 patients. The 9 long-term "medium" cholesterol Group A had a mean ±S.D. pretreatment cholesterol of 279.7±14.0; at 2 years, 228.1±22.0; at 3 years, 230.4±32.6 mg/dl. The 14 long-term "high" cholesterol Group B had a pretreatment cholesterol of 384.6±79.7; at 2 years, 288.8±39.8; at 2-1/2 years, 308.7±47.4 mg/dl. For Groups A and B, the 2 year cholesterol levels were 18.4% and 24.9% below baseline, respectively. Changes in weight status, triglyceride levels, hematological and non-lipid biochemical parameters (particularly uric acid, calcium, phosphorus) were not significant. Colestipol was effective in diet-resistant Types IIA and B HLP, familial and non-familial, with and without xanthomas. Only 3 of 51 patients showed a cholesterol decrease $< 15\%$.

DIFFERENT SYNTHESIS OF LIPOPROTEINS IN NORMAL AND CHOLESTEROL-FED RABBITS

D. Moltoni, M.R. Lovati, M. Marinovich, A. Catapano, G. C. Ghiselli, and C.R. Sirtori

Center E. Grossi Paoletti for the Study of Metabolic Diseases and Hyperlipidemias, University of Milan, Milan, Italy

Synthesis and interrelationship between plasma lipoproteins were determined in normal (N) and cholesterol-fed (HC) rabbits. Two groups of six animals, after 24 hrs of fast, were injected i.v. with an ^{3}H-labelled amino acid mixture. Plasma samples were drawn at intervals during the 8 hrs after injection, and the different lipoprotein fractions were separated by sequential ultracentrifugation.

Radioactivity incorporation into lipoproteins followed a strikingly different pattern in the two groups of rabbits. In particular, in N the earlier radioactivity peak was found in VLDL, similarly to humans and rats, followed by IDL, LDL and HDL peaks, suggesting a precursor-product relationship between VLDL and the other lipoproteins. Furthermore, the highest radioactivity was found in IDL at all successive intervals.

In HC rabbits, VLDL and IDL incorporated the bulk of the injected radioactivity, whereas only a minor fraction of radioactivity was incorporated in LDL and HDL. There was no obvious indication of a metabolic relationship of VLDL with IDL and the other lipoprotein fractions. The consistently higher radioactivity found in the VLDL fraction of HC rabbits suggests a reduced metabolic conversion to IDL in these animals, and confirms previous findings from our laboratory (Atherosclerosis 23: 73, 1976), indicating accumulation of these atherogenic fractions in HC rabbits.

Preliminary findings from rabbits treated with cholesterol-metformin will also be presented.

ABNORMAL LOW-DENSITY LIPOPROTEINS IN JUVENILE FAMILIAL HYPERCHOLESTEROLEMIA-EFFECTS OF LIPID-LOWERING RESIN THERAPY ON CONCENTRATION AND COMPOSITION

R. Mordasini, G. Schlierf, C.C. Heuck, P. Oster, B. Schellenberg, and H. Twelsick

Medizinische Universitatsklinik Heidelberg , 6900 Heidelberg, West Germany

In 20 children and adolescents with familial Type II hyperlipoproteinemia, serum lipoproteins were examined before and during treatment with lipid-lowering resins. The composition of LDL was compared to that of healthy siblings. The patients were given cholestyramine (0.6 g/kg body weight) and colestipol (0.5 g/kg body weight) in a cross-over study for 8 weeks each, after they had been under dietary treatment for at least 12 months. In 6 children, drug treatment had to be interrupted due to side-effects. The most common complaints were gastrointestinal discomfort and constipation.

Cholesterol, triglycerides and phospholipids were measured in whole serum and in isolated lipoprotein fractions after ultracentrifugation. Apo-B- was determined by radial immunodiffusion.

Mean cholesterol concentration in patients before drug therapy was 290 mg/100 ml, LDL-cholesterol was 230 mg/100 ml. HDL-cholesterol levels were significantly lower than in healthy children ($p<0.0005$). Apo-B was markedly increased in the patients. The Apo-B:cholesterol ratio in whole serum and in the LDL fraction was identical in the patients and in the controls. The LDL triglyceride:Apo B ratio, however, was 50% lower in the patients ($p<0.0005$).

The decreases of total- and LDL-cholesterol and Apo-B were similar with colestipol and cholestyramine (25-30%). HDL-cholesterol and LDL-triglyceride concentrations remained abnormally low. Thus, resin therapy did not normalize LDL composition in juvenile type II-hyperlipoproteinemia.

THE EFFECT OF HYPOLIPIDEMIC DRUGS ON CONCENTRATIONS OF SERUM LIPOPROTEINS IN THE RAT

K. Muller

Research Department, Pharmaceuticals Division, CIBA-GEIGY Limited, CH-4002 Basel, Switzerland

The lipoprotein spectrum differs significantly in the rat and in man. Testing hypolipidemic drugs in the rat is therefore of questionable value as long as total serum cholesterol is taken as the parameter. We have therefore investigated whether different hypolipidemic drugs induce similar changes in lipoprotein concentrations in rats to those observed in man.

Male rats were treated for 7 days with one of the following compounds: nicotinic acid, cholestyramine, L-thyroxine, clofibrate, nafenopin, tibric acid. Serum lipoproteins were separated by ultracentrifugation and analyzed for cholesterol, triglycerides, phospholipids and protein.

The shifts in VLDL-, LDL- and HDL-cholesterol caused by nicotinic acid, L-thyroxine, tibric acid were comparable in the rat and in man; in both species cholestyramine affected LDL-cholesterol and HDL-cholesterol and clofibrate VLDL-and LDL-cholesterol in a similar way.

In the rat, in contrast to man, VLDL-cholesterol was decreased by cholestyramine and HDL-cholesterol by clofibrate. Further changes will be discussed.

It is concluded that many hypolipidemic drugs produce similar changes in the lipoproteins of rat and man. The rat is thus an acceptable test animal, provided lipoprotein concentrations are used as parameters.

EFFECT OF CLOFIBRATE ON GLUCOSE, INDIVIDUAL FFA AND FIBRINOGEN IN HYPERTRIGLYCERIDEMIC SUBJECTS

H. Nakamura and M. Nagano

Department of Medicine, Tokyo Jikeikai Medical College, Aoto Hospital, Katsushika, Tokyo, Japan

Clofibrate has been known to improve glucose and lipid abnormality in diabetic patients. The present study was conducted to determine the change of the glucose, and fibrinogen level in the hypertriglyceridemic subjects with or without clofibrate. FFA were determined by GLC in order to avoid the interference on colorimetry by the drug during 50g oral glucose tolerance test.

The drug (1.5g daily for 4-5 weeks) reduced FFA and fibrinogen level. FFA and glucose responses to glucose ingestion prior to the drug administration were delayed without the drug, but their responses tended to improve on the drug.

Analysis of individual FFA showed the consistent decrease in every fatty acid on the drug. Percentage decrease in oleic acid responded to glucose ingestion was prominent. This decrement seemed to be related to the decrease in fibrinogen.

This study may suggest the possible metabolic link of the particular FFA with fibrinogen.

THE LDL-LOWERING EFFECT OF CHOLESTYRAMINE (QUESTRAN) GIVEN TWICE DAILY IN TYPE II HYPERLIPOPROTEINEMIA

A.G. Olsson

King Gustaf V Research Institute, Karolinska Hospital, S-104 01 Stockholm, Sweden

Because of practical problems of taking cholestyramine (Questran) 4 times daily as recommended by the manufacturer, the drug was given 8 g twice daily in 18 subjects with primary, asymptomatic type II hyperlipoproteinemia. Lipoprotein concentrations were estimated before and after 4 and 24 weeks treatment. Results: (mmol/l)

	VLDL		LDL		HDL		Total	
	TG	CHOL	TG	CHOL	TG	CHOL	TG	CHOL
Before	0.80	0.67	0.77	6.45	0.18	1.48	1.74	8.55
After 24 weeks	0.82	0.63	0.47***	4.87***	0.19	1.66**	1.53	7.20**

TG=triglycerides, CHOL=cholesterol, **=p<0.01, ***=p<0.001

The LDL cholesterol decrease was of the same magnitude as reported on 4g 4 times daily.

Constipation was noted in 2/3 of the patients after 4 weeks treatment, in about 1/4 after 24 weeks treatment (=4 dose regimen).

Conclusion: As the results are comparable to those in other studies where the same daily dose was given 3 or 4 times, the two dose regimen could probably be a satisfactory alternative.

INCREASE IN LOW AND HIGH DENSITY LIPOPROTEINS DURING TREATMENT OF TYPE IV HYPERLIPOPROTEINEMIA

A.G. Olsson, D. Ballantyne and L.A. Carlson

King Gustaf V Research Institute, Karolinska Hospital, S-104 01 Stockholm, Sweden

The rise in low (LDL) and high (HDL) density lipoprotein (LP) cholesterol known to occur during treatment of type IV hyperlipoproteinemia was studied in 30 type IV patients in a metabolic ward to relate LP changes to time. After 5 days on an isocaloric diet (P/S ratio 1.5/1) 1.5 g clofibrate or 1.5 g clofibrate + 0.025 g pyridyl carbinol or 4.5 g nicotinic acid were given daily. As no differences were seen in the effects of the drugs the results were pooled (Table). Very low density LP (VLDL) decreased on diet and diet + drug, LDL increased. The effects on VLDL and LDL occurred at the same time, reached maximum after 3 days on drug and remained throughout the study indicating a close metabolic relation. HDL was unaffected by the dietary treatment and did not rise until 7 days on drug, continued to rise until 23 days and then remained constant suggesting another underlying mechanism.

Day	0	5	8	12	70
Treatment	Pre-	Diet	Diet + Drug		
VLDL	2.46 ±0.28	1.67*** ±0.16	0.91*** ±0.09	0.95*** ±0.09	1.37*** ±0.21
LDL	3.68 ±0.19	3.99* ±0.18	4.22*** ±0.15	3.81 ±0.17	4.27* ±0.23
HDL	0.73 ±0.04	0.73 ±0.03	0.76 ±0.04	0.87** ±0.04	1.10*** ±0.06

Cholesterol,mmol/l.*, **, ***: p<.05, .01, .001

DOSE-RESPONSE STUDY OF BEZAFIBRATE (BM 15.075) ON SERUM LIPOPROTEIN CONCENTRATIONS IN HYPERLIPOPROTEINEMIA

A.G. Olsson, S. Rossner, G. Walldius, L.A. Carlson and P.D. Lang

King Gustaf V Research Institute, Karolinska Hospital, S-104 01 Stockholm, Sweden

In a previous study we showed that Bezafibrate (600 mg daily) is 20% more effective than clofibrate in reducing VLDL concentrations in hyperlipidemia. It also decreases elevated LDL concentrations. To establish optimal dose of Bezafibrate the serum lipoprotein lowering effect at doses 450, 900 and 1350 mg daily was studied in 20 patients with different types of hyperlipoproteinemia. After 1 month on placebo and 2 months on each dose lipoprotein concentrations were measured.

Results: (mmol/l)

	VLDL		LDL		HDL	
	TG	CHOL	TG	CHOL	TG	CHOL
Placebo	2.77	1.40	0.67	4.40	0.21	1.11
450 mg daily	1.31*	0.75*	0.48*	4.20	0.16*	1.45*

TG=triglycerides, CHOL=cholesterol, *=$p<0.05$

LDL cholesterol was the only lipoprotein that decreased further on 900 mg daily to 3.99 mmol/l ($p<0.05$).

No further mean changes of lipoprotein concentrations occurred at 1350 mg.

Subjective and biochemical side effects were few, tolerable and reversible.

Conclusion: Optimal effect of Bezafibrate is reached at the dose 450 mg daily for all lipoproteins but LDL cholesterol, for which it was 900 mg.

DIURNAL LIPID AND LIPOPROTEIN PROFILES WITH BEZAFIBRATE AND CLOFIBRATE

P. Oster, G. Schlierf, R. Mordasini, C.C. Heuck, H. Raetzer, and B. Schellenberg

Medizinische Universitatsklinik Heidelberg, D-6900 Heidelberg, West Germany

Fasting and as well postprandial lipids appear to be atherogenic. While a number of studies have been performed on diurnal effects of different diets, such information is lacking with regard to most lipid lowering drugs. We therefore tested clofibrate (halflife 15 hr) and the new compound bezafibrate (halflife 2 hr) in 30 hypertriglyceridemic patients on our metabolic ward; they received in randomized order either placebo (n=10), clofibrate (3 x 0.5 g/d) or bezafibrate (3 x 200 mg/d) for 10 days; body weight was kept stable with a fat modified diet. On the 10th day formula diet was given (35% fat, 15% prot., 50% CH) and blood was drawn 8 times till the next morning. Triglycerides, cholesterol, FFA, phosphatides and lipoproteins by means of ultracentrifugation were analyzed, drug intake was controlled by gas chromatography (as well in the 10 day period).

Despite low plasma levels during the night the lipid lowering effect of bezafibrate lasted 24 hours. While fasting lipid levels were similar after clofibrate and bezafibrate, 24 hour plasma triglycerides were lowest with bezafibrate. Only minor differences were noted on lipoprotein triglyceride and cholesterol content. Low fasting lipid values stay low postprandially under the influence of bezafibrate and clofibrate.

ENZYME KINETICS OF PURIFIED LIPASES FROM HUMAN POST-HEPARIN PLASMA AND BOVINE MILK

A.-M. Ostlund-Lindqvist and J. Boberg

Department of Medical and Physiological Chemistry, Uppsala University, BMC, S-751 23 Uppsala, Sweden

Salt resistant triglyceride lipase (SRL) and lipoprotein lipase (LPL) from human post-heparin plasma have been purified by affinity chromatography on one conventional and one modified heparin-Sepharose, which removed most of the plasma antithrombin. Affinity chromatography on anti-human antithrombin-Sepharose removed the rest of the antithrombin.

The enzyme preparations of SRL and LPL had specific activities of 120 and 400 micromoles fatty acids released per minute and mg of protein.

The enzyme kinetics of these enzyme preparations were compared with the kinetics of purified bovine milk LPL which had a specific activity of 600 micromoles fatty acids released per minute and mg of protein. A labelled soybean oil/phospholipid emulsion and purified apolipoprotein-C II was used. The enzyme kinetics for purified LPL from human post-heparin plasma and from bovine milk behaved in a similar way. Different amounts of clofibrate added to the assay system were tested *in vitro*. A slight increase of activity was found with high concentrations of clofibrate.

SITOSTEROL REVISITED

O.J. Pollak

9 Kings Highway, Dover, Delaware 19901, U.S.A.

Sitosterol has been used as cholesterol-depressant from 1952-1964. It fell into disuse because of a few erroneous reports resulting from ill-conceived studies, the broad acceptance of PUFA, and the introduction of hypocholesterolemic drugs. The argument that large doses of sitosterol are needed is wrong. High purity β-sitosterol powder taken with meals is effective in reasonably small doses. The need for continuous medication is common to all drugs or diets which act on the principle of interference with cholesterol absorption from the intestinal lumen. Objections that the response to sitosterol is unpredictable or too mild were based on results which had been averaged for unselected subjects, without consideration of the height of plasma cholesterol or the etiology of hypercholesterolemia. The results are quite predictable and acceptable for subjects with alimentary hypercholesterolemia. They also are comparable to results with drugs and diets used for this type of patient. Sitosterol is free of contraindications and adverse reactions of pharmaceuticals. It is not a drug but a natural substance present in small amounts in seed oils, fruits and vegetables. Reliable information about its low absorbability and mode of action, and comparison with diets and drugs led to renewed interest in β-sitosterol for clinical use.

EFFECTS OF NICOCLONATE, A NEW NICOTINIC ACID DERIVATIVE, ON PLASMA LIPIDS IN RATS

M. Prosdocimi, L. Caparrotta, P. Dorigo, R.M. Gaion and G. Fassina

Department of Pharmacology, University of Padua, Padua, Italy

Nicoclonate is an ester of nicotinic acid with p-chlorophenylisopropylcarbinol. It has been reported that this drug exerts hypolipidemic effect both in humans and animals. We have tested its action in rats both in basal conditions and after noradrenaline injection. The drug was given by gastric catheter (470 mg/kg or 940 mg/kg). The effect on blood lipids (total esterified fatty acids (TEFA); cholesterol; free fatty acids (FFA); glycerol) and blood glucose was controlled for 8 hours. As a comparison experiments were done with nicotinic acid in the same experimental conditions. Nicoclonate was able to lower basal TEFA until 8 hours after administration and cholesterol until 6 hours after administration.

Nicotinic acid has no effect on TEFA and cholesterol.

Noradrenaline was always given i.p. 30 minutes before sacrifice. Nicoclonate was able to antagonize the action of noradrenaline on FFA and glycerol blood levels. The maximum inhibitory effect (65 to 70%) was evident between the 4th and the 6th hour after administration of nicoclonate.

The hyperglycemic effect of noradrenaline was potentiated by nicoclonate which had been administered an hour before sacrifice. But after a longer period (6 and 8 hours) nicoclonate antagonized this effect of the catecholamine.

The clear antagonistic activity on noradrenaline-induced increase in FFA and glycerol levels and the long duration of the effect on TEFA and cholesterol levels in basal conditions suggests that nicoclonate could be studied as a future drug for the treatment of human dislipidemia.

THE EFFECT OF NICOTINIC ACID BOUND TO A POLYMER ON EXPERIMENTAL HYPERLIPEMIA

L. Puglisi, F. Maggi, R. Paoletti, P. Ferruti* and M.C. Tanzi

Institute of Pharmacology and Pharmacognosy, University of Milan, 20129, Milan; *Institute of Chemistry, University of Naples, 80134 Naples, Italy

The action of the hypolipemic drug nicotinic acid covalently bound to a high molecular weight polysaccharide matrix (P61) by ester bonds has been studied in rats and rabbits. P61 is effective in lowering plasma FFA when given by oral route, for a prolonged time (13 hrs) in comparison to an equal dose of free nicotinic acid (2 hrs). Since the plasma levels of nicotinic acid are very low after the administration of the polymer and remain constant up to 15 hrs, no rebound phenomenon was observed in FFA mobilization. Furthermore no cutaneous vasodilation has been observed in the auricle of the guinea pig up to 120 min whereas free nicotinic acid shows this side effect already at 20 min with the peak at 50 min. P61 is also effective in decreasing plasma cholesterol concentration in cholesterol-fed rats. The hypocholesterolemic activity of the macromolecular adduct appears to be more or at least equal to that of free nicotinic acid. The relationship between plasma cholesterol levels and extent of aortic lipid infiltration in cholesterol-fed rabbits will be discussed as well as the protective effects of the free and the bound nicotinic acid against dietary induced atherogenesis.

REGULATION OF HMG CoA REDUCTASE BY ATP AND NORADRENALINE

R. Ramasarma and R. George

Department of Biochemistry, Indian Institute of Science, Bangalore 560 012, India

The activity of hepatic microsomal 3-hydroxy-3-methyl glutaryl (HMG) CoA reductase is stimulated on treatment of rats with noradrenaline or agents that increase its intracellular concentration such as pargyline and 3,4-dihydroxy-phenyl serine. Noradrenaline-stimulated activity is insensitive to adrenergic blocking agents indicating intrahepatocyte action. The activity of the enzyme, depressed under conditions of starvation and cholesterol feeding, was partially restored on treatment of rats with ATP and other adenosine compounds and fully on simultaneous treatment with ATP and noradrenaline. The results with the neurotransmittor compounds and blocking agents suggested that the enzyme is under neuronal regulation with a possible interplay of adrenergic and purinergic systems.

EFFECTS OF PROCETOFENE (LIPANTHYL) ON SERUM LIPOPROTEINS IN HUMAN HYPER-LIPOPROTEINEMIA

S. Rossner and L. Oro

Departments of Internal Medicine, Karolinska Hospital and Ersta Hospital, and King Gustaf V Research Institute, Stockholm, Sweden

Serum lipids and lipoproteins were determined in 39 patients with IIa, IIb, III and IV hyperlipoproteinemia. After a screening period treatment was given with placebo and with 200, 300 and 400 mg procetofene (Lipanthyl). Each treatment period lasted one month. The drug was very well tolerated. The overall reduction of total TG was 54% and of cholesterol 24% on the 400 mg dose. In all types there was a dose-response effect for both TG and cholesterol irrespective of the lipoprotein type. In type IV 400 mg procetofene reduced both VLDL-TG and-cholesterol by 25%. In type IIa + IIb procetofene reduced LDL-cholesterol by 17%. HDL cholesterol did not fall in any group or at any dosage, but tended to increase. After treatment with 400 mg procetofene, 5 patients have been directly shifted to 2 g clofibrate daily. In these subjects total TG increased by 22% and total cholesterol by 15% compared to the last procetofene period. The results suggest that procetofene may be a useful drug in the treatment of hyperlipoproteinemia and exerts its lipid lowering effects mainly in VLDL and LDL.

EVALUATION OF PROCETOFEN HYPOLIPIDEMIC ACTIVITY AND TOLERANCE

J. Rouffy and B. Chanu

Centre de Recherche et d'etude des facteurs metaboliques de l'atherosclerose, Universite Paris VII C.H.U. Hopital St. Louis, 75010 Paris, France

Four hundred patients with essential atherogenous hyperlipoproteinemia resistant to dietetic regimens were treated by Procetofen at a dose of 200 to 400 mg/day. The treatment lasted from one to four years.

Procetofen induced a mean decrease of cholesterolemia, by 23% in types IIa and IIb, and of triglyceridemia by 35% in types IIb and IV. The hypolipidemic effect is proportionally related to the dose administered and no therapeutic escapes were observed.

Clinically, the hypolipidemic effect of Procetofen coincided with a stabilization and often with a regression of the extravascular lipid deposits (xanthelasma, tuberous and tendinous xanthoma) quantitatively estimated with repeated measurements.

The tolerance of the drug was excellent, with no observed side-effects on hepatic and hemopoietic functions. A slight increase in blood urea and creatinine levels was observed in some patients, but found to be reversible when treatment was withdrawn.

COMPARATIVE STUDY OF THE INHIBITORY EFFECTS OF CLOFIBRATE AND TIADENOL ON THE HEPATIC AND INTESTINAL BIOSYNTHESIS OF THE CHOLESTEROL IN THE RAT AND HAMSTER

F. Rousselet, G. Fredj* and M. Clenet*

Faculte de Pharmacie, 75006 Paris; *Centre de Recherches L. Lafon
BP 44, 94701 Maisons-Alfort, France

Hepatic biosynthesis of cholesterol from acetate 2-^{14}C was decreased in the rat and golden hamster under the effects of treatment with two hypolipidemic agents completely different from a chemical standpoint, clofibrate and tiadenol.

There was also a decrease in the biosynthesis of intestinal cholesterol under the same conditions.

A similar effect was seen _in vitro_, using homogenates of the livers of animals treated with these drugs.

By contrast, the utilization of mevalonate 2-^{14}C in the synthesis of cholesterol was not significantly altered under the influence of tiadenol, the inhibitory action of which is thus, situated during the first stages of the biosynthesis of cholesterol.

The substance has an action parallel to that of clofibrate with a degree which was found to be significantly greater.

COMPARISON OF THE EFFECTS OF CLOFIBRATE AND TIADENOL ON BILIARY AND FECAL EXCRETION OF CHOLESTEROL AND ITS METABOLITES IN THE RAT

F. Rousselet, G. Fredj* and M. Clenet*

Faculte de Pharmacie, 75006 Paris; *Centre de Recherches L.Lafon,
BP 44, 94701 Maisons-Alfort, France

Tiadenol, a new hypolipidemic drug, with an original structure decreases the blood concentration of cholesterol in the rat and in man. It was felt to be useful to compare its various types of activity with those of clofibrate.

The experiments reported here were aimed at demonstrating the mechanism of excretion of cholesterol in the bile and feces under the influence of treatment with clofibrate and tiadenol.

Initially, the biliary excretion of cholesterol ^{3}H was studied, followed by a study of fecal excretion.

In the three types of experiments, it was found that: a) bile output was increased under the influence of both forms of treatment. b) biliary output of radioactivity was increased under the influence of both drugs. This increase was more marked with treatment using clofibrate.

Fecal radioactivity was increased under the influence of both forms of treatment, this being more marked in the rats treated with tiadenol than in those receiving clofibrate.

The percentage of cholesterol metabolites in relation to total radioactivity was significantly greater under the influence of tiadenol than clofibrate.

Clofibrate tended to result in the excretion of more cholesterol in the non-broken down form than did tiadenol.

INHIBITION OF ARTERIAL CHOLESTEROL UPTAKE BY 7-KETOCHOLESTEROL

J.S.M. Sarma and R.J. Bing

Huntington Memorial Hospital, Hungtington Institute of Applied Medical Research, and University of Southern California, Pasadena, California 91105, U.S.A.

The cholesterol uptake by isolated arterial preparations from humans, pigs and rabbits, perfused with isologous plasma was inhibited significantly by an average of 90% in the presence of 7-ketocholesterol (700 nmoles/ml). Similar inhibition was demonstrated in the case of pig coronary arteries, perfused with a solution of either high or low density lipoproteins containing 7-ketocholesterol. Cholesterol uptake by rabbit aortas *in vivo* was only slightly inhibited, following multiple intravenous injections of 7-ketocholesterol, solubilized by sodium glycocholate. The injected 7-ketocholesterol was cleared rapidly from the animal's blood, with a maximal attainable plasma level of about 25 nmoles/ml. About 75% of the total blood 7-ketocholesterol was present in the erythrocytes. Using 7-keto-(4-^{14}C)-cholesterol as a tracer, it was shown that the steroid was biotransformed by the liver into a polar form, which was excreted mainly through the bile. Injections of 7-ketocholesterol into hepatectomized rabbits resulted in higher plasma levels (70 nmoles/ml) of the steroid, but no significant inhibition of aortic cholesterol uptake could be demonstrated. A competitive process between cholesterol and 7-ketocholesterol has been postulated but awaits confirmation.

EFFECT OF COLESTIPOL (ALONE OR PLUS PROCETOFEN) ON SERUM LIPIDS IN PRIMARY TYPE II HYPERLIPOPROTEINEMIAS

J.P. Sauvanet, L. Mejean, E. Wulfert, P. Drouin, and G. Debry

Departement de Nutrition, Universite de Nancy I, 54037 Nancy Cedex France

The lipid lowering effect of Colestipol given either alone or in association with Procetofen was studied in 55 patients affected by primary HLP type II (IIa, n=28; IIb, n=27). The methodology was as follows: Group I (n=22) was given diet for the first 3 months and diet + colestopol (15-30 g daily) for the next 9 months. Group 2 (n=33) was given diet for 3 months, diet + Procetofen (400 mg daily) for at least the following 3 months and diet + Procetofen + Colestipol for the last 9 months. Mean base-line levels before Colestipol therapy were:

	Group 1	Diet	Group 2	Diet	Diet + Procetofen
IIa	TC	4.02± 0.32	TC	4.32± 0.13	3.56± 0.10
	TG	1.02± 0.08	TG	1.18± 0.06	0.84+ 0.04
IIb	TC	3.99± 0.19	TC	4.16± 0.24	3.57± 0.18
	TG	1.72± 0.19	TG	2.68± 0.38	1.50± 0.18

The additional cholesterol lowering effect observed when Colestipol therapy was instituted was: Group 1: 11-18% (IIa), 20-23% (IIb), Group 2: 10-15% (IIa), 17-20% (IIb). Colestipol therapy did not affect the level of TG significantly. Colestipol tolerance was assessed according to standard clinical and biochemical methods. A special survey of cirulating levels of vitamins (A-B_{12}), folic acid, calcium, phosphorus and iron is reported. Plasma levels of Procetofen were controlled routinely during the trial. It could be demonstrated that Colestipol did not affect the bioavailability of this drug. These results demonstrate that Colestipol is effective in lowering TC and that Colestipol therapy did not affect serum TG significantly. Plasma levels of Procetofen were controlled routinely. No effect on blood levels could be demonstrated when Colestipol therapy was instituted. In conclusion, Colestipol is effective in lowering TC and the association of Colestipol + Procetofen appears to be very potent in the treatment of severe type of HLP (type II).

COMBINATION OF CHOLESTYRAMINE OR NEOMYCIN WITH EITHER CLOFIBRATE OR PENTAERYTRITOLTETRANICOTINATE IN THE TREATMENT OF TYPE II HYPERLIPOPROTEINEMIA

R.W.B. Schade, P. Demacker and A. van't Laar

Department of Internal Medicine, St. Radboud Hospital, University of Nijmegen, Nijmegen, The Netherlands

We previously found that cholestyramine (CH) and neomycin (N) are equally effective in the treatment of type II hyperlipoproteinemia (Acta Med. Scand.199:175, 1976). The additional effect of 2 g clofibrate (Cl) or 3 g pentaerytritoltetranicotinate (PETN), each given for 18 weeks, was analyzed in a cross-over study in 28 heterozygous type II patients already treated with CH or N and diet. Cl was tolerated well by all patients. PETN was not tolerated by 13.

Plasma cholesterol on diet alone was 445 ± 76 mg/100 ml (mean ± SD), on therapy with N or CH: 350 ± 64. Addition of Cl caused a further reduction of 10.7 ± 9.8% ($p<0.001$) to 311 ± 59 mg/100 ml. For those who could take PETN during 18 weeks, these data were respectively: 424 ± 56, 360 ± 70 and 323 ± 54 (9.5 ± 7.5%; $p<0.01$).

Lipoprotein isolation studies in another group of patients, treated with N or Cl or the combination of both, showed that N decreased LDL-cholesterol. Cl alone had no effect, but, added to N, it decreased LDL cholesterol. There was no effect on VLDL- or HDL-cholesterol.

It is concluded that the combination of CH or N with Cl is the therapy of choice in severe cases.

THE EFFECTS OF ESTROGEN ADMINISTRATION ON HUMAN LIPOPROTEIN METABOLISM

E.J. Schaefer, R.I. Levy, L.L. Jenkins and H.B. Brewer, Jr.

Molecular Disease Branch, National Heart, Lung, and Blood Institute, National Institutes of Health, Bethesda, Maryland 20014, U.S.A.

Five normal females (age 19-23) were studied for thirty day periods before and during daily administration of 0.1 mg of ethinyl estradiol (E). All subjects were maintained on an isocaloric, 300 mg cholesterol, normal P/S ratio, balanced diet. During E administration, plasma cholesterol and triglyceride levels increased 17% and 85% respectively. Plasma lipoproteins were fractionated into very low density lipoprotein (VLDL), low density lipoprotein (LDL), and high density lipoproteins (HDL_2, 1.063-1.125 g/ml and HDL_3, 1.125-1.21 g/ml). Protein, cholesterol, triglyceride, and phospholipid components of these fractions were quantitated.

E treatment was associated with a 16% increase in VLDL protein and a 75% increase in VLDL triglyceride, as well as a 17% increase in HDL protein and a 39% increase in HDL cholesterol. The major changes in HDL were in the HDL_2 subfraction. No significant changes were noted in low density lipoprotein levels.

VLDL and HDL apoprotein metabolism was studied utilizing autologous radio-iodinated lipoproteins. No significant changes in VLDL apoprotein B or HDL apoprotein A-I and A-II catabolic rate were noted. These studies indicate that E administration results in increased VLDL and HDL levels due to increased synthesis rather than delayed catabolism of these lipoproteins.

EXPERIMENTAL AND CLINICAL STUDIES WITH POLYUNSATURATED LECITHIN

G. Schettler and A.K. Horsch

Medizinische Universitatsklinik, 69 Heidelberg, West Germany

The effect of polyunsaturated lecithin (EPL), namely dilinoleylphosphatidylcholine on serum and aortic lipids in experimental animals and in man is reviewed.

Its influence on lipid metabolism and its serum lipid lowering effect have been shown in many species and in man. The prevention of experimental atherosclerosis has been observed and its regression has been suspected after EPL treatment, but the mechanism of action of this drug is widely unknown. *In vivo* and *in vitro* results suggest an interaction with lecithin-cholesteryl-acyl-transferase to form polyunsaturated cholesterolester that are more readily removed from the tissues, as well as alterations of other enzyme activities. Fatty acid and phospholipid synthesis in the arterial wall is depressed and esterification of cholesterol with saturated fatty acids seems to be decreased.

The relevance of these findings for the known effects of EPL is discussed.

EFFECT OF METFORMIN ON FFA - TRIGLYCERIDE INTERRELATIONS

J. Schonborn, J.G. Wechsler, H. Jaeger, K. Heim and H. Ditschuneit

Department fur Innere Medizin, Univ. of Ulm, 7900 Ulm/Donau, West Germany

Following pretreatment with an isocaloric diet (40% carbohydrate, 40% fat, 20% protein) the metabolism of plasma FFA and of plasma triglycerides was studied in hypertriglyceridemic subjects with maturity onset diabetes mellitus before and after administration of the dimethylbiguanide metformin for 1 week. Concentration and turnover of FFA were significantly reduced after administration of metformin. The reduction of the FFA rate constant indicated a decrease of the FFA clearance mechanisms. Simultaneously, the oxidation of FFA as determined by long-term infusion of 1-^{14}C-palmitate fell as well as the lipid oxidation being determined by indirect calorimetry. These changes were paralleled by a diminished transport of VLDL-triglycerides and a reduced concentration of insulin. Despite the reduced triglyceride transport an increased concentration of plasma triglycerides was observed in a minority of subjects, suggesting a decrease of triglyceride clearance mechanisms. It is suggested that the diminished oxidation and turnover of FFA are the decisive effects in the reduction of the triglyceride transport, while the decreased plasma insulin might reduce the triglyceride clearance.

LONG-TERM TREATMENT OF PATIENTS WITH HYPERLIPOPROTEINEMIA, CORONARY INFARCTION OR ANGINA PECTORIS WITH ETIROXATE

W. Schwartzkopff, H. Hoffmann, J. Njissen, V. Etzel, M. Zschiedrich

Medical Clinic, Free University, 1000 Berlin 19, West Germany

D,L-alpha-methylthyroxine-ethylester (40 mg/day) was administered to 40 patients with type IIa and 13 patients with type IIb hyperlipoproteinemia up to 390 days. Cholesterol decreased in type IIa at 23% or 83 mg/dl in the mean, in type IIb at 18% or 64 mg/dl. The lipid-lowering effect of Etiroxate was also studied in a double-blind cross-over trial in 183 patients with hyperlipoproteinemia. Most of them had a history of coronary infarction or suffered from coronary insufficiency. In comparison to the placebo phase (each period=12 weeks) cholesterol was decreased in 60% of all patients with type IIa or IIb by more than 10%. As regards the frequency of heart complaints, the consumption of nitroglycerol, and the heart rate at rest, there was no statistically significant differences between the placebo and Etiroxate period. Etiroxate did not have any unfavourable cardiac side effect in these patients.

ON THE MECHANISM OF THE LIPOLYTIC ACTION OF PTH IN HUMAN BEINGS

B. Simon and H. Kather

Medizinische Universitatsklinik Heidelberg, D-6900 Heidelberg, Germany

Parathyroid hormone has been shown to promote lipolysis in human adipocytes. A direct action of PTH on human fat cell adenylate cyclase has not yet been reported. We, therefore studied the effects of native bovine PTH and of the synthetic aminoterminal 1-34 fragment on the adenylate cyclase activity of human fat cell ghosts. Enzyme activity was determined according to Salomon _et al_ (Anal. Biochem. 58: 541, 1974).

Saturating concentrations of both hormone preparations (20U/ml) caused a significant increase of enzyme activity by about 200-300%. The guanosine nucleotide analogue GMP (PNP) (0.1mM) produced about a 3-fold enhancement of basal and parathyroid hormone-stimulated enzyme activity.

Activation by PTH was not influenced by β-adrenergic blockade in contrast to stimulation by epinephrine. The PTH-sensitivity of the enzyme system could, however, be selectively blocked by pretreatment of the fat cells with trypsin (1 mg/ml).

The results suggest that the lipolytic action of PTH is mediated via activation of the membrane-bound adenylate cyclase of human adipocytes.

PLASMA EXCHANGE IN THE TREATMENT OF HYPERCHOLESTEROLEMIA

L.A. Simons, J.P. Isbister and J.C. Biggs

Lipid Clinic and Hematology Department, St. Vincent's Hospital, Darlinghurst, NSW, Australia, 2010

Three subjects heterozygous for familial hypercholesterolemia have been treated by repeated plasma exchange using a continuous flow blood cell separator. The patients have attended for 15 exchanges over a 14 month period without significant side effects. Plasma lipids and lipoproteins and endogenous fecal steroid excretion have been studied at critical time points in the treatment. Coronary arteriography has been performed prior to the commencement of treatment and has indicated diffuse atherosclerosis. Each patient has achieved a reduction in plasma cholesterol concentration, (e.g. S.1, 430 reduced to 318 mg/100ml, S.2, 440 to 341 mg/100ml and S.3, 555 to 349 mg/100ml). Metabolic studies confirmed mobilization of tissue cholesterol as a result of plasma exchange but the procedure was limited in usefulness by the compensatory increase in endogenous synthesis of cholesterol which followed. All patients have recently started on drug therapy designed to suppress cholesterol synthesis. Clofibrate was only moderately effective in this role. Nicotinic acid 6 g/day appeared to be very effective in arresting the post-exchange rise in plasma cholesterol concentration. It is concluded that repeated plasma exchange plus drug therapy designed to suppress cholesterol synthesis is very effective in controlling severe hypercholesterolemia. Its effect on coronary atherosclerosis, if any, will be apparent in due course.

ORAL HYPOGLYCEMIC AGENTS: THEIR MODE OF ACTION ON LIPOPROTEIN METABOLISM IN 8 DIABETIC SUBJECTS

H.B. Stahelin, C. Keller, K. Mully, B. Reichlin and W. Berger

Geriatric Clinic, Lipid Laboratory, Department of Internal Medicine, Kantonsspital, 4000 Basel, Switzerland

In diabetes mellitus hyperlipoproteinemias play an important role as risk factor for atherosclerosis. In order to investigate the effect of oral hypoglycemic agents on lipid metabolism we compared in 8 diabetic subjects (mean age 66.8 years) the mode of action of sulfonylureas (SUA), biguanides (BIG), and placebo (PLA) on lipid metabolism. All tests were performed at the end of a three week treatment period. The VLDL turnover was estimated by labeling the apo-VLD *in vivo* with ^{75}Se-selenomethionine with subsequent isolation by prep. ultracentrifugation. In comparing SUA with BIG, the apparent apo-VLD turnover (and frac. turnover) was higher under SUA (54 vs 33 mg/h, $p<0.05$) as well as the plasma cholesterol (219 vs 192 mg/dl, $p<0.05$) and the β-lipoprotein fraction (58% vs 47%, $p<0.005$). Apo-VLD (23 vs 20 mg/dl) and plasma triglycerides remained unchanged (1.9 vs 2.0 mmol/l). Under PLA the apo-VLD turnover was 48 mg/h. The fract. turnover, cholesterol and triglycerides were similar under PLA and BIG. We conclude that SUA increase the *de novo* VLDL-synthesis and enhance the VLDL-catabolism thus increasing cholesterol and LDL-concentration. BIG on the other hand, appear to slow the VLDL synthesis without affecting the peripheral metabolism of VLDL. The observed effects of SUA may help to explain the reported increased incidence of coronary heart disease under SUA treatment.

EFFECT OF LIPANTHYL ON LIPID METABOLISM IN RATS

J.A. Story, S.A. Tepper and D. Kritchevsky

The Wistar Institute of Anatomy and Biology, Philadelphia, Pennsylvania 19104, U.S.A.

Male Wistar rats were fed a stock diet and given daily oral doses of 10 mg/kg of Lipanthyl (Procetofen) in gum tragacanth suspension; 30 mg/kg of Clofibrate (Atromid-S) or vehicle for 10 days. At the end of the feeding period serum and liver lipids, hepatic cholesterol 7α hydroxylase and hepatic lipogenesis were determined. Both drugs were hepatomegalic, increasing liver weight by 29% (Lipanthyl) or 48% (Clofibrate), respectively. The drugs lowered serum cholesterol levels by 11-14%. Liver triglycerides were increased 38% by Lipanthyl and 19% by Clofibrate.

Cholesterol synthesis from sodium 1-^{14}C acetate was inhibited by both drugs; 84% ($p<0.05$) by Lipanthyl and 62% by Clofibrate. Fatty acid synthesis from acetate was inhibited by 44% ($p<0.01$) in rats fed Lipanthyl and by 15% in those fed Clofibrate. Cholesterogenesis from 2-^{14}C mevalonic acid was inhibited (43%) by Lipanthyl ($p<0.05$) but not by Clofibrate. Cholesterol 7α hydroxylase activity was 32% lower than control in livers of rats fed Lipanthyl ($p<0.05$) and 34% lower in those of rats fed Clofibrate.

Lipanthyl at 10 mg/kg is slightly less hepatomegalic than Clofibrate fed at 30 mg/kg. The two compounds have similar effects on serum and liver cholesterol levels of rats. Lipanthyl inhibits hepatic lipid synthesis to a greater extent than Clofibrate.

PROSTAGLANDIN BIOSYNTHESIS IN PIGEON AORTA: DIFFERENCE BETWEEN SPONTANEOUSLY ATHEROSCLEROSIS-SUSCEPTIBLE AND RESISTANT BREEDS

M.T.R. Subbiah

Mayo Clinic, Rochester, Minnesota 55901, U.S.A.

Biosynthesis of prostaglandin E_2 (PGE_2) from 1-C^{14}-arachidonic acid was investigated in the aorta of spontaneously atherosclerosis-susceptible White Carneau pigeons and compared to that of atherosclerosis-resistant Show Racer breed. The PGE_2 formed was identified by converting PGE_2 into prostaglandin B_2 and thin layer chromatography. About 80% of the PGE_2 synthetase activity was located mainly in the microsomal fraction. The conversion was linear up to an hour and showed an optimum pH of 7.4. The formation of PGE_2 in the aorta of young White Carneau pigeons was significantly ($p<0.01$) higher than the age matched Show Racer pigeons (PGE_2 formed [pmole/mg/hr$\pm$SEM]: White Carneau 75.6 $\pm$ 6.0 vs 45.0 $\pm$ 2.3 in Show Racer). In vitro, PGE_2 strongly inhibited the cholesteryl ester hydrolase activity (51.6% inhibition at 4 x 10^{-7} conc.) in the supernatant. PGE_2 had no significant effect on the cholesteryl ester synthetase activity in the microsomes. The increased formation of PGE_2 in the aorta of atherosclerosis-susceptible pigeons and its effect on specific enzymes controlling cholesteryl ester concentration in aorta strongly suggest that PGE_2 (possibly other prostaglandins) could play a significant role in atherogenesis.

SOME ASPECTS OF HYPOCHOLESTEROLEMIC ACTIVITY OF PHYTOSTANOLS IN RATS

M. Sugano, I. Ikeda and H. Morioka

Laboratory of Nutrition Chemistry, Kyushu University School of Agriculture, Fukuoka-shi 812, Japan

The hypocholesterolemic activity of β-sitostanol (HS) in rats has been shown to be markedly greater than that of β-sitosterol (S). Dietary HS was almost completely recovered in feces and increased the excretion of dietary cholesterol significantly greater than did S, as determined by input-output analyses using chromium oxide as a marker.

Fecal recovery of labeled HS orally administered was over 97% as neutral steroids (88% with S) and the deposition into tissues was less than one-tenth that of S.

When labeled S or HS were given intravenously, about 25% of HS (10% with S) was excreted for 6 days as neutral steroids. Conversion of S and HS into bile acids seemed to proceed at a comparable rate though it was markedly lower than that of cholesterol. In comparison with S, deposition of HS into liver was significantly lower and turnover rate of serum HS appeared much faster. The ester ratio of labeled HS in liver and serum lipoproteins appeared considerably higher than that of S.

These data suggest that HS exerts its hypocholesterolemic activity throughout the absorptive process, but the post-absorptive effectiveness may not be excluded.

BINDING OF BILE ACIDS TO ANION EXCHANGING DRUGS IN VITRO

M. Thale and O. Faergeman

Second Department of Internal Medicine, Kommunehospitalet, DK-1399 Copenhagen, Denmark

Equal amounts of anion exchanger of the drugs Secholex, Colestipol, Cuemid and Questran, were incubated at 37°C with human duodenal fluid containing about 7 mM total bile acid. Binding of bile acid to Questran, which contains about 45% cholestyramine, was fastest: concentration of unbound bile acid after 2 hours was less than 3 mM compared to about 5 mM in the solutions incubated with the other drugs including Cuemid, which contains about 83% cholestyramine. After 24 hours, differences were less marked, but binding to Questran was still greatest. Glycocholic acid was least efficiently bound, especially to Secholex and Cuemid. The differences in rates of binding were unaffected by preincubation of the drugs with 1 N HCl to simulate stomach conditions.

Although differences between the cholestyramine components of Cuemid and Questran are not ruled out, it is possible that one or more of the other components of Questran significantly affect the *in vitro* binding of bile acids. Cholestyramine in the form of Questran may be the drug of choice in the treatment of hypercholesterolemia, in which reduction of the bile acid pool is desirable. In cholegenic diarrhea, however, one of the drugs with lower affinity for glycocholic acid may be preferable.

PRIMARY PREVENTION OF ATHEROSCLEROTIC DISEASES WITH AN ANABOLIC STEROID OF ETHYLNANDROL - RESULTS OF A 7 YEAR TRIAL

M. Tsushima, Y. Hata, T. Tsuchida, N. Irie and Y. Goto

Department of Medicine, Keio University School of Medicine, Tokyo 160, Japan

This study was designed to test whether the incidence of atherosclerotic vascular diseases could be reduced by lipid lowering drugs.

Out of three free-living populations, 320 subjects over 40 years of age were randomly selected and divided into two groups; the group treated with a lipid lowering drug of ethylnandrol and the control group on placebo.

The mean cholesterol and triglyceride levels of the treated group were significantly lower than those of the control group throughout the observation period.

Eight primary episodes of cerebral infarctions occurred in the treated group, while 9 of cerebral infarctions and 3 of myocardial infarctions in the control group. One out of 14 who had vascular diseases died within one month after episode in the treated group, while 7 out of 14 died in the control group. This difference was statistically significant. The major risk factors for the cerebral infarction were age, hypertension, obesity and hyperlipidemia, while those for the cerebral bleeding were hypertension, low protein and low fat intake.

We derived from the results the conclusion that a long term administration of a lipid lowering drug and dietary modification could alter the trend in the mortality and morbidity in atherosclerotic vascular diseases in a favorable direction.

EFFECT OF CI719 (GEMFIBROZIL) ON LIPOGENESIS IN LIVER CELLS GROWN IN TISSUE CULTURE

B.R. Tulloch and P.T. Iype

Departments of Medicine and Patterson Laboratories, University of Manchester, Manchester M13 9Wl, United Kingdom

The compound 2:2 dimethyl 5-(2,5 xyloxy)-valeric acid (CI719, Gemfibrozil) is an effective agent in lowering plasma triglycerides in experimental animals and in man. Its mechanism of action is however not clear.

Using cells cultured from normal rat liver for up to 26 weeks we have investigated the effect of C1719 on lipogenesis and lipoprotein synthesis. After addition at 10^{-7}M for 24 hours in serum-free Hams medium, CI719 results in a 50-100% increment in incorporation of ^{14}C acetate into fatty acids. Under similar incubation conditions, concentrations similar to those achieved in vivo (10^{-4}, 10^{-3}m) inhibit synthesis of both sterols and fatty acids to 5-20% of control levels. In medium enriched with 10% fetal calf serum, CI719 decreased ^{14}C amino acid incorporation into both VLDL and HDL lipoprotein fractions.

We conclude that CI719 has a biphasic effect on lipogenesis, with physiological concentrations affecting lipid, apoprotein and protein synthesis.

EFFECTS ON SERUM LIPOPROTEIN CONCENTRATIONS DURING LONG TERM TREATMENT WITH GEMFIBROZIL

B. Vessby, H. Lithell, J. Boberg, and I. Werner

Department of Geriatrics, University of Uppsala, Uppsala, Sweden

During short-term treatment gemfibrozil was shown to reduce serum cholesterol (S-Chol) by 19% and serum triglycerides (S-TG) by 43% corresponding to reductions of LDL-Chol by 14% and VLDL-TG by 49% (Proc. Royal Soc. Med. 69, Suppl. 2: 32, 1976). In the present study the effects of gemfibrozil during long-term treatment were investigated. Twenty-eight patients were, after an initial 6 week placebo period, treated with gemfibrozil during 48 weeks starting on 1200 mg daily. Patients who were still hyperlipoproteinemic after half the trial (n=9) increased the dose to 1600 mg daily. Twenty-six patients completed the trial but one was excluded because of irregular medication.

The S-TG decreased from 3.78 ± 1.49 ($\bar{x}$ ± SD) mmol/l on placebo to 1.79 ± 0.70 after 6 weeks on gemfibrozil (-49%, $p<0.001$), 1.90 ± 0.71 at 24 weeks (-45%, $p<0.001$) and 1.98 ± 0.73 at 48 weeks (-43%, $p<0.001$). The S-Chol decreased from 8.15 ± 1.90 mmol/l to 6.44 ± 1.32 at 6 weeks (-20%, $p<0.001$), 6.58 ± 1.61 at 24 weeks (-18%, $p<0.001$) and 6.53 ± 1.46 at 48 weeks (-18%, $p<0.001$). No further reduction of either S-TG or S-Chol was achieved by increasing the dose to 1600 mg daily. VLDL-TG, LDL-Chol and HDL-Chol were similar at 6, 24 and 48 weeks of treatment.

PAS-C[R] AS A SERUM LIPID LOWERING COMPOUND. A DOUBLE-BLIND CROSS-OVER STUDY

B. Vessby, H. Lithell, J. Boberg, and I. Werner

Department of Geriatrics, University of Uppsala, Uppsala, Sweden

A double-blind cross-over trial was undertaken to study the efficacy of PAS-C in lowering serum lipoprotein concentrations in 30 patients treated with a lipid lowering diet. The patients were prescribed PAS-C 6 g daily or placebo in randomized order during two consecutive 4 week periods.

The serum triglyceride (S-TG) concentration decreased by 28% ($p<0.001$) during treatment from 2.82 ± 1.28 ($\bar{X}$±SD) to 2.03 ± 0.81 mmol/l. The serum cholesterol (S-Chol) concentration was reduced by 12% ($p<0.001$) from 294 ± 48 to 259 ± 49 mg/100 ml. The decrease of S-TG corresponded to a reduction of VLDL-TG by 40% ($p<0.001$), of LDL-TG by 10% ($p<0.1$) and of HDL-TG by 15% ($p<0.05$). VLDL-Chol and LDL-Chol decreased by 46% ($p<0.001$) and 6% ($p<0.05$) respectively. HDL-Chol did not change during treatment. In hyperlipoproteinemia type II (n=10) the LDL-Chol reduction was 14% ($p<0.001$). In type IV (n=15) VLDL-TG decreased by 47% ($p<0.01$).

Serum insulin concentrations and glucose tolerance did not change during treatment. The lipoprotein lipase activity decreased slightly in spite of the pronounced reduction of S-TG.

The study indicates that PAS-C is effective in reducing not only increased LDL-Chol but also VLDL-TG concentrations. By increasing the dosage a more pronounced lipid lowering effect may be achieved.

COMBINATION OF CLOFIBRATE AND PHENFORMIN IN THE TREATMENT OF ENDOGENOUS HYPERTRIGLYCERIDEMIA IN A RANDOMIZED CROSS-OVER DESIGN

K.H. Vogelberg, I. Cicmir, Th. Koschinsky, E. Greiser

Diabetes-Forschungsinstitut an der Universitat Dusseldorf,
4000 Dusseldorf, West Germany

The lipid-lowering effect of clofibrate in combination with phenformin was studied in 2 groups of patients: (1) 15 out-patients with endogenous hypertriglyceridemia (HTG) (7 with subclinical diabetes, mean age 44 years, Broca-index 105) were treated in randomized periods of 3 months with placebo, clofibrate (1.5 g/day) or clofibrate (1.5 g/day) + phenformin (0.15 g/day), placebo and (2) 11 in-patients with HTG and stable maturity onset type diabetes (mean age 55 years, Broca-index 114) were treated in randomized periods of 10 days with placebo, phenformin (0.15 g/day) or phenformin (0.15 g/day) + clofibrate (1.5 g/day), placebo. All patients observed an isocaloric balanced diet without weight changes during the treatment periods. VLDL-, LDL- and HDL-triglycerides (TG) and -cholesterol (CH) and blood lactate were determined by established methods.

Studies applied demonstrated (1) that the total TG (-54%) and CH (-18%) lowering effect of clofibrate was increased in combination with phenformin by an additional 10% reduction of VLDL-TG and by an inhibition of the known clofibrate induced LDL-CH-increase, and (2) that at the same time clofibrate inhibited the known phenformin induced lactate increase.

Therefore, the combination of clofibrate + phenformin in the treatment of HTG could increase the lipid-lowering capacity avoiding at the same time unwanted side effects of both drugs.

INVERSE RELATIONSHIP BETWEEN ADIPOSE TISSUE LIPOLYSIS AND FATTY ACID INCORPORATION INTO HUMAN ADIPOSE TISSUE (FIAT) DURING TREATMENT WITH BM 11.189 AND NICOTINIC ACID

G. Walldius

King Gustaf V Research Institute, S-104 01 Stockholm 60, Sweden

In previous studies we have found an inverse relationship between lipolysis and FIAT in human adipose tissue (HAT) when lipolysis was stimulated *in vitro* by addition of isoprenaline or theophylline or inhibited by addition of nicotinic acid or PGE_1. In the present study the effects of BM 11.189 *in vitro* on lipolysis in HAT obtained by needle biopsy specimens were studied. Both basal and isoprenaline stimulated lipolysis were significantly inhibited in doses of 10-100 μg/ml. Eight patients with hypertriglyceridemia ($\bar{x}$=5.4 mmol/l) were then treated in a metabolic ward first by standardized diet to stabilize lipids and then for one week with BM 11.189 (per os, 10 mg x 3). Needle biopsies were taken before and after treatment and FIAT, lipolytic rate and serum triglycerides were measured. In all patients the fractioned FIAT(^{3}-H fatty acid incorporation into adipose tissue glycerides) decreased ($\bar{x}$ before 121, $\bar{x}$ after 88 nmol x g^{-1} x h^{-1}, $p<0.01$) whereas lipolysis increased ($\bar{x}$ before 334, $\bar{x}$ after 600 nmol g^{-1} x h^{-1}, $p<0.01$). These results suggest that there may be a rebound phenomenon in adipose tissue of increased lipolysis induced by BM 11.189 also decreasing the removal of fatty acids into adipose tissue as a likely explanation why the level of serum triglycerides remained uninfluenced ($\bar{x}$=5.5) during this short study. The results are in contrast with the findings of increased FIAT during long term treatment with nicotinic acid in which serum triglycerides are reduced due to decreased rate of lipolysis and increased FIAT activity. Results from these studies will also be presented.

PLASMA LIPIDS AND LIPOPROTEIN CONCENTRATION AND COMPOSITION IN HYPERLIPIDEMIAS TYPE IIb and IV UPON TREATMENT WITH BEZAFIBRATE

J.G. Wechsler, V. Hutt, H.U. Kloer, H. Jaeger, J. Schoenborn, and H. Ditschuneit

Department Innere Medizin der Universitat Ulm, 7900 Ulm, Germany

Twenty-six patients with hyperlipidemias Type IIb and IV were treated with a diet rich in polyunsaturated fatty acids until stable lipid levels were reached. Twenty-six patients with type IIb and IV were given 450 mg of Bezafibrate (2-[4-(Chlorbenzoyl-amino-ethyl)-phenoxy]-2-methylpropionic-acid) for 12 weeks and 600 mg daily for another 12 weeks. A placebo period of 8 weeks preceeded and followed the drug period.

During therapy with 450 mg Bezafibrate daily plasma triglycerides showed a decrement of 43.5% in type IV and 42% in type IIb. During treatment with 600 mg Bezafibrate daily they showed a 46% decrement in type IV and 43% in type IIb.

Treatment lowered the total cholesterol level by 5% in both types of hyperlipidemias. There were no differences between therapy with 450 and 600 mg of Bezafibrate daily.

The concentration of triglycerides, esterified cholesterol, free cholesterol, phospholipids and protein was determined in VLDL, LDL and HDL before and after therapy, after treatment with the lower dosage and after therapy with the higher dosage.

The composition of the lipoprotein classes was identical in the pre-treatment and post-treatment placebo phase in type IIb and IV. All VLDL constituents decreased upon treatment by about 40% in both types. The higher dosage had no significantly greater effect on the lipoprotein constituents. The LDL and HDL constituents did not change significantly.

Bezafibrate, a new clofibrate analogue, thus seems to have a good triglyceride lowering potency. However, its cholesterol lowering capacity does not appear to be much greater than that of clofibrate in types IIb and IV.

EFFECTS OF BETA-PYRIDYL CARBINOLE AND XANTINOL NICOTINATE ON PLASMA LIPIDS AND LIPOPROTEIN CONCENTRATIONS IN HYPERLIPOPROTEINEMIAS TYPE IIa

J.G. Wechsler, V. Hutt, H.U. Kloer, H. Jaeger, J. Schoenborn, and H. Ditschuneit

Department Innere Medizin der Universitat Ulm, 7900 Ulm, Germany

Ten patients with hyperlipidemia type IIa were treated for 16 weeks with 900 mg β-pyridyl carbinol daily. Another 10 patients received 3 g of Xantinol nicotinate for 16 weeks. A placebo period of 8 weeks preceeded and followed the drug period. All patients were given a diet rich in polyunsaturated fatty acids before, during and after therapy. On therapy with 900 mg β-pyridyl carbinole daily total cholesterol showed a decrement of 23% and plasma triglycerides were lowered about 10%.

During treatment with Xantinol nicotinate total cholesterol decreased by about 7%, but plasma triglycerides remained unchanged. Before, on and after administration of the respective drugs the concentrations of free and esterified cholesterol, triglycerides, phospholipids and protein were determined in VLDL, LDL and HDL.

The composition of the lipoprotein classes in the pre-treatment and post-treatment placebo phases was identical under both medications. All LDL constituents decreased upon treatment with β-pyridylcarbinol by about 30%. VLDL and HDL constituents remained nearly unchanged.

On 3 g Xantinol nicotinate daily constituents and composition of the lipoprotein classes did not change significantly.

The greater lipid lowering potency of β-pyridyl carbinole may at least in part be due to the fact that the administration of this ester of nicotinic acid led to somewhat higher plasma levels of nicotinic acid than those obtained when a threefold amount of Xantinole nicotinate was given.

IN VITRO STUDIES ON THE INFLUENCE OF ESSENTIAL PHOSPHOLIPIDS (EPL) ON LECITHIN:CHOLESTEROL ACYLTRANSFERASE IN MAN

A. Weizel and A. Horsch

Medizinische Universitatsklinik, 69 Heidelberg, West Germany

Lecithin:cholesterol acyltransferase (LCAT) activity was determined after incubation of normal serum with EPL, DOC/EPL (DOC: deoxycholate), and DOC. Normal LCAT activity (Stokke/Norum) was 151 ± 3.4 μmol/l/h. Incubation with a mixture of DOC/EPL (230μg/20μl, 460 μg/20 μl, 1150 μg/20μl) was followed by a marked decrease of LCAT activity (22.40 ± 3.50, 7.40 ± 1.83, 14.10 ± 3.75 μmol/l/h).

Almost the same degree of inhibition was achieved by *in vitro* incubation with DOC alone in 3 concentrations (230 μg/20 μl, 460 μg/20 μl, 1150 μg/20 μl). LCAT activity under these conditions was 44.80 ± 2.24, 28.6 ± 2.63, 46.20 ± 4.26 μmol/l/h.

Incubation with EPL alone did not change LCAT activity.

Conclusion: LCAT activity *in vitro* is inhibited by DOC and EPL/DOC, incubation with pure EPL does not change the LCAT activity.

SPECIFIC NEUROGENIC REGULATION OF LIPID METABOLISM (A MECHANISM OF ACUPUNCTURE)

C.-C. Wu

Taiwan University Hospital, Taipei, Taiwan

The author reported that selective acupuncture (SA) may enhance bile acid excretion in feces and decrease rabbit hypercholesterolemia in 1976. To find further detail mechanism this research was undertaken. Three groups of hypercholesterolemic rabbits, control, SA and sedative SA (S.SA) were needled at nonsite and a specific point except SSA group which was injected with 1% novocain at the specific point before needling for 3 weeks in experiment 1. Three groups of normal rabbits control, SA and SSA were fed on 2% cholesterol diet accompanied with needling for 2 weeks as above in experiment 2. Cholesterol, triglyceride and cyclic AMP levels of serum, liver and aorta were measured. ^{14}C or ^{3}H cholesterol were injected in each group and the radioactivity was corrected to d.p.m. Stimulation of sensory nerve at the specific point (SA) significantly reduced hypercholesterolemia, whole liver cholesterol, total activity of ^{14}C total and free cholesterol of serum and liver, but anesthesia of the same nerve (SSA) increased serum cholesterol and total activity of ^{14}C cholesterol of serum and liver in experiment 1. Stimulation and sedation of the same nerve induced a significant reduction of serum cholesterol and total activity of ^{3}H cholesterol and an increase of liver cholesterol in experiment 2.

Lipid metabolism may be regulated by the specific nerve positively or negatively.

ACTIVITY OF 3-HYDROXY-3-METHYL-GLUTARYL CONEZYME A REDUCTASE FROM RAT AND GUINEA-PIG LIVER. LIGAND SPECIFIC INHIBITION STUDIES AND AFFINITY CHROMATOGRAPHY

E. Wulfert

Centre de Recherches, Laboratoires Fournier, 21300 Chenove, France

The activity of rat hepatic 3-hydroxy-3-methyl-glutaryl Coenzyme A reductase (EC 1.1.1.34), the rate limiting enzyme of cholesterol synthesis, is inhibited in vitro by Procetofenic acid. The inhibitory effect varied widely with an average K_i of 5×10^{-7} M which was observed to be purely non-competitive. The property of high affinity towards Procetofenic acid allowed partial purification of active protein on a Procetofen-Agarose column (Pc-A). Low density lipoproteins ($d \leqslant 1.063$) inhibited enzyme activity and abolished the affinity towards Pc-A. The inhibition was competitive with regard to substrate. HMG-CoA reductase from guinea-pig liver however was not affected by Procetofenic acid, nor was bound on Pc-A. These data suggest the presence of a specific allosteric site for inhibitory ligands on hepatic rat HMG-CoA reductase. They also indicate a difference between rat and guinea-pig enzyme at the molecular level.

THE EFFECT OF BEZAFIBRATE ON PLATELET FUNCTION, FIBRINOLYSIS AND DRUG INTERACTION WITH PHENPROCOUMON

R. Zimmerman, P.D. Lang, A. Hoffrichter, E. Walter, W. Ehlers, K. Andrassy, G. Schlierf and E. Weber

Medizinische Universitatsklinik, 69 Heidelberg 1, West Germany

In addition to their effect on lipids, clofibrate and related drugs can influence platelet function and fibrinolytic activity. Interaction of these drugs with coumarin anticoagulants may induce hemorrhagic complications. Therefore the effect of a new hypolipemic agent (bezafibrate) on blood coagulation and components of the fibrinolytic enzyme system was investigated. Fifteen patients on long-term treatment with phenprocoumon received bezafibrate (450 or 600 mg daily) for 4 weeks. Evaluation of platelet function demonstrated a reduced platelet aggregation induced by collagen ($p < 0.05$) and prolongation of bleeding time ($p < 0.05$), depending on the given dose. Plasma fibrinogen was reduced moderately. Examination of the fibrinolytic activity yielded a shortened euglobulin clot lysis time ($p < 0.05$) but no change of inhibitors. Serum levels of phenprocoumon and bezafibrate were determined to obtain data about the mechanism of drug interaction. After reduction of the phenprocoumon dose by 22.6 or 34.8% the serum phenprocoumon levels decreased by 12.8 and 35.3%, respectively. Hypoprothrombinemia was maintained. The results support the hypothesis that hypolipemic drugs such as bezafibrate augment the anticoagulant response to phenprocoumon by increasing the affinity of the receptor site for coumarin and not by affecting the rate of metabolism.

AUTHOR INDEX

SUBJECT INDEX